Resilience in Pa
Care – Achievement in
Adversity

Resilience in Palliative Care – Achievement in Adversity

Edited by

Barbara Monroe
St Christopher's Hospice
London
UK

David Oliviere
St Christopher's Hospice
London
UK

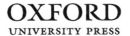

OXFORD
UNIVERSITY PRESS

OXFORD
UNIVERSITY PRESS

Great Clarendon Street, Oxford OX2 6DP

Oxford University Press is a department of the University of Oxford.
It furthers the University's objective of excellence in research, scholarship,
and education by publishing worldwide in

Oxford New York

Auckland Cape Town Dar es Salaam Hong Kong Karachi
Kuala Lumpur Madrid Melbourne Mexico City Nairobi
New Delhi Shanghai Taipei Toronto

With offices in

Argentina Austria Brazil Chile Czech Republic France Greece
Guatemala Hungary Italy Japan Poland Portugal Singapore
South Korea Switzerland Thailand Turkey Ukraine Vietnam

Oxford is a registered trade mark of Oxford University Press
in the UK and in certain other countries

Published in the United States
by Oxford University Press Inc., New York

© Oxford University Press 2007

The moral rights of the authors have been asserted

Database right Oxford University Press (maker)

First published 2007

British Library Cataloguing in Publication Data

Data available

Library of Congress Cataloging in Publication Data

Data available

Typeset by Cepha Imaging Private Ltd., Bangalore, India
Printed in Great Britain
on acid-free paper by
Biddles Ltd., King's Lynn

ISBN 978–0–19–920641–4

10 9 8 7 6 5 4 3 2 1

Foreword

Nathan Cherny

There is an underlying optimism at the heart of palliative care. It underscores the personal and professional investment in attempting to address intense human suffering in the context of impending death. In taking on this task, we, as healthcare providers, willingly expose ourselves to physical, emotional and existential distress on a daily basis. We seek not only to alleviate, but, in our infinite optimism, to elevate the experience of the patient, their loved ones and ourselves. At the very least, we seek to make the unbearable, tolerable; and, at best, to make this a personally enriching experience for all involved.

I do not romanticize dying or death. The transition between living with an incurable, progressive, life-threatening disease to dying is often slow and protracted. It commonly involves agony, fear, debilitation, deep sadness, and anger. Often it involves putrid secretions, awful disfiguration and humiliating debilitation. Parents leaving orphaned children, spouses losing partners, parents losing their offspring are all part of the daily routine. The pain and distress reverberate between the patients and their loved ones; often with one amplifying the distress of the other.

Caring for patients and their families in this context day after day (and, in many cases, for years on end), challenges us. We are challenged as professionals and as individuals; each with our own families, needs and outside stressors. We are challenged as healthcare teams; the differential stressors borne by members of the care team can strain and challenge even the best of collaborative relationships.

As caregivers, resilience is the quality that enables us to withstand and to develop despite the tidal surge of suffering that we dare to confront with skills, dedication, and good intentions. As teams, resilience is the flexible, binding matrix that keeps us working constructively together despite forces of team stress, conflict, interpersonal frictions and grievances that would potentially fragment or undermine our ability to deliver care.

By virtue of self-selection, clinicians choosing to enter into a career of palliative care often have a strong perception of personal resilience. We have, for the most part, chosen our work and we are thus self-interested partners in developing and preserving our ability to function, to contribute, and to rise above the suffering we help relieve. Not all, however, who work in palliative care, do so by choice. Interns, resident staff, nursing students, administrative and support staff often find themselves in palliative care by consignment rather than by choice. For those without innate resilience or good supports, this can be a high stress challenge that can only be endured if given support, understanding, and an environment that helps foster coping and resilience.

The patients and families we seek to help have not chosen their fate. How they cope, or are helped to cope, hinges on both meticulous care and on the fostering and supporting of resilience in the patient, the individual family members and of the family as a unit. Some come with rich sources of personal and family resilience. Many, however, come to us overwhelmed and bereft. Beyond the relief of physical symptoms, the processes of adaptive coping and of psychological and spiritual healing all demand this special quality that is the focus of this volume.

For many of us, palliative care is more than just about relieving suffering, it is about personal and family growth through the shared experience of accompanying a loved one or a patient to the end of life and then of the surviving family members through their grief experience. Irrespective, if we are to strive for the lofty ideal of personal growth through the experience of death, understanding of the factors that can facilitate this sort of human resilience is essential to our task.

As an oncologist and palliative care clinician, practising in a region of conflict, in a relatively impoverished healthcare system, I breathe this subject daily.

I am reminded of the visual allegory of Shalom Aleichem's 'Fiddler on the Roof', scratching out joyous and beautiful music in the most precarious positions as he dances on a fragile shanty Rooftop in the Pale of Russia.

What is resilience? From where is it derived? Why are some so blessed with it and others, so apparently, bereft? What is the history of resilience research? How can this characteristic be fostered and developed in individual clinicians, in teams, among our patients and their family members? These are among the issues addressed in *Resilience and Palliative Care. Achievement in Adversity*.

I extend my thanks and blessings to the editors, Barbara Monroe and David Oliviere, who have brought together a wonderful collection of reflections and advice from sociologists, psychologists, psychiatrists, and bedside clinicians.

I commend and recommend this warmly.

With gratitude, affection and respect
Nathan Cherny
Shaare Zedek Medical Center
Jerusalem, Israel

Contents

Acknowledgement

The year 2007 is St Christopher's 40th year of endeavour in improving end-of-life care. We dedicate this book to the resilience of dying people and those close to them and the staff and volunteers who seek to support them.

Contributors

Amanda Bingley
Research Fellow
International Observatory on
End of Life Care
Institute for Health Research
Lancaster University
Lancaster
UK

Kerry Bluglass
Consultant Psychiatrist,
Senior Clinical Lecturer,
Department of Psychiatry,
University of Birmingham
Birmingham
UK

Nigel Hartley
Director of Creative Living
Resource Centre
St. Christopher's Hospice
London
UK

Timothy Jackson
Nurse Director
Creative Living Resource Centre
South East London
Cancer Network
Guy's Hospital
London
UK

Allan Kellehear
Professor of Sociology
Department of Social &
Policy Sciences
University of Bath
Bath
UK

David Kissane
Alfred P. Sloan Chair and Chairman
Department of Psychiatry &
Behavioral Sciences
Memorial Sloan-Kettering Cancer
Center, and Professor of Psychiatry
Weill Medical College of Cornell
University
New York
USA

Linda Machin
Visiting Research Fellow
Research Institute for Life Course
Studies
Keele University
Staffordshire
UK

Joan Marston
Advocacy Co-ordinator
Hospice Palliative Care
Association of South Africa
Pinelands
South Africa

Elizabeth McDermott
Lecturer in Applied Social Science
Department of Social Policy &
Social Work
University of York
York
UK

Barbara Monroe
Chief Executive
St Christopher's Hospice
London
UK

David Oliviere
Director of Education & Training
St Christopher's Hospice
London
UK

Malcolm Payne
Director of Psychosocial &
Spiritual Care
St Christopher's Hospice
London
UK

Sheila Payne
Help the Hospices Chair in
Hospice Studies
International Observatory on
End of Life Care
Institute for Health Research
Lancaster University
Lancaster
UK

Stephen Regel
Principal Behavioural
Psychotherapist
Centre for Trauma,
Resilience and Growth
Nottinghamshire Healthcare NHS
Trust & University of Nottingham
Nottingham
UK

Phyllis Silverman
Scholar in Residence
Women's Studies
Research Center
Brandeis University

Waltham
MA
USA

Peter Speck
Revd Prebendary
Honorary Senior Lecturer
(Palliative Care),
King's College
London
UK

Julie Stokes
Consultant Clinical Psychologist
& Founder
Winston's Wish
The Clara Burgess Centre
Cheltenham
Gloucestershire
UK

Adrian Tookman
Medical Director
Marie Curie Hospice, Hampstead
Consultant Royal Free Hospital
NHS Trust
London
UK

Stefan Vanistendael
Deputy Secretary General
Bureau International Catholique
de L'Enfance (BICE),
Geneva
Switzerland

Max Watson
Consultant Palliative Medicine
Northern Ireland Hospice, Belfast
Research Fellow
Belfast City Hospital
Adviser to the Hospice Friendly
Hospitals Programme
Dublin

Barbara Young
Volunteering Consultant &
Community Development Officer
Hume Palliative Care Consultancy
Team, Ovens & King Community
Health Service,
Wangaretta
Victoria
Australia

Talia Zaider
Research Fellow,
Department of Psychiatry &
Behavioral Sciences
Memorial Sloan-Kettering Cancer
Center
New York
USA

Introduction: unlocking resilience in palliative care

Barbara Monroe and David Oliviere

Resilience has been described as a 'universal capacity which allows a person, group or community to prevent, minimise or overcome damaging effects of adversity' (Newman 2004). It is not just about re-forming but about the possibility of growth. We believe that the concept of resilience is important to the future delivery of end of life care and the significant challenges it faces. It offers a unifying concept to both retain and sustain some of the most significant understandings of the last four decades of palliative care and to incorporate more effective investment in a community approach and a public health focus. This integration is vital if we are to resolve the ever-increasing tension between the rhetoric of choice and equity coupled with the demands of rising healthcare expectations in ageing populations, and the inevitably limited availability of informal and professional caregivers and financial resources. These Western world challenges are compounded by the huge needs of resource-poor countries. Extending effective palliative care is vital to prevent millions of people each year suffering unnecessarily painful and undignified deaths.

Resilience is receiving increasing research attention as we seek to explain the complexities and variety of human response to difficult circumstances and our recent understanding that many more individuals than initially thought can continue to thrive despite adverse experiences and compounding risk factors. Indeed it is increasingly clear that everyone needs opportunities to develop coping skills and that individuals should not be excessively sheltered from the situations that provide such challenges. Professionals working in palliative care regularly testify to the many examples of ordinary people achieving extraordinary things in the face of impending loss. Resilience is inextricably linked to risk in an interactive process occurring over time and influenced by individual and family variables, social context, and social structure. Resilience moves us towards a more sophisticated assessment that recognizes that many of these variables are crosscutting and can be positive or negative in impact. As Machin comments in her contribution to this book, 'family, religion and culture may provide a coherent background to beliefs ... or present dissonant voices and variable pressures to react to loss in different ways'.

Work on disadvantage and exclusion links to this agenda. As Garmezy (1994) reports, 'the danger to children lies in the cumulation of adversities that exist in many families but are evident disproportionately in the poor.' The difficulty in delivering effective responses to issues of social inequality may have contributed to the current emphasis on individual therapeutic interventions. We are at risk of losing the founding ethos of the hospice movement that sought to empower and promote the strengths and resources of patients within their family and friendship networks and their communities. Mirroring this, is the need to strengthen the resources of health and social care professionals and volunteers in their teams and organizations. Also beginning to be apparent is a return to the privileging of a narrow medical definition of palliative care, 'The central aspect of palliative care is symptom control delivered humanely with adequate information ... Undue emphasis on attending to families is demanding of resources which might be better devoted to a wider population of patients.' (Randall and Downie 2006). However, some of the economic realities of modern healthcare are drivers in another direction. In a recent systematic review of factors influencing death at home in terminally ill patients with cancer, Gomes and Higginson (2006) emphasize the need to explore family support and empowerment and the role of prevention and public education. It is important for the future development of end of life care that health and social care issues remain integrated and that the concepts of risk and resilience are used to inform rather than to polarize policy and practice (see Figure 1). As Rutz (2001) asserts, 'we must avoid the counter-productive split between mainstream medicine, promotion and prevention ... by acknowledging that factors promoting health are also factors preventing disorder.'

St Christopher's Hospice held a series of 10 study days in 2005 on various aspects of palliative care from a resilience perspective. The themes that emerged from the analysis of 29 papers presented by an international faculty of speakers included: secure attachments, meaning and sense, hope, coherence, creativity, good memories, public education and community support, cultural awareness, internal locus of control, well-being, self-esteem, one supportive person and learned optimism (Oliviere and Monroe 2006).

Insights from the field of bereavement also underline the importance of balancing vulnerability and health-promoting factors. Stroebe and Schut (1999) have examined the healthy 'oscillation' between a future-facing, action-oriented focus and rumination on the loss. Neimeyer's (2005, 2006) and Nadeau's (1997) work on the beneficial power of narrative and meaning-making suggests ways of supporting individual and family stories to integrate and surmount difficult experiences and underlines the importance of narratives that can distil benefit out of adverse events. Boss (2006) looks at the value of family work in helping cognitive restructuring; working with family belief systems to

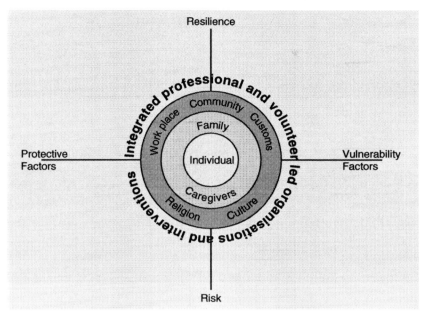

Figure 1 Risk Resilience Paradigm.

reframe and relabel events that cause guilt and shame and sometimes assisting in the reattribution of the cause. Kissane's work (2004) on families reminds us that the adaptation following bereavement is associated with personal growth for many people, 'Self awareness, increased empathy, appreciation of family relationships, independence, reprioritised goals and values, deepened spirituality and increased altruism can all result from positive reappraisal'. At its best palliative care has always been about preventive healthcare, helping the next generation to approach death and loss, less afraid. Studies on 'hope' in end of life care emphasize the value of reminiscence therapy, humour, and the nurturing of independence (Herth 1989, 1990; Buckley and Herth 2004). There are links here to Tookman's insights in this book on the importance of rehabilitation. The value placed by patients on creative therapies also demonstrates how palliative care can increase the resources of individuals for use at time of threat, even within the limited time frame of a dying trajectory (Kennett 2000; Hartley 2005). Resilience work also supports the concept of brief, focused interventions designed to avoid pathologizing and to boost confidence, coping, and action (Kissane 2002; Monroe and Kraus 2004). Such approaches fit both the need for cost-effective care and the shortened time frames of terminal illness.

The insights described are linked to evidence from the fields of psycho-immunology and psychophysiology that positive emotions, imagery, and thoughts are linked with positive action. As Watson reports in this book, we are beginning to gain a clearer understanding of the psychobiological basis of behaviour and its links to resilience (Charney 2004). Fredrickson (2001) and Tugade and Fredrickson (2004) note that the resilient people are able to find positive meaning within stressors and have greater access to stored positive information that enables them to avoid being overwhelmed by the negative experiences and emotions that everyone goes through.

Adopting a resilience approach encourages the integration of current practices in end of life care and resists the drift towards increasing professional stratification. Indeed social and demographic change, including geographic mobility and ageing populations, will mean that professional care alone cannot expand to meet the needs of all the dying and the bereaved. Palliative care must work in partnership with the communities in which people live and empower those communities to respond sensitively and supportively to the dying and bereaved. Kellehear (1999, 2005) has expounded the importance of a health-promoting palliative care that seeks to alter community attitudes. An example of a community-based approach to palliative care is the project to develop support for terminal illness in the workplace, funded by the Australian Government's Care in Communities project (Tehan 2004). The model aims to support employers' risk management responsibilities and to encourage compassionate and sensitive workplace policies and practice. Field (2000) also argues that the values and attitudes of society (including those of professional helpers), affect the ways in which people cope with loss and their capacity to respond with resilience. Walter (1999) emphasizes the importance of shared ritual and social support in grieving and suggests that the lack of a community of mourners often experienced in modern society has resulted in the preponderance of models of private grief and the perceived need for personal therapy.

Palliative care has long used professional education and training as mechanisms to extend its messages beyond its immediate sector; seeking to influence the practice of family doctors, teachers, funeral directors, clergy, the police and others that dying and bereaved individuals will meet in their everyday lives. School linked programmes (Rowling 2003) and attempts at wider public education are emerging. Social marketing and information strategies will become more important as we attempt to find the right balance between expert professional interventions and general loss education that promotes protective personal and social learning. Existing public receptiveness to internet-based resources demonstrates some of the possibilities (Aitken 2004). Studies of user involvement in palliative care (Payne *et al.* 2005) demonstrate the positive therapeutic impact of engagement. Group work emerges as a valuable tool in interventions for carers, patients, and the bereaved; reducing feelings of isolation, increasing social connectedness and providing opportunities to give as

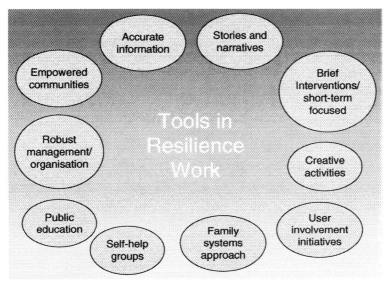

Figure 2 Tools in Resilience Work.

well as to receive help (Monroe and Kraus 2004; Harding *et al.* 2002). Physical environments can be designed to reduce barriers to social engagement and to create opportunities for community. The future will hold new forms of mutual help groups and volunteering (Silverman 2004; Sinclair 2004).

This book attempts to understand and review how health and social care professionals can identify, promote, and work with resilience (see Figure 2). It is 'work in progress'. We present the emerging evidence from research and practice to identify what works in promoting healthy coping, empowerment and prevention, and how to integrate work with individuals, families, organizations, and communities.

References

Aitken A (2004) Webwatch—a new style of mourning. *Bereavement Care* **23**(3), 37.

Boss P (2006) Resilience and health. *Grief Matters* **9**(3), 52–57.

Buckley J, Herth K (2004) Fostering hope in terminally ill patients. *Nursing Standard* **19**, 33–41.

Charney DS (2004) Psychobiological mechanisms of resilience and vulnerability: implications for successful adaptation to extreme stress. *American Journal of Psychiatry* (**161**)2, 195–216.

Field D (2000) *What do we mean by 'psychosocial'?* Briefing Paper No. 4 March. London: National Council for Palliative Care.

Fredrickson BL (2001) The role of positive emotions in positive psychology: the broaden-and-build theory of positive emotions. *American Psychologist* **56**, 218–226.

Garmezy N (1994) Reflections and commentary on risk, resilience and development. In: *Stress, Risk and Resilience in Children and Adolescents: Processes, Mechanisms and Interventions* (eds Haggerty RJ, Sherrod LR, Garmezy N, Rutter M). Cambridge: Cambridge University Press.

Gomes B, Higginson I (2006) Factors influencing death at home in terminally ill patients with cancer: systematic review. *British Medical Journal* (**332**), 515–521.

Harding R, Leam C, Pearce A, Taylor E, Higginson IJ (2002) A multi-professional short term group intervention for informal caregivers of patients using a home palliative care service. *Journal of Palliative Care* **18**, 275–281.

Hartley N (2005) Love …. Actually?—attempting to articulate the heart of hospice. In: *Music Therapy at the End of Life* (eds Dileo C, Leowy J). Cherry Hill, NJ: Jeffrey Books.

Herth K (1989) The relationship between level of hope and level of coping response and other variables in patients with cancer. *Oncology Nursing Forum* **16**, 67–72.

Herth K (1990) Fostering hope in terminally ill patients. *Journal of Advanced Nursing Forum* **15**, 1250–1259.

Kellehear A (1999) Health promoting palliative care; developing a social model for practice. *Mortality* **4**, 75–82.

Kellehear A (2005) *Compassionate Cities. Public health and end of life care.* Milton Park: Routledge.

Kennett C (2000) Participation in a creative arts project can foster hope in a hospice day centre. *Palliative Medicine* **14**(5), 419–425.

Kissane DW (2004) Bereavement. In: *Oxford Textbook of Palliative Medicine*, 3rd edn, pp. 1135–1154 (eds Doyle D, Hanks G, Cherny N, Calman K). Oxford: Oxford University Press.

Kissane DW, Bloch SF (2002) *Family Focused Grief Therapy.* Buckingham: Open University Press.

Monroe B, Kraus F (eds) (2004) *Brief Interventions with Bereaved children.* Oxford: Oxford University Press.

Nadeau JW (1997) *Families Making Sense of Death.* Newbury Park, CA: Sage.

Neimeyer R (2005) Grief, loss, and the quest for meaning—narrative contributions to bereavement care. *Bereavement Care* **24**(2), 27–30.

Neimeyer R (2006) Meaning making in the midst of loss. *Grief Matters* **9**(3), 62–65.

Newman T (2004) *What Works in Building Resilience?* Ilford: Barnardo's.

Oliviere D, Monroe B (2006) *Resilience and Palliative Care.* Abstract. 3rd Research Congress of EAPC, May, Venice.

Oliviere D, Hargreaves R, Monroe B (1998) Working with groups. In: *Good Practices in Palliative Care. A Psychosocial Perspective*, pp. 71–93. Aldershot: Ashgate.

Payne S, Gott M, Small N, Oliviere D (2005*) User Involvement in Palliative Care—a scoping study.* Sheffield: Palliative and End of Life Care Research Group, University of Sheffield.

Randall F, Downie R (2006) *The Philosophy of Palliative Care—Critique and Reconstruction.* Oxford: Oxford University Press.

Rowling L (2003) *Grief in School Communities: effective support strategies.* Buckingham: Open University Press.

Rutz W (2001) Mental health in Europe: problems, advances and challenges. *Acta Psychiatrica Scandinavica* **104**, 15–20.

Silverman PR (2004) *Widow to Widow*, 2nd edn. Hove: Brunner-Routledge.

Sinclair S (2004) Crossing the great barrier grief. In: *Brief Interventions with Bereaved Children*, pp. 227–240 (eds Monroe B, Kraus F). Oxford: Oxford University Press.

Stroebe M, Schut H (1999) The dual process model of coping with bereavement: rationale and description. *Death Studies* **23**, 197–224.

Tehan M (2004) *Developing a Best Practice Support Model for Terminal Illness in the Workplace*. Proceedings Palliative Care Victoria Conference, November, Victoria.

Tugade MM, Fredrickson BL (2004) Resilient individuals use positive emotions to bounce back from negative emotional experiences. *Journal of Personality and Social Psychology* **86**, 320–333.

Walter T (1999) *On Bereavement. The Culture of Grief*. Buckingham: Open University Press.

1

Resilience and its narratives

Kerry Bluglass

Rockabye baby on the tree top,
When the bough bends the cradle will rock
When the bough breaks the cradle will fall,
Down will come baby, cradle and all
Old English Nursery Rhyme

What is resilience? Is it important? Why? Is it merely a modern 'buzz word'?

In the mid twentieth century studies of disadvantaged children who avoided delinquency gave rise to the concept (originally referring to the properties of materials) and many definitions now exist, adopted by different disciplines. Not all of these are obviously relevant to human behaviour. Usually a connecting thread can be perceived, however, even in the material world—'malleability, capacity to absorb energy and to bounce back' suggesting characteristics of survival in difficult or adverse situations.

In physics and engineering, resilience is defined as the capacity of a material to absorb energy when it is deformed elastically and then, upon unloading to have this energy recovered. It is represented by the area under the curve in the elastic region in the stress–strain diagram. Modulus of Resilience, U_r, can be calculated using the following formula:

$$U_r = \frac{\sigma^2}{2 \times E} = 0.5\sigma_\varepsilon = 0.5\sigma \times \left(\frac{\sigma}{\varepsilon}\right)$$

Resilience is the process of, capacity for, or outcome of successful adaptation despite challenging or threatening circumstances.

Masten et al. (1990)

Resilience is predicated on exposure to significant threat or adversity, and on the attainment of good outcomes despite this exposure.

Luthar et al. (2000)

Resilience is the act of rebounding or springing back after being stretched or pressed, or recovering strength, spirit, and good humor.

Webster's New Twentieth Century Dictionary of the English Language

The term 'resilience' is reserved for unpredicted or markedly successful adaptations to negative life events, trauma, stress, and other forms of risk. If we can understand what helps some people to function well in the context of high adversity, we may be able to incorporate this knowledge into new practice strategies

Fraser et al. (1999)

What accounts for the enormous increase (75% in 1 year is suggested) in references in the last few years in articles, papers, and books, or indeed the near overuse of the word in journalism? It is now freely, and rather loosely, used in almost every context, in everyday speech and newspapers, with no apparent need for explanation or definition. The assumption is that all listeners or readers will understand the term. Hence a casual reference to the calm state of the recently recovered survivor of a disaster or a kidnap victim might be appropriate, if premature, but when applied to a disappointed, defeated, but still cheerfully determined football team in the World Cup, its use may be more questionable.

Allusions in print journalism include financial investments and the state of the stock market, organizations, systems and institutions, the environment, ecology, industrial safety, ethnic identity, anthropology and even a cosmetic remedy ('resilience cream') for wrinkles.

The word is clearly a victim of 'definitional drift', as well as convenient shorthand as a means to express more or less complex issues.

In the psychosocial field it is sometimes rather loosely used as a 'marker'[1] of the absence of post-traumatic stress disorder, 'a delayed and/or protracted response to a stressful event or situation (either short- or long-lasting) of an exceptionally threatening or catastrophic nature, which is likely to cause pervasive distress in almost anyone (e.g. natural or man-made disaster, combat, serious accident, witnessing the violent death of others, or being the victim of torture, terrorism, rape, or other crime)' (ICD-10 1992).

Like describing an elephant to a person who has never seen one, resilience is sometimes difficult to describe exactly but it is assumed that 'you will know it when you see it'.

---

[1] 'With a 'checklist' points systems, according to which a score over a certain point indicates post-traumatic stress disorder and below which the individual is said to be 'resilient'. This seems to be an extrapolation of its original sense to a quite specific situation.

I have deliberately included some of these references to resilience in other fields as they illustrate the extent to which borrowing from the physical, material world has been useful; indeed the more varied those definitions the more we find useful concepts and ideas; for example, 'springiness', 'absorbing energy', 'elasticity', change and strengthening through stress/pressure, 'impact stress', and others. They not only describe the innate qualities of the individual but also imply that strengthening can be fostered, encouraged, and developed. This is important when we remember that we are all subject to adversity.

Mid-twentieth century definitions and psychosocial applications first attracted professional attention in the child psychiatry studies of Anthony and Koupernik (1974), which suggested that some highly disadvantaged, vulnerable children at risk of delinquency and other difficulties could achieve better eventual social and emotional adjustment. In other words those certain children, without pills or potions or 'therapies,' could have better than expected lives.

Early work focused on the relationship between childhood resilience and the ability to withstand extremely adverse social, family, and educational disadvantage. More recently this focus has also extended to other age groups and the prevention or avoidance of depression and anxiety, self-harm, and resistance to or coping with psychological injury following war, natural and man-made disasters. There is now an extremely large and complex scientific literature (Fonagy *et al.* 1992) concerning the prevention of difficulties in later life following adverse events.

Appreciation of the concepts as well as the scope of the research evidence may be helpful in understanding and balancing positive or negative outcomes for children at risk (Bluglass 2003, pp. 491–511), and their possible application to promote resilience in other areas of human experience, such as the focus of this book, namely palliative care and bereavement, including patients, families, staff, and communities.

Many of the most relevant studies in this rapidly expanding literature come from social work and psychology, stress and trauma. For children, of course, the interest, research, and applications continue widely, as in the International Resilience Project (Grotberg 1997).

Perhaps a relative absence from adult mental health literature is explicable by the focus on the medical model and on pharmacological treatments for the more acute conditions. Huge research efforts in psychobiology, especially, with better techniques in neuroimaging and genetic contributions to vulnerability (to serious mental illness) are yielding impressive results (Castle and Murray 2002; Kington and Murray 2003; McDonald *et al.* 2004). However, resilience theory and psychobiology do already interact: in psychoneuroimmunology where exciting research is demonstrating surprising resistance of some individuals to disease, for example, long survivors of AIDS (Solomon 1993; Ironson *et al.* 1995). Is this also one of the biological keys to resilience? And how does the individual's genetic structure determine either vulnerability or resistance to hazard and adversity, or vice versa?

Professional pessimism about outcomes for disadvantaged children originated in clinical studies of 'clinic' populations, individuals with 'pathology', who sought help. In the United States the prevalence of psychoanalytical thinking pre- and post-World War 2 influenced child psychiatry training and practice.

As in the medical model, this approach was biased towards treatment and intervention for illness, abnormality, and deviation from the norm. This differed diametrically from positive, preventive or protective aspects or of health promotion, for which the model was a 'Public Health' one with its emphasis on prevention of communicable disease and secondary disability.

Furthermore, despite the great enthusiasm of child care professionals, there was often a perceptible air of defeatism and pessimism. Achieving improvements in environmental circumstances, employment, housing and the relief of poverty were usually seen as the only possible remedies for change. When local or government agencies seemed indifferent or impotent some professionals, aiming for social change, chose political careers. It is therefore not surprising that many Liberal and Socialist politicians in the United Kingdom have had a social work or child psychiatry background.

Now, however, perhaps for the first time, with the notion of 'resistance' to, or 'overcoming', or 'resilience' in adversity, it was possible to see the glass of a child's future as, at the very least, half full rather than irrevocably half empty.

The distinguished English child psychiatrist Professor Sir Michael Rutter pursued this theme:

> The related notion of 'resilience,' the term used to describe the positive pole ... of individual difference in people's responses to stress and adversity. For many years the phenomenon had been put aside as largely inexplicable and therefore of little interest ... However, the issue of individual differences would not go away, and [...] a growing appreciation that it was a key topic in risk research and that understanding the mechanisms involved should throw crucial light on the processes involved in risk itself, as well as having implications for prevention and intervention.

Rutter (1990)

In the past few years, since the turn of the twentieth century, ideas about resilient children have attracted interest in Europe (Vanistendael 1998; Cyrulnik 1999, 2000; Manciaux 2004; Vanistendael and Lecomte, 2000), although in France more than 30 years of significant American and English research appeared to be unknown or ignored. It certainly existed in French dictionaries in the eighties in relation to 'mechanics', and the translation of the subdefinition, 'impact strength' is quite useful. Generally, definitions applied to human beings were more general ('Children are more resilient than adults') than psychological.

The highly accessible book of Cyrulnik, a French child psychiatrist, 'Un Merveilleux Malheur' (1999) popularized the concept and had a huge impact in France, widely available even in supermarkets as well as in bookshops. French Television took up the baton; Cyrulnik's name became 'mediathique' and suddenly it seemed that the word 'resilience' was everywhere in the French speaking media, although it was still often hard to find in its psychological application in dictionaries.

Until quite recently there was apparently no Castillian Spanish equivalent, the words 'elasticidad' or 'resistencia ante la adversidad' serving instead. South American Spanish now has 'resiliencia', German has 'Resistenz' and Norwegian the charming concept 'loevetannbarn' or 'dandelion children', resistant little plants that grow in the most unpromising conditions, and also spread their seeds as resilient people influence others in their environment (Vanistendael 2000, pp. 18–19).

The fundamental importance of the 'critical periods', the first few years, remained unchallenged. Yet for years the evidence of exceptions has been there: Clarke and Clarke (2000), and their more recent book (2003) for instance. They confirm that even after extremely disadvantaged beginnings more positive outcomes were possible.

One of the most striking examples, first described by Koluchova (1972, 1976) was that of grossly deprived, abused twins. When found in a cellar aged 7, they were virtually mute and retarded. Professionals doubted that they could develop beyond the level of severe mental disability. The recent update documents their unexpected progress from institution to devoted fostering, and to their current independent living and working.

Rutter (1990) also suggested that:

> resilience could not be thought of as an attribute born into children or even acquired during development. It is the indication of a process which characterizes a complex social system at a moment in time ... Resilience cannot be seen as anything other than a series of social and intrapsychic processes which take place across time given felicitous combinations of child attributes, family, social and cultural environments. In principle all the psychosocial processes which underpin healthy development may be involved.

During World War 2, many Jewish children were hidden by altruistic Christians (Bluglass 2001, 2003). Subjected to separation, displacement, and deprivation, despite compensatory kindness, affection, and mutual attachment from some of their rescuers, the literature on long-term outcomes suggested almost uniform pessimism (Bluglass ibid, pp. 68–93). As this was consonant with my training and experience with traumatized patients, discovering the existence of some psychologically robust individuals was surprising and stimulating. This consequently led me to explore their lives in more depth, (Bluglass, ibid, pp. 491–591).

Vaillant (1993, p. 298) advanced some explanations for 'surviving well' and I could identify numerous examples in surviving Hidden Children's personal reflections on their lives.

- Cognitive strategies
- Attributional style
- Temperament
- Social supports
- Ability to internalize social supports
- Psychosocial maturity
- Hope and faith
- Social attractiveness
- Ego mechanisms of defence
- Absence of risk factors and presence of protective factors
- Luck, timing and/or context
- Self-esteem and self-efficacy.

Vaillant's attribution of resilience in successful adults to the existence of 'mature defence mechanisms' is an attractive and persuasive way of understanding their survival of difficult childhood experiences:

> Mature coping mechanisms are common in healthy individuals between the ages of twelve to ninety and include:
> Altruism: vicarious but constructive and productive service to others.
> Humour: overt expression of ideas and feelings without individual discomfort and without unpleasant effect upon others.
> Suppression: the conscious or semiconscious decision to postpone paying attention to a conscious impulse or conflict.
> Sublimation: indirect or attenuated expression of instincts without either adverse consequences or marked loss of pleasure.

An awareness of the existence of these 'mature defences' helped to understand how well these potentially damaged individuals had survived, and indeed thrived. As Vaillant says:

> Defenses are healthy. However disordered, sick, sinful, or unreasonable defenses may appear to the observer, they reflect an adaptive response and an intact working brain. By themselves defenses are not evidence of illness. As in the case of immune mechanisms, however maladaptive the results, defenses are deployed in the service of coping.

The distinction between 'defending' and 'coping' are quite as arbitrary as the distinction between the unhealthy pus of acne and the healthy ingestion by our white corpuscles of intruding bacteria. The situations that call forth defenses and those which call forth white corpuscles are perilous; we cope as best we can. The distinction between adaptive and maladaptive is often in the eyes of the beholder.

Ibid (1993)

He advocates illustrating the 'wisdom of the ego' in successful survivors, by studying their 'biography' to demonstrate that defences reflect health and creativity and not illness, using vignettes (or narratives) from the lives of potentially disadvantaged people. He points out that longitudinal studies of normal adult development showed that defences are important to well-being as immune mechanisms; that as the body grows during childhood, the human ego is capable of maturation during adulthood.

Some writers see resilience as a balance sheet of relative absence of risk factors and the relative presence of protective factors. Rutter (1990) has cautioned, however, that it is not a matter of a simple equation, that if some succumb to the 'sum of accumulated risk factors minus the sum of accumulated positive experiences ... it appears inadequate to account for the phenomena.' Rutter also believes that 'process' is a more apposite term than 'factor'.

Positive attributes include good intellectual ability, attractive appearance, and easy temperament. One can see how important these attributes would have been in bonding the Hidden Children to their new caregivers. In the exceptionally difficult and dangerous times of Occupied Europe such children were usually swiftly concealed with little preparation for child or rescuer. They were a drain on scarce food resources and represented an enormous threat and danger to the rescuing families.

Humour and high intelligence are also believed to be important. A sense of humour, wit, and high intelligence were evident on meeting men and women survivors. The capacity to find humour in past and present events is perhaps among the most important keys to living positively.

Bettine

A former hidden child (Bluglass 2003, pp. 413, 415) whose separation from her family and subsequent life, hidden in wartime France, were miserable and deprived, recounts with much humour the fruitless attempts of staff in an orphanage to rid her of the ubiquitous head lice, and how callously hitting her on her head for some misdemeanour an orphanage teacher was enveloped in 'lice powder'. She was able to endure many of her traumatic experiences by using a detached, ironic and humorous stance, has used humour creatively all her life, eventually becoming a successful comedy actress. She works voluntarily with elderly Holocaust survivors.

Much of what they had to tell me about their childhood was sad, solemn, tragic; they neither dismiss nor deny these aspects, nor avoid the expression of the emotions they evoke. We shall see how encouraging some of these approaches have relevance for patients, families, staff and communities in palliative care.

Altruism can take many forms. Many successful survivors have become educators, doctors, therapists, and social workers. Although some writers such as Langer (1991) dispute the possibility of finding any 'meaning' (Frankl 1989), after the Holocaust, many survivors do cite it as a powerful driving force. For others, helping and healing may be a practical contribution to *tikkun olam* (healing the world). Most of my interviewees care passionately about educating the young to combat prejudice and racism and to reflect on the lessons of the Nazi era, together with its relevance for contemporary conflicts and genocides, and they have proved to be sensitive, inspiring, and effective teacher.

Sylvie

Sylvie is a confident, charming and resolute Belgian voluntary worker in a national organization.

Her frightening early years could have destroyed the adjustment of many. She was a capricious, cosseted little girl until her life was dislocated by the arrest of her parents and she was hidden by a couple already grieving the deportation of their own son for resistance activities.

Although witty and assertive now, her perception of the events of the Holocaust and their contemporary relevance to racial prejudice and hatred are deeply felt. She describes how she uses these in a gentle, creative, but at the same time, determined way when she works with school children of different cultures. She believes that surviving positively has given her, and others like her, an enormous capacity to grow as an individual, and she is determined to use this as a force for good.

The capacity to live well with mature, coping mechanisms despite repeated adversity demonstrates their use, even as adults, of the patterns suggested by Vaillant, in measures neither too much, too little, but 'just right'.

Are there additional components to resilience that we have not as yet considered, especially in the field of palliative care and bereavement? What weight should we place on the concepts of 'suffering' and of 'courage'? Are they essential experiences in resilience or in its development? Is being courageous a manifestation of resilience? Can resilience occur without suffering?

Samuel Pepys, the seventeenth century diarist, rose by hard work and his talent for administration to be the Chief Secretary to the Admiralty under King James II. He was one of the first to apply methodical research and careful record keeping to the business of government, and his influence was important in the early development of the British Civil Service. Yet this highly successful and resourceful man endured from childhood the most appalling physical pain and suffering from urinary tract and bladder calculi (stones) at a time when the only remedy was surgery without anaesthetic. He was almost never without pain and other symptoms.

In 1657, Pepys took the brave decision to undergo surgery, an operation known to be especially painful and hazardous. The procedure, being 'cut of the stone', was conducted without anaesthetics or antiseptics, and involved restraining the patient with ropes and four strong men; the surgeon then made an incision along the perineum about three inches (8 cm) long and deep enough to cut into the bladder. The stone was removed through this opening with pincers (Tomalin 2003). Pepys' stone was successfully removed and was described as being the size of a tennis ball. However, he made a good recovery and determined to celebrate on every anniversary of the operation. On Monday 26 March 1660, he wrote, in his diary: 'This day it is two years since it pleased God that I was cut of the stone at Mrs. Turner's in Salisbury Court. And did resolve while I live to keep it a festival, as I did the last year at my house, and for ever to have Mrs. Turner and her company with me'.

Much courage must have been necessary for such patients, then as now; although in Western, developed countries we have increasingly come to hope for adequate pain relief; sadly this expectation of sophisticated analgesia in childbirth, medical, postoperative and end of life care is not universally met. In some parts of the world analgesia has not advanced much beyond that of Pepys' time. Courage, 'fortitude', the ability to confront fear, pain, danger, uncertainty, can be divided into physical courage in the face of pain, hardship, fear of death—and 'moral courage'—in the face of shame, scandal and discouragement.

Reflecting on the lives of those young hidden children (Bluglass, ibid, 2003, 2007) now in their late sixties and seventies who demonstrate undoubted lifelong resilience, it is clear that their experiences involved substantial suffering. Admitting to 'courage' might be harder for these modest people, for they felt that they usually had no choice but to endure.

Janek

Neither Janek nor his wife (also a hidden child) have ever considered that their adjustment to life required professional help. He does become understandably emotional when recounting some facts, particularly when he talks about his father, but his psychological stability is evident in all dimensions of his life. He is a successful business man, loving husband, father, valued colleague and friend, and all of this is the more remarkable, considering his clandestine confinement for two and a half years of his early childhood, in the locked room of a house behind the German barracks on the outskirts of Krakow. He had reached the family after his parents arranged for him to be smuggled out of the Ghetto in a suitcase.

He accepts that the family who sheltered him were necessarily strict with him. Hiding a Jewish child put their own lives and those of their own children at risk. Unlike some people, whose parenting, or lack of it, has seemed to them to underpin later psychological illness or difficulties, he fully recognizes the role of his brave rescuers who risked their lives to conceal him, and succeeded in obtaining a posthumous award[2] for the family, celebrating their acts of heroism.

He is a living example of the tenet that 'When bad things happen to good people', they are not inevitably destroyed (Kushner 2001).

In some cases, indeed, they had even more difficult events to navigate after the war. Rehabilitation to such relatives as survived was often difficult; leaving their rescuers involved further separation; anti-Semitism was still evident and displacement and relocation to other countries and the need to absorb new languages were further hurdles.

Josia

One of the difficulties Josia had to endure, not unusual for hidden children, was the conflict between the 'hiding mother' and her own mother who survived to claim her after the war. To some extent they have never been able to resolve this. Her mother who herself endured separation and hiding during the war was, and remained, intensely jealous. Her personality has probably always been a rather difficult one. Josia, now settled in Israel with her family, including her mother, tries to maintain a balance between expressions of affection to her large 'hiding family' still in the Netherlands, and her own ageing mother. She exemplifies those hidden children who experienced the 'loyalty conflict' on the return of a parent or other surviving family member. She remains nevertheless a balanced, mature and affectionate wife, mother and grandmother dealing with these problems with equanimity and compassion.

Patients, staff, and families are of course no strangers to suffering. However, sometimes the sheer size of the task or other current circumstances can cause

---

[2] Righteous Gentiles ... Awards from Yard Vashem.

any of us to lose confidence in our own abilities, and learning from the tasks that resilient, 'hardy' people have surmounted can often help individuals, groups and organizations to regroup their psychological forces and to find potential untapped strengths.

Some of the current resilience literature indeed suggests that stress or threat is not necessarily to be avoided, for mastery may make us stronger and more resilient, in other words the route to achieving resilience may be by way of learned, often painful or stressful experience; for example, the response of a sizeable number of the bereaved (Kissane 2004). Rutter has also used the analogies of 'tempering 'steel to strengthen it by stressing it, and cited the well known benefits of 'nasty-tasting medicine', which makes us well.

For exploration of the nature, existential meaning and significance of 'suffering', and the stoical philosophies of other religions, see Chapter 7 (Resilience and spirituality).

Increasing interest in the concept of resilience and creative applications to other aspects of human existence led to an imaginative series of conferences at St Christopher's Hospice in 2005. Stimulated by the learning potential for staff and patients, relatives and organizations in palliative care settings, the first conference brochure proposed: 'Drawing on the concept of "well-being" and the worldwide research on resilience, components of resilience and their connections to palliative care will be identified. Listening to resilient Holocaust survivors may help us to revise our views of the negative effects of major crisis, loss and trauma'.

There was also an historical connection between thinking about 'positive psychology and well-being' and the Hospice's educational activities. In June 1982 St Christopher's hosted an international conference in London at which Martin Seligmann, in a keynote paper on 'Helplessness' discussed the connections between cognition and depression, giving up, and hopelessness. His seminal work (1992) on 'Learned Helplessness' (with repeated exposure to inescapable aversive events, the person or animal learns that escape is impossible. In subsequent circumstances where escape or avoidance is possible). The identified cognitive components of depression, loss, and trauma and was influential in practical treatment approaches. It led naturally to the contemporary focus on fostering positive attitudes in overcoming adversity, the concept of 'Learned Optimism' (Seligman 1991), the lessons of which can be practised and learned: for example, Seligman and his colleagues taught learned optimism to 40 cancer patients and produced a very sharp increase in the activity of natural killer cells, the cells that kill foreign invaders in the body, such a viruses, bacteria, and tumour cells. Optimism:

- inoculates against depression
- improves health.

These concepts are linked to the understanding of 'explanatory style', individual thinking that attributes events in optimistic or pessimistic ways, thinking that can be successfully challenged in interventions.

'Locus of control', another important concept in understanding how individuals regard their ability to influence events around them, refers to a continuum, ranging from external to internal; for example, an individual believes that his/her behaviour is guided by his/her personal decisions and efforts. With an external locus of control, the individual believes that external factors are responsible for events and that he has no effect or control over them. In general, it seems to be psychologically healthy to perceive that one has control over those things that one is capable of influencing. A more internal locus of control is generally seen as desirable. Having an internal locus of control can also be referred to as 'self-agency', 'personal control', 'self-determination'.

From an understanding of those concepts has come development of 'positive psychology', (Masten and Redd 2004), the 'Happiness and Well-being' movement, and, in the therapeutic sphere, Cognitive Behavioural Modification. These areas of understanding of human cognition influencing behaviour are significant contributors to the field of positive psychology, the scientific study of optimal human functioning.

The American psychologist and philosopher William James, in *The Varieties of Religious Experience* (1902) argued that happiness is a chief concern of human life and those who pursue it should be regarded as 'healthy-minded.' 'Happiness' means several different things, for example, joy, satisfaction. Consequently, many scientists prefer the term 'subjective well-being.'

It is fascinating to note that this now coincides with improvements in 'healthy eating' advice; encouragement to reject previous pessimistic, deterministic acceptance of one's lot (or fate), and instead to take some initiative and autonomy for one's own well-being.

The consequences of the former, defeatist, approach can be seen especially in the United States and has been shown persuasively by Whybrow in his critique of the 'more' generation (2005). Possibly, one would hope, the recent recognition of the growing importance of healthy psychological as well as physical and physical states may augment future well-being in general. So the questions posed at the beginning of this chapter 'What is resilience? Is it important? and Why?' begin to elicit a response.

The significance of this to palliative care, as well as to other fields, is that there is now a powerful basis for individuals and groups to capitalize on existing resources, emphasizing the potential for the exercise of choice and control in illness, difficult circumstances, chronic and palliative care. Of course those familiar with the origins and practice of hospice care may feel that from its early days these principles, together with the essential drive towards effective symptom control, were there already, avant la lettre; but despite wide dissemination and recognition, achieving this beyond specialised teams has been a longer trajectory. As Monroe and Oliviere (2006) point out resources are finite, and having reached the present levels of competence, it will also be important to harness the wider resources of the community. In our present emphasis on technology we may have de-skilled some with untapped psychological resources to offer. An understanding of the potential of resilience can lead to exploration, encouragement and development of positive aspects and individual strengths, another way of expressing the notions of vulnerability, and resilient survival. Where professionals often experience despondency and anxiety about outcomes, more hopeful possibilities can be evaluated, fostered, encouraged, and promoted.

In the first St Christopher's Resilience Conference in 2003 and in the year-long series that followed, we hoped that experiences of adversity with healthy outcomes could illustrate a new and different dimension, and possibly challenge current thinking of staff working in particularly difficult specialized areas such as palliative care and bereavement. In such work the potential for growth and recognition of resources and strengths had perhaps been relatively unremarked by some, because of an emphasis on inevitability and acceptance.

Egan (1993) challenged the assumption that burnout is primarily an organizational phenomenon, suggesting that the individual worker's own self and world view was also influential, advising managers and educators to foster workers' sense of self-mastery and self-esteem to prevent burnout. The strengths perspective has also been a unique contribution to the understanding of the helper–client relationship. Bell (2003) explored its utility as a conceptual framework for research in a qualitative study with counsellors of abused women.

> An emphasis on strengths allowed the researcher to identify strategies and resources that prevented symptoms of secondary trauma in the majority of counsellors. These strengths include a sense of competence about their coping, maintaining an objective motivation for their work, resolving their own personal traumas, drawing on early positive role models of coping, and having buffering personal beliefs.

This has obvious relevance for practice, education and research and in other areas of intervention in stressful work. Retrospective studies have drawbacks, but can be complementary to prospective ones as Gilgun (2005) points out, highlighting the importance of qualitative, descriptive work. Despite the weight attached to quantitative studies, qualitative ones are now attracting recognition for their particular insights; descriptive, narrative accounts give us a unique opportunity to examine the subsequent lives of individuals once considered very vulnerable and at risk (Vaillant, ibid). Their insight into the older adult many years after adverse childhood experiences can be instructive. Green (2002) has illustrated the insights that listening to Holocaust survivors can give workers in order 'to promote client resilience and coping strategies'.

Henry Greenspan (1998), psychologist and author has described and dramatized the narratives of Holocaust survivors, insisting that listening is the most important part of the process. It is true that nothing has more power to make us reflect than hearing authentic voices. There is no substitute for the personal account of the lived experience: the subjective narrative of the emotions felt at the time, eye witness descriptions (the terror experienced, the vivid visual images, the paradoxical contrast between the elegant appearance of the Gestapo officers and the inhumanity of their actions in the Krakow Ghetto); the terrifying effect on the child witness clearly has an immediate impact.

Janina

One of the most extreme experiences, so far removed from contemporary child care, was that endured by Janina.[3]

Following a harrowing escape from the Krakow ghetto when her elder brother pushed her into a sewer, to escape the Nazis, throughout the harsh winter of 1943, this frail 12-year-old child had to survive completely alone, in remote Polish countryside, offering casual work on farms and smallholdings, managing to exist, on the run for 2 years, with abscesses and bleeding gums, covered in vermin and undernourished.

This was the mode of survival of several other Polish children 'on the run' at the time. Not all survived their ordeal.

As a neglected, solitary, and parentless child she was deprived of appropriate nurturing and education for years. She could well have become a completely unsocialized individual, perpetuating in peacetime her wartime survival strategies. Instead she struggled to complete her education, and today is a cultivated, competent, and attractive woman.

What is apparent in the live presentation by a resilient survivor is not a forced Polyanna-ish cheerfulness, nor a manic, defensive denial of difficulties, but the evident stability of the individual, the wisdom gained, the ability to reflect and express a normal range of appropriate emotion: loss, grief, sadness, resignation even, but without all-consuming self-destructive bitterness: the bough, to use the nursery rhyme analogy, has bent but it has not broken. That in our terms is a live manifestation of resilience. That is why we need to

---

[3] For the full story of Janina's journey from then to the present, her survival and her talents, see *Have You Seen My Little Sister?* (Fischler-Martinho 1998), and a discussion of the effects of privation on her and other Hidden Children, in Bluglass (ibid, pp. 175–206).

encourage listening to the narratives, exploring the strategies, internal worlds and cognitive processes of people who have developed such inner strength. This is in striking contrast to 'ordinary', less resilient people blaming their much less arduous lives, exemplifying the Polish expression, *mialam ciezkie dziencinstwo bo chidzialam do szikoly pod gorkedzie* (I had a difficult childhood; when I was a child, I was obliged to walk uphill to school).

Other applications concern mental health, the prevention of depression, improving educational outcomes and the mastery of traumatic memories.

From much of this work, then, we see that from simply becoming aware that resilience exists, identifying its characteristics and trying to understand it (Vanderpol 2002), we are now moving towards fostering, encouraging it (Vanistendael 1996, 2000), and promoting it (Egan, ibid), in the same way as physical health promotion and illness prevention. For, as the eighteenth century writer humorist Laurence Sterne pointed out in *Tristram Shandy* (1992), the physical and the psychological are linked, entwined, 'A man's body and his mind are like a jerkin and a jerkin's lining. Rumple the one and you rumple the other'.

Lise

Lise had lived happily with her parents until the arrival of the German Occupation in Belgium. Her father was an immigrant Polish furrier and thus an easy target for Gestapo activity and deportation. Her mother, who did not survive the war had to find a hiding place for her. Many children in hiding were well cared for despite the exigencies of the time, but she was sent to live with a cold and uncaring woman in a dark basement with inadequate food. She was exploited at the age of eight as a laundry maid. Her only link with the outside world was a Resistance worker who came to give her some lessons from time to time.

She emerged at the end of the war, undernourished and fearful; her strange host used to taunt her, 'I'll tell the Gestapo to come and collect you!' and would tell her that she would never see her family again, 'they are all burnt'. Significantly, though, as has been indicated in the lives of many resilient individuals and in many of the works on resilience there was also in her deprived existence an important supportive figure, the kind resistance worker who used to visit to give her Catholic instruction, helped her with literacy, and was sometimes able to bring her a little food. This woman was her model, her mentor, and she attributes much of her later capacity for endurance to her example. After the Liberation she remained in touch and Lise regarded her as a surrogate mother. She helped her a little educationally and with moral support, almost certainly contributing to her remarkably successful personal survival. A mark of Lise's overcoming adversity and absence of bitterness for a lost childhood was her ability to feel some compassion for the other woman (who had agreed to hide her but who had so ill treated her), to visit her in hospital and attend her funeral. 'After all', she said, 'she had saved my life'. After she was married and living in Britain, Lise felt that she responded positively to everything. She constantly felt how wonderful it was to be free, and from an isolated and neglected child she became a sociable, welcoming woman, making a supportive circle of friends. Despite Lise's own serious illnesses she remains strong. She feels that her kind mentor fostered her significant inner strengths.

Danuta

Danuta was smuggled out of the Warsaw Ghetto and hidden by a Catholic family. Her first years were a long succession of orphanages and children's homes, in miserable and deprived conditions, cold winters, poor food, and all the illnesses of war, inadequate nutrition and poverty.

Her parents and grandparents were never seen again.

Danuta believed herself to be a Catholic war orphan. At the age of ten she was 'adopted' by a traumatized Jewish camp survivor trying unsuccessfully to replace her own lost family. Danuta painfully learned of her own Jewish identity in post-war Poland where anti-Semitism was still much in evidence. The 'adoption' failed. She eventually trained as a nurse but kept her true identity secret, even from her Catholic husband and his family until, many years later she succeeded in leaving Poland for France with her young daughter. Only then was she able to acknowledge her origins to her own child.

Her early life was deprived and harsh, but the post-war years were even more difficult. She lived with a confusion of religion, identity, and constant deception. Concealment was a constant struggle. Yet she has become a lively, open trustworthy person, capable of giving and accepting affection, understanding the vicissitudes of the past without bitterness, with a brilliant professional career.

In short, the early lives recounted here have, at first sight, all the ingredients of later psychological disturbance, shaken confidence and self-esteem, depression, difficulty in making relationships, trusting, even honesty, perhaps. The fact that they are today such remarkably stable individuals, the French expression '*bien dans leurs peaux*' even more apt than 'well-adjusted', overturns our preconceptions of 'damage' from childhood adversity, unless we take account of human resilience. When I listened to each of these resilient survivors it was hard not to be powerfully affected by the immensity of the hurdles they had had to overcome. Some of the positive as well as negative contributions to their lives were striking:

- The influence of early attachment.
- Coping with fear and loss.

- Patterns of survival, for example stealing, lying and subterfuge as opposed to more 'socialized behaviour', and how the former could be given up for the latter.

- A 'good outcome': ability to overcome adversity to achieve a balanced life, without major physical or psychological pathology, to be able to 'to work, love, and play' (the three instinctual human drives suggested by Freud) appropriately.

- Attitudes to their own roles as future parents: mastering the fear of future losses and disrupted attachments.

- Self -perception as competent, able, and well adjusted; comparisons with attributions of help-seeking individuals to adverse childhood experiences.

How can such resilience, such 'impact strength' be encouraged? Of course looking at the different experiences and life paths of those who are innately 'resilient' and those who are not, it would be simple (and expensive), if we could simply prescribe and liberally apply the soothing and no doubt deliciously fragrant 'resilience cream' described in the beauty pages of the colour supplements, and then present them with T-shirts bearing the logo of the resilience formula illustrated above, for all to recognize and acknowledge.

It is not, unfortunately, quite so simple; indeed, as Vanistendael (2000) has pointed out, we should not expect that everyone will be resilient all of the time. However, teaching techniques and playing to the innate strengths of the individual, studying the lessons of Seligman's 'Learned optimism' should give us, as professionals, a new springboard for helping and healing.

Where do we place the relevance of resilience theory to good quality end of life and palliative care? We can apply this understanding to what we have learned; for example, that there is a capacity of individuals to grow stronger in crisis; development of new, unexplored opportunities; using humour effectively and other constructive, positive defences; challenging negative ideas and focusing on positive ones; promoting hope; not 'catastrophising' thoughts. Some people are innately more able to function in this way, but very often gloomy pessimists can be supported with skilled intervention. They can be encouraged, often with reference to their past achievements and strengths to see their own potential, which they often underestimate. The positive psychological aspects of patient care are as important as, and highly complementary to, the material and physical ones.

It may not seem immediately easy to apply, or to teach, resilience principles in palliative and end of life care, but our experience of this work teaches us that patients and families grow and can exhibit or can acquire such character-istics, for example:

- stoical, philosophical attitudes
- 'denial', in the healthy, protective sense
- recognition of achievements in the present despite current or past adversity, e.g. enjoying small, short-term goals
- capacity to learn, unburdened by negative past experience
- capacity to grow through crisis, an opportunity for change, reconciliation, reflection, and closure
- use or acquisition of 'healthy' defences, including humour
- hope, whether or not mediated by faith.

It is perfectly true, as the philosophers say …
Life can only be understood by looking backwards, but they forget to add that it also has to be lived forwards.

Søren Kierkegaard (1996, *Journals*)

References

Anthony JE, Koupernik C (1974) (eds) *The Child in His Family*, Vol. 111: *Children at Psychiatric Risk*. New York: Wiley.

Bell H (2003) Strengths and secondary trauma in family violence. *Social Work*, **48**(4), 513–522(10).

Bluglass K (2001) Surviving well: resistance to adversity. In: *Remembering for the Future: The Holocaust in an Age of Genocide*, pp. 47–62. Vol. 3(Memory), (eds Roth JK, Maxwell E). New York: Palgrave and Macmillan.

Bluglass K (2003) *Hidden from the Holocaust: stories of resilient Hidden children who survived and thrived*. Westport, CT: Greenwood.

Bluglass K (2007) Relative values: attachment between host family children and their hidden 'siblings'. In: *Beyond the Camps and Forced Labour* (eds Steinert JD, Weber Newth, I). Osnabrueck: Secolo Verlag.

Castle DJ, Murray RM (2002) Schizophrenia: aetiology, genetics and risk factors. In: *Principles and Practice of Geriatric Psychiatry*, 2nd edn, pp. 503–508 (eds Copeland JRM, Abou-Saleh MT, Blazer DG). Wiley: Chichester.

Clarke AM, Clarke ADB (2000) *Early Experience and the Life Path*. London: Jessica Kingsley.

Clarke A, Clarke ADB (2003) *Human Resilience: a fifty year quest*. London: Jessica Kingsley.

Cyrulnik B (1999) *Un merveilleux malheur*. Paris: Editions Odile Jacob.

Cyrulnik B (2000) *Les vilains petits canards*. Paris: Editions Odile Jacob.

Egan M (1993) Resilience at the front line: hospital social work with AIDS patients and burnout. *Social Work in Health Care* **18**(2), 109–125.

Fischler-Martinho J (1998) *Have You Seen My Little Sister?* London: Valentine Mitchell.

Fonagy P, Steele M, Steele H, Higgett A, Target M (1994) The theory and practice of resilience. *Journal of Child Psychology and Psychiatry* **35**(2), 231–257. (The Emanuel Miller Memorial Lecture, 1992.)

Frankl VE (1989) *Man's Search for Meaning: An Introduction to Logotherapy.* New York: Washington Square Press.

Fraser MW, Richman JM, Galinsky MJ (1999) Risk, protection, and resilience: Toward a conceptual framework for social work practice. *Social Work Research* **23**(3), 131–143.

Gilgun JF (2005) Evidence-based practice, descriptive research and the resilience-schema-gender-brain functioning (RSGB). *British Journal of Social Work* **35**, 843–862.

Green RR (2002) Holocaust survivors: a study in resilience. *Journal of Gerontological Social Work* **37**, 13–18.

Greenspan H (1998) *On Listening to Holocaust Survivors: Recounting and Life History.* Westport, CT: Praeger.

Grotberg E (1997) The International Resilience Project: findings from the research and the effectiveness of interventions. In *Psychology and Education in the 21st Century: Proceedings of the 54th Annual Convention. International Council of Psychologists,* 118–128. (eds Bain B, Janzen H, Paterson J, Stewin L, Yu A). Edmonton: ICP Press.

ICD-10 (1992) *Classification of Mental and Behavioural Disorders.* Geneva: World Health Organization.

Ironson G, Solomon G, Cruess D, Barroso J, Stivers M (1995) Psychological factors related to long-term survival with HIV/AIDS. *Clinical Psychology and Psychotherapy* **2**(4): 249–266.

James W (1902) *The Varieties of Religious Experience.* New York: Random House.

Kierkegaard S (1996) *Papers and Journals: a selection* (Trans. A. Hannay). Harmondsworth: Penguin.

Kington J, Murray RM (2003). Schizophrenia: the new evidence. *The Mental Health Review* **8**(3), 31–33.

Kissane DW (2004) Bereavement. In: *Oxford Textbook of Palliative Medicine,* 3rd edn (eds Doyle D, Hanks G, Cherny N, Calman K) Oxford: Oxford University Press.

Koluchova J (1972) Severe deprivation in twins; a case study. *Journal of Child Psychology and Psychiatry* **13**, 107–104.

Koluchová J (1976) Severely deprived twins after 22 years observation. *Studia Psychologica* **33**, 23–28.

Kushner HS (2001) *When Bad Things Happen to Good People,* Twentieth Anniversary edn. New York: Schocken Books.

Langer LL (1991) *Holocaust Testimonies: The Ruins of Memory.* New Haven: Yale University Press.

Luthar SS, Cicchetti D, Becker B (2000). The construct of resilience: A critical evaluation and guidelines for future work. *Child Development* **71**, 543–562.

Manciaux M (2004) *La resilience: resister et se construire,* 3eme tirage. Geneva: Medecine et Hygiene.

McDonald C, Bullmore E, Sham P, Chitnis X, Wickham H, Bramon E, Murray R (2004) Genetic risks for schizophrenia and bipolar disorder are associated with specific (grey) and generic (white) brain structural phenotypes. *Archives of General Psychiatry* **61**, 974–984.

Masten AS, Redd MGJ (2004) Resilience in development. In: *Handbook of Positive Psychology* (Chapter 6) (eds Snyder CR, Lopez SJ). Oxford: Oxford University Press.

Masten AS, Best KM, Garmezy N (1990) Resilience and development: contributions from the study of children who overcome adversity. *Development and Psychopathology* **2**, 425–444.

Monroe B, Oliviere D (2006) Resilience in palliative care. *European Journal of Palliative Care* **13**, 22–25.

Rutter M (1990) Psychosocial resilience and protective mechanisms. In: *Risk and Protective Factors in the Development of Psychopathology*, pp.181–214 (eds Rolf J, Masten AS, Cicchetti D, Nuechterlein K, Weintraub S). Cambridge: Cambridge University Press.

Seligman MEP (1991) *Learned Optimism*. New York: Alfred A. Knopf.

Seligman MEP (1992). *Helplessness, Depression and Death*. New York: Freeman.

Solomon GF, Benton D, Harker JO, Bonavida B, Fletcher MA (1993) Prolonged asymptomatic states in HIV-seropositive persons with 50 CD4 T-cells/mm3: Preliminary psychoneuroimmunologic findings. *Journal of AIDS* **6**, 1173.

Sterne L (1992) *Tristram Shandy*. London: Palgrave Macmillan.

Tomalin C (2003) Samuel Pepys. *The Unequalled Self*. Harmondsworth: Penguin.

Vaillant GE (1993) *The Wisdom of the Ego: Sources of Resilience in Adult Life*. Cambridge, MA: Harvard University Press.

Vanderpol M (2002) Resilience: the missing link in our understanding of survival. *Harvard Psychiatric Review* **10**, 302–306.

Vanistendael S (1998) *Growth in the Muddle of Life: Resilience: Building on people's strengths*, 2nd edn. Geneva: International Catholic Child Bureau.

Vanistendael S, Lecomte J (2000) *Le bonheur est toujours possible: construire la resilience*. Paris, Editions Bayard.

Whybrow P (2005) *American Mania: When more is not enough*. Norton.

2

Resilience and the psychobiological base

Max Watson

Even though conditions such as lack of sleep, insufficient food and various mental stresses may suggest that inmates were bound to react in certain ways, in the final analysis it becomes clear that the sort of person the prisoner became was the result of an inner decision, and not the result of camp influences alone

Frankl (1946)

Frankl's reflections from the Auschwitz concentration camp mimic those of others who from the earliest times have witnessed how individuals adapt to adverse events very differently. The capacity or incapacity to function despite having to deal with emotional, physical, and social stressors is variously called courage/cowardice, strength/weakness or resilience/helplessness. Repeated use of such words in the collective societal manner of the newspaper leader writer, 'Brave toddler fights leukaemia', packed with human value judgements, can make critical understanding of the individual biological processes involved particularly difficult to unpack. On the other hand the use of the highly specific language of the neuroendocrinologist or psychiatrist can cause other problems. By seeking to avoid both pitfalls this chapter sets itself up for 'double failure'.

In reviewing psychobiological research into resilience this chapter provides an outline framework, explores the useful concepts of allostasis and allostatic load, and then details some of the psychobiological processes that have been identified connecting mind, brain, and behaviour as they collectively and interactively adapt to change.

Framework for studying psychobiological resilience

> Psychobiologial resilience is the efficient blending of psychological, biological and environmental elements that permits human beings ... to transit episodes associated with significant periods of stress and change successfully

Flach (1990)

Flach's definition of psychobiological resilience underscores the reality that resilience is an ever-changing dynamic process and not a static capacity. In addition it emphasizes that resilience cannot exist without environmental challenge, for it is forged in the process of adapting to change. '... more than just the 'flip side' of a risk factor the notion of resilience encompasses psychological and biological characteristics, intrinsic to an individual that might be modifiable and confer protection against the development of psychopathology (or indeed other pathology) in the face of stress' (Hoge *et al.* 2007).

Opportunities to study the impact of severe trauma, abuse and stressful events are unfortunately all too many. Research has tended to be focused among vulnerable groups such as children, women, caregivers, victims of violence, and combatants.

One organizational framework for conceptualizing resilience suggests that it is valuable to consider both internal and external factors. 'Internal factors include biological and psychological processes. External factors are related to the nature and quality of relationships within or outside the family group' (Mandleco and Peery 2000).

This chapter will focus on the internal factors, though it is clear that both internal and external are constantly interacting and impacting on each other and the importance of the role of each factor will vary according to the situation.

Within these internal psychobiological processes, research into resilience has identified several themes including:

◆ acute stress and allostasis
◆ adaption and allostatic load
◆ neurobiological transmitters impacting on resilience
◆ acute adaptive processes
◆ chronic adaptive processes
◆ fear conditioning and memory
◆ future research.

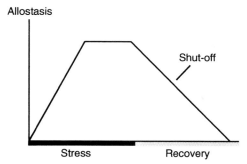

Figure 2.1 Allostasis in the Autonomic Nervous System and the Hypothalamic-pituitary-adrenal Axis. Allostatic systems respond to stress by initiating the adaptive response, sustaining it until the stress ceases, and then shutting it off (recovery). *Reprinted from (McEwen, 1998a) by permission from the New England Journal of Medicine. Copyright 1998 Massachusetts Medical Society. All rights reserved.*

Acute stress and allostasis

The body responds to the external and internal environment by producing hormonal and neurotransmitter messengers, and, at a cellular level, cytokines that set in motion physiological processes throughout the body. The measurement of such responses allows the opportunity to look at the connection between exposure to change and the development of effects resulting from that change including the development of resilience as well as, conversely, physical or psychological damage.

This exposure to change is often termed 'stress', and the popular understanding is that 'stress' is always a bad thing. This is far from biological reality.

The 'stress-mediating' hormones, including cortisol and catecholamines, are constantly varying in their basal concentrations with a diurnal pattern co-ordinated by the light/dark cycle. Without the constant 'stress tone' that they provide throughout the day, it would be impossible to conduct normal human activities, such as walking or standing. Of course, they are also associated with the much more acute, 'fright flight fight' response to danger, which is also termed 'stress' and is caused by the activation of the autonomic sympathetic nervous system.

To get round the ambiguity of the word 'stress', the term 'allostasis' (Fig 2.1) is increasingly being used by those involved in resilience research: 'Allostasis is the process of achieving stability, or homeostasis, through physiological or behavioural change. This is normally carried out by the hypothalamo-pituitary–adrenal (HPA) axis hormones, the autonomic nervous system, cytokines or other systems and is generally adaptive in the short term' (McEwen and Wingfield 2003; McEwen 1998b).

While homeostasis involves the regulation of the body around a single point of balance (i.e. if a person is hot the body will try to reduce heat through sweating) allostasis is a much more complex process of adaption to change that involves the dynamic balance of multiple systems, as well as behavioural processes in an effort to maintain function in the face of change. (That men have been able to walk on the moon and on the bottom of the ocean is testament to our powers of 'allostasis'.)

However, for all its adaptability, the human cannot maintain changes too far from the norm for very long without consequences—the allostatic load.

Adaption and allostatic load

The allostatic load (Fig 2.2) refers to the wear and tear that the individual experiences due to repeated cycles of allostasis as well as the inefficient turning on or shutting off of these responses

McEwen and Stellar (1993); McEwen (1998a)

In short, what is beneficial in meeting the short-term crisis can cause serious damage if that acute response is maintained.

A businessman in the cut and thrust of his work will make regular use of his acute allostatic responses, including raised levels of cortisol and other catecholamines. However, if these acute adaptive responses are not adequately turned off this will lead to long-term cortisol excess, the potential impacts of which include atherosclerosis, obesity, type 2 diabetes, raised blood pressure, inflammatory and autoimmune disorders, fatigue, and so on.

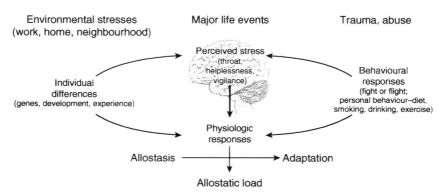

Figure 2.2 Allostatic Load.

Bruce McEwan and Teresa Seeman (1999) summarize the four key features of the allostatic model.

1. The brain is the integrative centre for co-ordinating the behavioural and neuroendocrine responses to challenges.

2. Some of the differences in resilience between individuals are based on interacting genetic, developmental, and experiential factors. A genetic predisposition in association with critical developmental events such as childhood abuse may combine to predispose the individual to over-react physiologically and behaviourally to events throughout life.

3. Neuroendocrine and behavioural responses are set to be protective in the short term but controlling such responses efficiently and appropriately is crucial to reduce the accumulation of allostatic load.

4. There are a vast number of factors contributing to the allostatic load including genes, development, and learned behaviours reflecting life-style choices such as diet, exercise, and smoking.

Neurobiological transmitters impacting on resilience

While the general concepts of allostasis and allostatic load are useful in understanding resilience it is also helpful to understand some of the specific physiological and cellular changes involved in processes that are thought to contribute.

Acute adaptive processes

The mediators of allostasis include the hormones controlled by the HPA axis such as adrenal steroids, including **cortisol** and **noradrenaline** and other hormones such as dihydroepiandrosterone (DHEA). These mediators produce both an immediate effect through direct action on receptors in key organs such as heart, muscle, and lungs (the 'fright, flight, fight' response) and long-term effects through their ability to promote metabolic changes and gene expression at the cellular level.

DHEA is secreted in response to the same stimuli that activates the HPA hormones. DHEA has an antiglucocorticoid action in the hippocampal neurons of the brain. It has an important role to play in switching off the acute response. *Interestingly soldiers with low levels of DHEA have been shown to be more likely to develop post traumatic stress disorder (PTSD) and depression.* (Unpublished work by Rasmussen *et al.* quoted in Charney 2004.)

Corticotrophin-releasing hormone (CRH) is the crucial mediator of the individual's response to stress and the HPA axis. Release of CRH from the hypothalamus leads directly to the activation of the HPA axis and an increase in circulating adrenal steroids and DHEA. CRH is also found in the amygdala, that part of the limbic system in the brain concerned with the panic response and the processing and memory of emotional reactions. Persistent elevation of CRH levels has been correlated with higher levels of PTSD (Bremner *et al.* 1997; Nemeroff 2002).

Neuropeptide Y (NPY) is a small peptide found in the hypothalamus that appears to have functionally opposite actions to CRH, thus it can reduce the activation of the HPA axis and also impact on the storage of distressing memories. Soldiers with high levels of NPY have been shown to demonstrate better performance under challenging conditions than those with normal or low levels (Morgan *et al.* 2000a,b). (It is perhaps worth speculating that too much resilience encouraging NPY may not actually promote survival in soldiers who but for their unnatural 'resilience' would have retreated!)

Galanin is another small peptide found in ascending neural pathways, which can reduce anxiety levels by decreasing the activity of the locus coeruleus (Bing *et al.* 1993), a part of the brain stem responsible for physiological responses to panic.

Dopamine is a neurotransmitter found in different sites throughout the brain. Increases in dopamine concentrations in certain areas brought about through responses to challenging stimuli can impede cognitive function. In other areas of the brain insufficient dopamine can lead to delay in the extinction of conditioned fear responses with a noted clinical impact of increased incidence of PTSD (Hamner and Diamond 1993; Lemieux and Coe 1995).

Dopamine is also involved in the reward systems of the brain. Preservation or hypersensitivity of the reward system is an important factor contributing to resilience. An example is the capacity to enjoy a beautiful sunset despite being in the middle of a distressing traffic jam.

Serotonin, like dopamine, has several different actions. Depending on which serotonin receptors are being activated, serotonin can work as both an anxiolytic and anxiogenic neurotransmitter.

Blocking the function of 5HT1a receptors in very early life in mice produces long-term abnormalities in the regulation of anxiety behaviours in adulthood, which cannot be improved if these receptors are later reactivated (Gross *et al.* 2002). 5HT1a receptors are inhibited by adrenal steroids. Thus stress in early life reduces the density of the 5HT1a receptors. This allows speculation on a possible biopsychological mechanism to explain how long-term predisposition to dysfunctionality in the presence of anxiety can have its origins in exposure to stress-mediating steroids during the crucial window period when long-term management skills for dealing with anxiety are developing (Charney 2004).

GABA

Neuroimaging studies show that cortical and frontal cortex and possibly hippocampal benzodiazepine (GABA) receptor binding is reduced in patients with PTSD (Nutt and Malizia 2001). (In other words these individuals have impeded ability to take advantage of the brain's 'natural valium'.)

Fear conditioning and memory

A very important safety mechanism to protect humans involves being able to recall unpleasant experiences so that the risks of repeating such experiences are reduced. However, if fear conditioning is inappropriately 'set' within the brain it may encourage unnecessary avoidance behaviour, or undermine resilience processes by fear memories.

Central to this process is the amygdala, which regulates the storage of fear memories and also categorizes and consolidates traumatic memories stored elsewhere in the brain (McGaugh 2002; McGaugh *et al.* 2002). If one of the catecholamines, noradrenaline, is infused into the amygdala it enhances memory consolidation. Thus in the acute allostatic situation when the stress mediators are being activated the amygdala will be particularly enabled to consolidate memories. (McIntyre *et al.* 2002).

How a memory is stored early on will thus be influenced by the chemical milieu at the time of the event. The more CRH and noradrenaline (anxiogenic), the more vivid the memory, while high levels of NPY (anxiolytic) will downgrade the vividness and impact factor of the memory. Whether such reasoning would be encouraging or discouraging of acute crisis debriefing to reduce the risk of PTSD, or distressing flashbacks developing will require further study.

The way forward

While the above psychobiological processes working individually or in combination are helpful in understanding how resilience or vulnerability may develop, it is important to place them within the wider context of overall allostatic load.

It has become the cornerstone of modern preventative medicine that it is the cumulative effect of modest derangements of multiple body systems that lead to the major impacts on physical health (McEwen and Stellar 1993). As yet the major research on allostatic load has been on markers of physical health, including such things as:

1. Overnight cortisol, noradrenaline, and adrenaline urinary excretion.
2. Serum DHEA levels.

3. Average systolic and diastolic blood pressure.

4. Waist–hip ratio circumference.

5. High-density lipoprotein cholesterol and ratio total cholesterol to high-density lipoprotein.

6. Blood glycosylated haemoglobin.

Such an approach offers a way forward for a better understanding of resilience. In physical health the cumulative effect of multiple abnormalities in different systems has been found to be significantly more accurately prognostic than individual markers on their own. It is unlikely to be different in psychobiological systems.

Charney calls for an analogous research model to be adopted looking at the neurobiological risk factors related specifically to psychopathology and resilience (Charney 2004). He speculates that a resilient profile will be characterized by individuals in the highest quartiles for measures of DHEA, NPY, Galanin, 5HT1a receptors and benzodiazepine receptor function, and the lowest quartile for HPA axis, CRH and brain noradrenaline activity.

Should this model be proved by research then interventions aimed at moderating dysfunctional responses to change and encouraging the development of resilience across a range of psychobiological parameters could prove a rich vein of study for future interventions. That some of these parameters are shared by both physical and psychobiological systems suggests that physical in combination with psychological interventions, may prove to offer the most valuable strategies in promoting resilience.

Conclusions

Having spent much of this chapter outlining psychobiological processes connected with the reduction of allostatic load it would be tempting to feel that it will soon be possible to explain Victor Frankl's Auschwitz resilience observation entirely through a psychobiological model. Such hubris would be dangerous.

Twin studies from Vietnam (True et al. 1993) report that inherited factors contribute only up to 32% of variance in developing PTSD. Thus, those of us aware of our own lack of resilience cannot claim that genetic factors are totally responsible, nor be absolved from the knowledge that we can each make significant impact on our own resilience by reducing our exposure to allostasis, and the hormones of acute adaption.

The belief that it is impossible to promote resilience is as much a myth as to believe that all resilience is just a matter of 'pulling ourselves together'.

References

Bing O, Moller C, Engel JA, Soderpalm B, Heilig M (1993) Anxiolytic-like action of centrally administered galanin. *Neuroscience Letters* **164**, 17–20.

Bremner JD, Licinio J, Darnell A, Krystal JH, Owens MJ, Southwick SM, Nemeroff CB, Charney DS (1997) Elevated CSF corticotropin-releasing factor concentrations in post-traumatic stress disorder. *American Journal of Psychiatry* **154**, 624–629.

Charney DS (2004) Psychobiological mechanisms of resilience and vulnerability: implications for successful adaptation to extreme stress. *American Journal of Psychiatry* **161**, 195–216.

Flach F (1990) *The Resilience Hypothesis and Post Traumatic Stress Disorder*. Washington DC: American Psychomatic Press.

Frankl VE (1946) *Man's Search For Meaning*. Vienna. Originally 'Ein Psycholog erlebt das Konzentrationslager'. Published as 'Man's Search For Meaning' 1963. New York: Washington Square Press.

Gross C, Zhuang X, Stark K, Ramboz S, Oosting R, Kirby L, Santarelli L, Beck S, Hen R (2002) Serotonin1A receptor acts during development to establish normal anxiety-like behaviour in the adult. *Nature* **416**, 396–400.

Hamner MB, Diamond BI (1993) Elevated plasma dopamine in posttraumatic stress disorder: a preliminary report. *Biological Psychiatry* **33**, 304–306.

Hoge EA, Austin ED, Pollack MH (2007) Resilience: research evidence and conceptual considerations for posttraumatic stress disorder. *Depression and Anxiety* **24**, 139–152.

Lemieux AM, Coe CL (1995) Abuse-related posttraumatic stress disorder: evidence for chronic neuroendocrine activation in women. *Psychosomatic Medicine* **57**, 105–115.

Mandleco BL, Peery JC (2000) An organizational framework for conceptualizing resilience in children. *Journal of Child and Adolescent Psychiatric Nursing* **13**, 99–111.

McEwen BS (1998a) Protective and damaging effects of stress mediators. *New England Journal of Medicine* **338**, 171–179.

McEwen BS (1998b) Stress, adaptation, and disease. Allostasis and allostatic load. *Annals of the New York Academy of Science* **840**, 33–44.

McEwen BS, Seeman T (1999) Protective and damaging effects of mediators of stress. Elaborating and testing the concepts of allostasis and allostatic load. *Annals of the New York Academy of Science* **896**, 30–47.

McEwen BS, Stellar E (1993) Stress and the individual. Mechanisms leading to disease. *Archives of Internal Medicine* **153**, 2093–2101.

McEwen BS, Wingfield JC (2003) The concept of allostasis in biology and biomedicine. *Hormones and Behaviour* **43**, 2–15.

McGaugh JL (2002) Memory consolidation and the amygdala: a systems perspective. *Trends in Neuroscience* **25**, 456.

McGaugh JL, McIntyre CK, Power AE (2002) Amygdala modulation of memory consolidation: interaction with other brain systems. *Neurobiology of Learning and Memory* **78**, 539–552.

McIntyre CK, Hatfield T, McGaugh JL (2002) Amygdala norepinephrine levels after training predict inhibitory avoidance retention performance in rats. *European Journal of Neuroscience* **16**, 1223–1226.

Morgan CA, 3rd, Wang S, Mason J, Southwick SM, Fox P, Hazlett G, Charney DS, Greenfield G. (2000a) Hormone profiles in humans experiencing military survival training. *Biological Psychiatry* **47**, 891–901.

Morgan CA, 3rd, Wang S, Southwick SM, Rasmusson A, Hazlett G, Hauger RL, Charney DS (2000b) Plasma neuropeptide-Y concentrations in humans exposed to military survival training. *Biological Psychiatry* **47**, 902–909.

Nemeroff CB (2002) Recent advances in the neurobiology of depression. *Psychopharmacological Bulletin* **36** (Suppl. 2), 6–23.

Nutt DJ, Malizia AL (2001) New insights into the role of the GABA(A)-benzodiazepine receptor in psychiatric disorder. *British Journal of Psychiatry* **179**, 390–396.

True WR, Rice J, Eisen SA, Heath AC, Goldberg J, Lyons MJ, Nowak J (1993) A twin study of genetic and environmental contributions to liability for posttraumatic stress symptoms. *Archives of General Psychiatry* **50**, 257–64.

3

Resilience and bereaved children: helping a child to develop a resilient mind-set following the death of a parent[1]

Julie Stokes

Introduction

This chapter will consider a variety of factors that can help a bereaved child to develop a resilient mind-set. We will see that these interrelating factors come from:

- within the individual child
- their parent(s)
- their community
- the society in which they live.

The chapter begins with a general discussion of resilience in relation to children with a focus on the cognitive processes involved in building a resilient mind-set. It identifies the spectrum of risk factors that can complicate a child's response to a parental death. Particular attention is given to resilience in relation to vulnerable and violent communities, looked after young people and trauma, and also the relevance of gender issues. Guidelines for practice are outlined and the chapter continues by addressing the vital role of a surviving parent in nurturing resilience and the role of emotionally intelligent schools. Finally, the importance of understanding memory processes in developing a healthy connection between the child and the parent who has died is discussed.

---

[1] All the case scenarios and quotes are from families that have been involved in the Winston's Wish service and responded to service evaluations. Names and some identifying details have been changed or simply omitted to preserve confidentiality. The term 'parent' is used to include parent, step-parent or other key carer in a parental role.

Resilience and children

A resilient child is not a child in a certain set of circumstances, but rather a child with a certain set of attitudes.

A 5 year old watches helplessly as his younger brother drowns. In the same year glaucoma begins to seriously impair his vision. His family are unable to fund the medical care that may save him from becoming blind. Both parents later die during his teenage years. Eventually he is taken into care and not permitted access to leisure activities, including music. Given the obstacles he faces one would not easily predict he would become a world renowned musician.

This man's name was Ray Charles. His life story is similar to many other individuals who have faced great emotional, physical, and environmental adversities. They show that some children do survive and even thrive. Yet, others face ongoing struggles, often finding themselves as educationally underachieving adults with a series of failed and abusive relationships, living in deprived conditions with a range of mental health problems. In reviewing the literature on resilience and bereaved children we need to ask what exactly do the survivors do that enable them to succeed? How do they think? What kinds of experience do they have that may be absent in the lives of those who are not successful? How much of their survival can be predicated by genetics, parenting, education, mentoring, temperament, and mental health? (Goldstein and Brooks 2005).

The concept of resilience can be understood as the means by which children thrive emotionally, behaviourally, academically, and interpersonally either in the face of risk and adversity or not. A resilient child will be able to rebound from disappointments, mistakes, trauma, to develop clear and realistic goals, to solve problems, to mix comfortably with others and to treat him/herself and others with respect and dignity. Brooks and Goldstein (2001, 2002) put forward the concept of building stress hardiness by helping children to develop a **'resilient mind-set'**. Resilient children are not simply born that way nor are they made from scratch by their experiences. Thus, the question is no longer whether and to what degree genes or environments matter, but how genes and environment work together to produce resilient children and adults.

Cognitive ability is a strong and consistent predictor of resilience in childhood and adolescence. In particular, thoughts about the self and control over things that threaten self-safety are crucial. Self-efficacy is the belief that goals can be accomplished. Self-esteem stems from feeling valued by and valuable to other people. Good outcomes are also associated with a resilient mind-set. Those who believe that the worst will happen are less likely to adapt well when difficult circumstances arise. In contrast those who are optimistic are more able to save and use their resources when they need them and be protected from subsequent stresses (Aspinwall 2001).

For example, an adolescent with a pessimistic thinking style who fails a test at school may say to themselves 'I'm stupid, I can't do science'. Equally if they did well on the test they might think 'The test was easy; that's why I did well'. The student expects failure to continue and believes that there is nothing he or she can do to improve performance (i.e. they have a low internal locus of control). Over time these patterns of thinking become more overwhelming and entrenched. The young person feels passive, hopeless, and despairing. Depression and anxiety are often linked to such thinking styles.

There are potentially damaging consequences of viewing resilience simply as an 'individual' trait. Adaptation is embedded within the context of multiple systems of interactions including families, schools, community, and culture. A child's resilience is therefore also dependent upon other people and other systems of influence (Roberts and Masten 2004). The degree of success the child has in overcoming obstacles is a complex combination of personal strengths and vulnerability as well as ongoing interactions with their families, friends, and community networks. At best these can work in harmony to build a resilient mind-set.

Resilience when a parent dies

The International Resilience Project, which surveyed almost 600 eleven-year-old children, described the most commonly mentioned adversities reported by children. Top of the list was the death of a parent or grandparent (Grotberg 1997). A child who is adapting to the death of a parent is unlikely simply to recover quickly. If they did 'bounce back' immediately it may suggest an ambivalent or inhibited grief reaction. Moreover, the child will be adapting to major family change, which often involves many secondary losses alongside all the natural reactions of grief. Additionally, their surviving parent may be significantly impacted by the death themselves and the child's everyday relationships with friends may feel awkward.

Jenny

Jenny (now 23), who was bereaved as a teenager, struggled to find her inner resilience.

> After my mum died I was in a kind of wilderness often drinking heavily to escape. At times I felt quite reckless and irresponsible, it took me a while to get my head straight and decide what I wanted to do in life. Sometimes I look around at other people my age who are faffing around mindlessly... I think 'just get on with it, go for it, don't worry about failure and all that stuff'. I guess I know that I have coped with something terrible and perhaps that gives me an inner confidence.

All children bereaved of a parent, will generally experience a better outcome when they:

1. have a secure attachment and positive relationship with at least one competent adult (ideally their surviving parent if they have one)

2. maintain a healthy connection to the dead person

3. engage well with their peers

4. have an area of competence valued by themselves and by society.

If we want to maximize opportunities in the lives of a child who has been bereaved then together we must help them build a resilient mind-set. However, the reality is that no single factor will account for a successful outcome. Table 3.1 describes different factors that may all have an impact on a bereaved child's capacity to rebuild their life. The factors expand on 'a short-list' drawn up by Masten (2001) relating to all children.

Table 3.1 Factors that impact positively on the resilience of a bereaved child

Child

Social and adaptable temperament in infancy

Characteristics valued by others and self (talented, physically attractive, sense of humour etc.)

Makes and maintains peer friendships

Has strategies to regulate emotions and behaviour

Good problem solving skills

Sets goals that are achievable

Has a feeling of control over his/her life

Positive view of self (self confidence, high self esteem, self efficiency)

Shows a balanced acceptance and understanding of self, acknowledging both limitations and strengths

Hopeful outlook on life and has faith in the future.

Family

Stable and supportive home environment

Authoritative parenting style (high on warmth, boundaries, and monitoring)

Parent involved in child's education

Higher education of the parents

Socioeconomic advantages

Faith and religious affiliation

Supportive connections with family and friends

Parent or main carer confident to accept support for the bereaved child and themselves

Parent or carer had a positive relationship with the person who has died

Extended family able to offer practical and emotional support that is valued by the parent.

Community

Lives in a quality neighbourhood (safe, non violent, affordable housing, recreation centres, clean air and water)

Effective schools academically and in terms of their capacity to respond to bereavement

Table 3.1 Community (continued)

Employment opportunities for parents and young people
Quality health and emergency care services
Availability of accessible specialist child bereavement services where they can meet other
    children who have been bereaved.

Cultural/societal

Society has a low acceptance of physical violence, drug misuse, poverty, health and social
    inequality
The government sets protective and preventative child policies
Policies are backed by long term funding contracts for both the voluntary and state sector
The death of parent or sibling is accepted as a primary risk factor for all children
Government and society value and direct resources to develop community child bereavement
    services.

Stephen

In a recent evaluation, parents who had experienced a child bereavement service were asked if they felt that their child showed any indication of resilience.
This was Stephen's mother's response:

> Steve has said so many things that indicate increased resilience, things about moving
> on, learning to live with sadness and still have fun, about remembering always in a
> way that enriches his life. He says 'Dad would like this, Dad would be proud, I know
> he is with me'. He has even helped his Grandfather cope with the loss of Steve's Gran.
> 'My dad said to me later "I am taking a leaf out Stephen's book; there is still a lot to
> live for, remember and move on."'

It is encouraging to read this mother's comments on her son's perceived
increased resilience. However, in relation to the factors that predispose children
to develop a resilient mind-set to life, this particular child clearly had a good start.
Prior to his father's death, his parents appear to have experienced a solid relationship, creating a secure and loving home environment for Stephen. In addition
there was a close and respectful relationship between mother and son. Steve was
an intelligent child both intellectually and emotionally, popular with adults and
peers alike—often demonstrating good social skills and a strong sense of feeling
in control. He had a great sense of humour and a number of sport and creative
skills, which he valued, and others around him regularly praised him for. He
received clear messages about the importance of maintaining relationships in a
healthy way with somebody who has died. Indeed one of the things his mother
chose to do following her husband's death was to have a tiny shoulder tattoo
made of a humming bird to represent her husband's connection with Trinidad,
as well as being a symbol of the permanence of their relationship. Steve's mother
also actively sought help for her son and herself in terms of accessing a specialist
child bereavement service that was over 200 miles away.

The case study below shows a somewhat different experience for a child of a similar age who needed coaching to help him develop a more resilient mind-set following his father's death by suicide (Love 2006).

Jack

Jack and his mother required substantial intervention. His father had died by hanging following a long and complicated mental health history. Following the assessment, individual work was offered to his mother who felt extremely angry and embittered towards her husband who had been both abusive and unfaithful throughout their marriage. His suicide occurred the day after she had finally decided to leave him. After six sessions she was more able to accept that despite her own feelings of great ambivalence towards her husband it was important for her son to be able to construct a relationship with his father that was not damaging. Jack also understood that he needed help to firmly differentiate himself from his father's psychiatric illness and his suicide. Before attending a group intervention, both mother and son were together encouraged to complete a 'memory jar' that specifically directs them to focus on more positive memories (Stokes 2004, p. 114). They were given five categories that began with the following headings:

- A special time we spent together …
- Something we enjoyed, or laughed at together …
- A memory that offers me some comfort …
- Something I liked about him …
- One thing I valued about our relationship …

They then shared their memories with each other. It was only possible to complete this kind of work having given both mother and son plenty of opportunities to express their considerable ambivalent feelings of anger and resentment towards the father. Jack, who was musical, created a metaphorical 'anger mountain' making sounds from African drums. After a particularly exhausting drumming session, he collapsed and sobbed 'why did my dad have manic depression?' A small, yet significant step towards expressing his true feelings and thus starting to build a more resilient mind-set.

Jane

Another parent recounted her beliefs several years after the family was bereaved. In many ways it serves as a window into the way one parent has changed her thinking in order to survive as a lone mother with three children.

> We all became more resilient as a result of meeting the others—some would say that we are frighteningly so seven years on! What did we learn?

1. Terrible things happen. They are not fair, can't be explained, and you have to carry on
2. Things that other people fuss about are not worth the emotional energy
3. Be thankful for what we DO have
4. No matter how resilient we are, it still hurts like crazy and the pain changes as you get older
5. The death wasn't the end of our lives but the beginning of a new phase of it
6. We all wish he hadn't died but are increasingly proud of how well we are doing as a family
7. It is sometimes hard to be resilient, especially when we are around people who haven't had to learn to be so
8. It is a quality my children will carry with them always, no matter what and a great strength, albeit hard to have acquired so young.

Parent's Evaluation (2006)

Bereaved children at risk

In a climate where resources for child mental health are limited, it is crucial to recognize that **the death of a parent or sibling is a primary risk in itself**. Thus, even children such as Stephen on page 43, who may be perceived as resilient, will still benefit from child bereavement services.

Table 3.2 reflects the experience of children referred to Winston's Wish over the past 15 years. In excess of 300 children each year receive a direct service (assessment, individual and group work with ongoing open access). A further 8000 are supported annually via a national helpline and many more make contact via the website 'ask' section. Recent evaluations focusing on particularly vulnerable children show that most will need significant outreach work to ensure a referral actually takes place. However, the majority of bereaved children referred benefit from early intervention (within 6 months of the death) and there is increasing evidence to demonstrate that these services actively promote resilience for a moderate resource investment (Stokes 2004). Some particularly vulnerable children are unlikely to benefit from child bereavement services until their primary needs of safety, hunger and homelessness are addressed.

Vulnerable and violent communities

Many urban and disadvantaged communities struggle with a subculture that promotes violent solutions to bereavement and condones the abuse of drugs, alcohol, and sex. In the United States it is estimated that 73% of deaths among youths are due to behavioural causes (accidents, murder, manslaughter and suicide, and alcohol and illegal substances are often involved) (Goldstein and Brooks 2005). It is widely recognized that almost 20% of all children in the UK live in poverty. Poverty is associated with multiple risk factors and long-term

Table 3.2

10%	Child is **highly resilient** prior to the death and has a supportive parent. Access to Child Bereavement Service: Easy to engage. Positive, proactive referral by parent. Only need core aspects of service, the child copes well with future transitions and change. These children provide an excellent 'return on the investment' of early intervention.
75%	Child is **moderately resilient** prior to death and has a supportive parent. Access to Child Bereavement Service: Reasonably easy to engage, parents likely to be prompted to access the service by a professional, usually school or palliative care. There may be complications surrounding the way the person died that will require individual work before group work. Re-referral likely when the child faces future transitions. Intervention likely to build resilience and prevent further risk. For this group a modest investment within the first year of a death can have a great impact on preventing future mental health issues and reduce the risk of the child showing their grief in anti-social ways.
15%	These children are **highly vulnerable** and their capacity to be resilient will be affected by a variety of social and psychological factors. (See Tables 3.1 & 3.3) There may be family instability and severe deprivation. They may have experience of being excluded from school and/or involvement in criminal behaviour. Drug and alcohol abuse within the family and amongst peers may be common place. Some will be in local authority care already or enter care due to the death of a lone parent. Those that have a surviving parent are likely to experience inadequate parental support. Initially outreach community and schools work will be essential to engage these children. Partnership working with frontline agencies is crucial so they can encourage families to consider assessment. In some cases primary needs (e.g. housing, safety, nourishment etc.) will need to be addressed before a child bereavement agency can be effective. If an agency is to form meaningful relationships which address the complexities of the grief reaction, insecure attachment histories and so on, then modifications to existing programmes will be required. Longer term relationships with a key worker need to be agreed. In some cases it will not be possible to engage a parent. However, these factors should not prevent the child accessing a service.

stresses that threaten development including exposure to violence, lack of appropriate medical education and psychological care and poor nutrition (Thomas and Hocking 2003).

Finding ways of consistently reaching these particularly vulnerable groups living in vulnerable and deprived communities is of growing concern to child bereavement service providers trying to help such disadvantaged children develop a resilient mind-set. A study of 12 000 adolescents suggested that the best single predictor of resistance to high-risk behaviour (e.g. violence, substance abuse, suicide, etc.) is having a good relationship with one adult such as a teacher, parent, or mentor (Resnick *et al.* 1997).

Looked after young people

A significant number of children in care will have been bereaved and it is essential that we develop awareness and outreach programmes to ensure they can access support at the time the death happens (Penny 2007).

Most children and young people looked after by local authorities will have suffered abuse, neglect, experienced bereavement, disability or serious illness in one or both parents (The Mental Health Foundation 2002). More than 60 000 children are currently in care in the United Kingdom. Of the 6000 who will leave care this year, 4500 will not have even one GCSE qualification. Within 2 years, 3000 of those 6000 will be unemployed; 2100 will be mothers or pregnant; 1200 will be homeless, at least 1500 will be in prison and just 60 will make it to university (Longfield 2006).

> We are already spending £40k per year on each child in care. In addition there is the unknown cost of failure … it is nonsensical to save money on, for example, foster care only to spend a fortune later on the failed care leaver … Millions of pounds are being spent at the wrong time and on the wrong things.
>
> Sergeant (2006, p. 121)

Youth justice

In one study (Liddle and Solanki 2000) it was found that 22% of young offenders from an outer London borough had experienced the death of a close relative. This contrasts sharply with the estimated rate of 4% of 5–15 year olds in the general GB population thought to have experienced the death of a parent (Green 2004). Often significant life events such as a family death are omitted from the individual's case history and more immediate problems such as violence or crime are the prime focus. In 2003 the Youth Justice Trust (UK) concluded that 'crime prevention would follow when grief, loss and rejection issues were acknowledged and attended to'.

Lyon (2000) identified that young people aged 15–20 in youth offending centres or prison were 13 times more likely to have been in local authority care. One young person currently coming to the end of a 6 month placement in a secure unit for driving offences, reported:

Ben

> I have been fostered 3 times, 2 children's homes, kicked out of school and now I am in this unit. This all started when our mum died. I was 10 years old, there was no help. I was just left to get on with it, no one asked me what I felt like or how life changed after mum died. I am still not even sure why she died. It was in the middle of the night, she was gone in the ambulance when I woke up, I never saw her again or went to the funeral. At first the crack and cider took the pain away …

At a recent case conference to plan Ben's future care there were 17 different professional agencies invited, eight attended. He said that no one (other than his grandmother) had known him at the time of his mother's death 4 years before. Indeed at the case conference no one other than his now desperate maternal grandmother placed any significance on the fact that one of his closest childhood friends had recently died aged 17, from leukaemia. Significantly, Ben had not been allowed to be involved in his palliative care or to attend the funeral. Equally, not even his grandmother knew of another friend, Keith, who Ben had met in the secure unit. Ben looked up to Keith who had befriended him. A week after his release Keith (who had previously worked as a rent boy to fuel a heroin habit) was found murdered in Cardiff. No one actually told Ben; he heard about it from one of the other boys who were joking in a derogatory way about how he died. He hit out in response. He said there was no point explaining why he was angry, no one would listen. 'Unreasonable and violent behaviour' were cited as reasons why he was recommended to be detained for a further 6-month period.

There remains a major piece of work to educate policy makers on the relevance and need for early and long-term intervention for particularly vulnerable children who have been bereaved.

Resilience and trauma

Traumatized children rarely discuss their fears and traumas spontaneously (Pynoos and Nader 1990). They also have little insight into the relationship between what they do, what they feel and what has happened to them (Dyregrov and Mitchell 1992). Many bereaved children are suffering from complex trauma and attachment histories. The child and often their parent require therapeutic intervention on an individual basis (McIntyre and Hogwood 2006). A bereaved parent can often feel so emotionally depleted from their own grief that it is a continual struggle to embrace the need to be loving, accepting, curious, empathetic, and playful with their child. These qualities are key to parenting traumatized attachment resistant children and helping them to develop a resilient mind-set (Hughes 1997). The following case study illustrates the importance of attachment theory (Bowlby 1980) and narrative therapy (Freeman et al. 1997) when working with bereaved children.

Emily

An appreciation of different attachment styles was needed to understand 9-year-old Emily and also her mother's capacity to provide effective parenting for a complex and often violently angry child. Emily was adopted when she was 5 years old. Her early years had been punctuated by severe neglect and physical abuse. Emily's natural mother died from a heroin overdose when Emily was 3. Her adoptive parents knew they faced a significant hurdle in helping her to trust them. Her adoptive father was made redundant when Emily was 7 and his mental health subsequently deteriorated. He started to drink heavily, which provoked violent mood swings. When Emily was 9 she was repeatedly told by her adoptive father that she had brought harm to their family. One afternoon having returned from school, Emily and her adoptive mother found him semi-conscious, having taken a toxic mix of alcohol and antidepressant medication. She witnessed traumatizing images of her father in severe pain followed by desperate attempts by her mother at resuscitation before he died. Six months later, Emily and her mother attended regular sessions to work on their own deteriorating relationship. The sessions initially aimed to develop a more secure attachment between Emily and her mother. This was necessary before any grief work could be done in relation to her father. A year later they both attended a residential weekend for 20 children and 12 parents bereaved by suicide (Alilovic 2004; Love 2006).

Given her attachment history it had taken Emily a long time to trust and to risk sharing her true feelings of rage and rejection. Naturally, having made a relationship, Emily was also apprehensive about closure. The transfer to secondary school (or more relevantly the leaving of primary school) resulted in three further sessions that Emily herself requested. Mum also decided to return to work part-time and this process also needed careful planning for Emily to cope with the changes to routine and fear of separation from her mother. This change was negotiated carefully through a helpline call with mum and a 'therapeutic letter' (White and Epston 1990), which mum wrote to Emily.

Emily's story highlights the barriers that can impede the development of a resilient mind-set in a traumatized and emotionally vulnerable bereaved child. Timely and targeted support can be pivotal in reversing a potential downward spiral—in order to maximize the optimism, hope, and resilience Emily possesses.

What bearing does gender have on resilience in children?

In an analysis of families receiving a bereavement service, 75% of parental deaths are fathers, 25% are mothers. (Stokes 2004). Therefore the majority of children who come to child bereavement services will do so to remember a father. The importance of male role models for boys has been well documented (Lucinda 2007). It is also recognized that the majority of workers who tend to be attracted to child bereavement work both on an employed and voluntary basis are females, typically aged between 35 and 65. Therefore planning to create an effective gender and ethnic balance is particularly important for child bereavement services.

The more we can sustain a healthy vulnerability in boys, the more resilient they will become and remain. Resilience is a new hallmark of emotional well-being for boys and young males. Boys often show what Pollack (2004) calls a 'pseudo resilience' and this often fools adults and children themselves into believing the stoical mask is real rather than risk an interface with the boy's deeper, hidden pain. The cult film 'Stand by Me' (Columbia Pictures 1986) provides a brilliant insight into the minds of four adolescent boys, and in particular shows one boy's real struggle with grief since his brother's death. The film powerfully demonstrates the healing and understanding provided by his peers. This is in stark contrast to the atmosphere at home and distance that particularly grows between the surviving child and his embittered father. To justify his absence from home he reassures his friends that all will be OK, 'I am now the invisible child at home since Danny died'.

The 'boy code' as defined by Pollack pushes boys towards extremes of self-containment, toughness, and separation (Pollack 1998). In society, boys are subtly encouraged to feel ashamed if they express certain emotions and to deny feeling weak or helpless. The standards for maturity involve being independent, self-reliant, and autonomous. Many boys feel a sadness and disconnection they cannot even articulate. Boys frequently experience intense sadness, vulnerability, and a troubling sense of isolation, disconnection, and despair (Pollack 2000). While many bereaved boys are in deep emotional pain, their suffering often remains difficult to detect, sometimes almost invisible.

On the outside, a boy may seem cheerful, playful, and resilient but on the inside he may actually feel lonely, afraid, and desperate, because of the pressure society places on boys to act tough, follow a strict code of masculinity and hide their emotions at all costs. It is often hard to notice when boys are failing to reach their potential at school, when their friendships are not working out, when they are feeling depressed or even suicidal. We are too often fooled by the seemingly robust cheerfulness and ruggedness boys project on the outside (Pollack 2004). Often there is a short window when grief arising from a family death will be acknowledged; afterwards a boy's disruptive behaviour is the most likely thing to be noticed.

We know from the adult bereavement literature that there are gender differences around grieving (Stroebe *et al.* 2001). McLaren (2005) specifically provides an insight into the gender differences following the death of a child. It is therefore crucial that we design child bereavement interventions and printed resources that will also appeal to fathers and boys, male practitioners, and male volunteers. An initiative at Winston's Wish has been to take bereaved teenagers on an Outward Bound weekend. The programme is adventurous, challenging, and physically demanding and led by clinicians and volunteers with an interest and experience in sport and outdoor activities. We have found that such an intervention has particularly appealed to teenage boys, a subgroup often deemed 'hard to reach'. The 'I Can' 3-day programme embraces the shared experiences of a family death during adolescence (Nugus 2006).

Opportunities for connection and honest emotional expression lead boys to feel greater self-confidence, have a clear sense of who they are, diminishes fear, and harnesses optimism and personal success. The emotionally engaging 'candlelight ceremony' sometimes used in group interventions (Stokes 2004, p. 112) has been effective in helping boys to safely share their feelings. However, this therapeutic process relies heavily on the physical activities that are planned earlier in the day.

It is also important when we train volunteers to work on child bereavement programmes that we actively seek to recruit and train young male role models from culturally diverse backgrounds.

Hassan

A 15-year-old Muslim boy whose father had been murdered said:

> All that seems to matter is how my mother is feeling, every day she cries then shouts, then cries holding my father's photo. In the family no one asks or even notices if I am having a bad day. My teacher at school is great though, he has a list of important dates like my birthday, my dad's birthday, the day he died, and religious days when I miss him most. Meeting the other boys at the camp has been cool, one friend I email at least once a week, and I use the chat board. At last I feel like I belong somewhere and someone is noticing my sadness.

So what are the characteristics of a resilient mind-set?

Resilient children possess qualities and ways of viewing themselves and the world that are not apparent in children who have not been successful in meeting such challenges (see Table 3.3). The death of a parent or sibling is obviously a key challenge for any child to cope with. Similarly, the beliefs that children have about themselves influence both the behaviours and skills that they develop. In turn, these behaviours and skills influence this set of beliefs, so that a dynamic process is constantly operating to deliver strength and optimism.

An understanding of the features of a resilient mind-set can provide parents and other adults with guideposts for nurturing inner strength and optimism in children who have had their world shattered by a significant bereavement and all the secondary losses that may follow. A resilient mind-set clearly requires a child to have hope for the future. It also requires them to have the capacity to trust others and risk forming secure attachments. A capacity to talk about the person who has died in a way that brings comfort and worth to the relationship is also a key resilience building block. Above all, the child will need to find a way of creating an overall meaning for life and death issues that allows future growth.

Natalie

The following case study reflects how the **circumstances** of a death can adversely complicate a child's beliefs and the meaning they construct following a family death. The meaning will have a significant relationship with their ability to develop a resilient mind-set.

Natalie was going to school. At breakfast she asked her mum to iron her skirt. Her mum was annoyed at this late request and even more frustrated when Natalie decided the skirt was not short enough and now wanted her trousers ironed instead! A fairly normal encounter between an indecisive,

Table 3.3

To build resilience a (bereaved) child needs to:-

- Be secure, safe, loved – to feel special and appreciated
- Have learned a set of realistic goals and expectations of themselves
- Believe they have the ability to solve problems and make sound decisions
- Be able to view obstacles as challenges and mistakes as something to learn from
- Know that coping strategies encourage personal growth
- Be aware of their weaknesses but view them as areas for improvement rather than unchangeable flaws
- Recognise and enjoy their strong points and talents
- See themselves as confident
- Feel comfortable with others and have good interpersonal skills with their peers and adults. This enables them to seek out guidance and support readily
- Be able to define the aspects of their lives over which they have control. Then they need to be able to focus their energy on these rather than on factors they have little or no influence over
- Have at least one parent who examines his/her own beliefs and actions in order to nurture such characteristics in their children. It is well established that the basic foundation of resilience is the presence of at least one adult (hopefully several) who believe in the goodness of the child. This becomes even more relevant in the case of a bereaved child who has experienced the death of a lone parent.

---

self-absorbed adolescent and a busy working mum who was running late. However, the 'meaning' of this encounter later led to extreme episodes of self-harm and a severe depression during which Natalie was admitted as an inpatient for several weeks because her mother died in a road traffic accident on her way to work.

Such cognitive disconnections can occur in a climate of shame. Shame moves people into isolation and disempowers and immobilizes people. Shame is the experience of feeling unworthy of love (Jordan 1989). This was certainly the case for Natalie and had a profound impact on her capacity to feel resilient following her mother's death. It was 5 months before she was even able to say the destructive words '*I killed my mother*', and a further 8 months and several sessions of cognitive-behavioural therapy before she modified her belief to. '*I really regret having that row with mum over breakfast because that was the last time we spoke, I never meant for her to die, I loved her and I know she loved me, I miss her so much it hurts*'.

In isolation we repeat patterns caught in persistent negative thinking and are often disempowered as a result. This was true for Natalie and as part of her 'recovery', she desperately needed to meet other teenagers who were struggling to make sense of a parent's death.

Resilience implies energy, creativity, and flexibility to meet new situations. Sometimes it involves courage and the capacity to move into situations when we feel fear or hesitation. Attending a teenagers group organized by a specialist child bereavement service was a big step. Natalie found comfort in the fact that other teenagers had ambivalent relationships with their parents before they died. Natalie said she felt good having spent time with another young person who was deeply troubled and confused by her mother's death. The prohibition of anger for girls (Miller 1985; Jordan 2005) is often a great obstacle to developing resilience. Natalie and her group made use of a graffiti wall (www.winstonswish.org.uk). They began to recognize that the anger was a signal of the hurt and Natalie began to recognize that she did not really hate her father with whom she regularly argued nor herself.

Meeting other bereaved young people gave Natalie the opportunity to offer support to her peers as well as to receive it. The social support literature demonstrates the benefits of giving to others (Luks 1982; Love 2006). We find meaning when contributing to the well-being of others but also need to feel cared for, given to and treated with respect. Creating an effective balance is an important focus for child bereavement services aiming to support adolescents in a group setting (Wood 2004).

Before she left for college, Natalie was able to construct a set of beliefs that laid stronger foundations for the next part of her life journey. The beliefs she eventually generated at the end of six sessions of cognitive-behavioural therapy are outlined in Table 3.4.

Table 3.4

I believe that........

1. I can continue to have a close relationship with my mum for the rest of my life

2. Its ok to cry, its ok to laugh, its not ok to feel shame or self hate

3. I am not responsible for my mother's death, even though we argued and I nagged her to do the ironing for me, I never intended that she should die

4. I can see that my attitude to things, even really bad things, makes a big difference to how I feel

5. Now I can share stories and memories of mum with people who can listen without becoming very upset or very angry

6. I have met others who feel and think the same as me so I know that this painful stuff is natural when someone you care about dies

7. If my dad meets someone I do not have to choose. I can relate to both my mum and a new step mother, if that happens

8. I now believe that life is for living. Mum would have wanted me to sort out the things I want to do, so I have made a list of my top ten goals and now I am going to go for it.

Natalie
03.10.04

Practice guidelines to enhance resilience in bereaved children

Given the ongoing reality for a bereaved child, there is clearly a compelling need for child bereavement services to act as a direct advocate; offering support to children, parents, and the communities in which they live. Such support will nurture the resilience required to survive not only the first years after a family death, but also the lifelong journey a bereaved child will face.

What are the factors that help some children and young people appear to bounce back from bereavement while others become overwhelmed with feelings of helplessness and hopelessness? Some achieve considerable success that could never have been predicted, somehow finding the inner strength to overcome obstacles in their paths. Table 3.5 shows the 10 priorities for practitioners, which can guide practice to enhance resilience.

Every child who survives and thrives will be unique, yet all will have some common strengths and skills as shown in Table 3.1. Services specifically designed to nurture these strengths and skills may be more relevant rather than services to simply eradicate problem behaviours. This may be especially relevant to the children who are at an elevated risk due to known complicating factors, for example the state of the surviving parent's mental health; the cause of death may have been traumatic; the child may have had difficulties prior to the death and so on. Timely and targeted child bereavement services may therefore serve to

Table 3.5

1. Enable a child to construct a **coherent narrative** (story) that they can tell with emotional integrity throughout the lives (Lichter *et al.* 1993; McIntyre and Hogwood 2006). Recognize that the story will grow and develop with the child, often resulting in a re-referral and the need for open ended child bereavement services.

2. Develop cognitive and behavioural strategies to help a child **rewrite negative scripts.** Negative scripts are those beliefs or behaviours that are followed daily with predictable negative results.

3. Help the child to develop effective **communication** strategies to use with their family and friends on the subject of their bereavement and the confidence to own their story and communicate it with those they trust.

4. Ensure the child has an age-appropriate understanding of the **dual process model** creating a mind-set that allows a healthy oscillation between 'loss' and 'restoration' to take place (Stroebe and Schut 1999). Explain by using age-appropriate language and using examples to give them a framework to accept the thoughts, feelings and behaviours associated with their individual grief journey. In particular it will help them manage the isolation of feeling upset at one moment and the need to distract themselves with other task-focused activities in the next moment.

5. Provide opportunities for bereaved children to develop empathy and have **positive connections with others who have been bereaved**. Offer this both directly (e.g. day groups, residential weekends), and indirectly (e.g. through books, websites, newsletters, films, etc.).

6. Create non-pathological services that are **appealing to children**. Even a child bereavement 'club' can be experienced as fun, vibrant, cool, and non-judgemental.

7. Help children who have been bereaved to feel understood and confident with their peers and with teachers at **school.**

8. Always include **services for parents or carers** of children who have been bereaved.

9. Create services that **build family cohesion and adaptability**. Helping families to cope with the immediate overwhelming nature of the loss, together with current and future secondary losses (e.g. a house move, new partners, step-children, etc.).

10. Provide a range of age-appropriate activities that encourage children to **secure and maintain continuing attachments** to a parent, brother, or sister who has died. Recognize that these activities will need to change and be reoffered as the child matures and develops.

prevent a significant number of children or young people being referred to mental health, youth justice, educational welfare, or social services.

A realistic thinking style and positive coping skills promote resilience and may buffer bereaved children from internalizing problems. It is therefore crucial that child bereavement services provide a range of cross-cutting interventions for the individual child and others who may have a positive influence on their thinking for example, family, teachers, friends, and other bereaved children (Stokes 2004). It is the responsibility of the children's workforce to complete comprehensive assessments of children and families so that limited resources can be channelled to promote resilient mind-sets in children who have been bereaved. An excellent summary of brief interventions is presented in Monroe and Kraus (2005).

The role of a surviving parent in nurturing resilience

The quality of a child's support system, particularly the quality and nature of the child's interaction with the surviving parent (see Table 3.6), is the factor which most strongly influences his or her adjustment to the death (Furman 1974).

There has been a growing awareness over recent years of the importance of a family centred model of care, to meet the needs of families involved with palliative care services and to maintain continuity of support into bereavement (Kissane 1998). As Zaider and Kissane articulate in Chapter 4, a death within the family requires the family to modify its rules, roles, and leadership. Family flexibility is incredibly important for fostering resilience in a bereaved child. Flexible relationships allow for discussion between parent and child, rules that can change according to their developmental appropriateness and roles that are shared among family members. At the other extreme, a chaotic relationship is defined as one devoid of consistent leadership, and ultimately unsupportive of the child developing a resilient mind-set.

> The functioning level of the surviving parent is the most powerful predictor of the child's adjustment to the death of a parent. Children with a less well functioning parent will show more anxiety and depression and sleep and health problems
>
> Worden (1996)

There are parents who can intuitively understand and fortify in their children the different characteristics of a resilient mind-set. Such parents believe in their children and convey unconditional love. They provide their children with opportunities to confirm their strengths and feelings of self-worth and dignity (Brooks 2005). However, assuming such a role can be particularly

Table 3.6

Foundations of good parenting

1. Being empathetic, having a secure and trusting relationship with their child

2. Communicating effectively and listening actively

3. Changing negative scripts

4. Loving children in ways that help them feel special and appreciated

5. Accepting them for who they are and helping them to have realistic goals

6. Nurturing their strengths

7. Helping children realise mistakes are experiences from which to learn

8. Developing responsibility, compassion and a social conscience by providing children with opportunities to contribute

9. Teaching children to solve problems and make decisions

10. Using discipline in ways that promote self discipline and self worth

challenging for a grieving parent who will be faced with their own emotional and practical mountain to climb after the death of a partner or child.

Since it opened in 2001, a UK Helpline for anyone concerned about a bereaved child has received over 20 000 calls (Stubbs 2004). Seventy-five per cent of these calls are from a parent or close family member. An independent evaluation clearly demonstrated that the majority of parents are seeking guidance, reassurance, empathy, and practical advice when calling the helpline (Eddershaw 2006). Confidence is often particularly low in bereaved parents who are frequently trying to discriminate between conflicting advice from friends and relatives. The need to 'do the right thing' and 'protect' their children from further harm can leave a parent feeling unskilled and unable to maintain control (Sandler *et al.* 2003). A parent who had been encouraged to develop a more positive communication style with her child said '*Using these techniques I learnt that as surviving parent I can be part of the solution for my child rather than adding to the problem. Before I just felt that the wrong parent had died and I was simply making matters worse*'.

Resilience enhancing schools

In order for schools to foster resilience in bereaved children, it is first necessary for staff to understand what makes a positive difference for the bereaved child. One Head Teacher called to complain because she felt a practitioner had inappropriately asked a member of her teaching staff to provide what she described as 'counselling' to a 5 year old who had witnessed his father's murder at home. During the home assessment with his mother, it had emerged that James was frequently calling out in class, '*My daddy has been shot, My daddy has been shot*'. Mum said the current practice in class was to ignore his outbursts and to distract him on to an educational agenda. At his mother's request, a practitioner spoke to the class teacher and explained that it might help to simply endorse James statement by saying 'Yes James, your daddy was shot', gently explaining that this was both very unusual and terribly sad, and then moving him back to his school work. However, on this occasion the Head Teacher remained adamant, stating that '*It was not their job to meet the emotional needs of children in school*'.

'*I didn't mention it, as I didn't want to upset him*'. This comment was from a Primary School teacher, calling the Winston's Wish helpline, 2 days after a child in her class had returned following an absence of 10 days due to his father's sudden death from throat cancer. The child quickly realizes through these subtle communications that dad's death is a subject that can not be openly discussed or acknowledged, even by a trusted teacher. Fortunately this somewhat defensive response is becoming replaced by an increasing acceptance that bereavement can and needs to be part of the emotional tool kit for all schools (Rowling 2003).

Clearly the needs of bereaved children and their parents cannot be segmented or packaged so that just specialist child bereavement agencies respond, somehow insulating everyone else from the need to take responsibility for their role in building resilience. There are now many positive examples of other teachers who would have readily abandoned the curriculum to respond to children like James or the boy mentioned above. They may have even initiated circle time enabling the other children to support their friend and in turn modelling emotionally intelligent social skills for the entire class.

In the UK, schools are now required to have a crisis management plan that is put in place following the death of a pupil or teacher. The inclusion of this in the school's critical incident plans has encouraged more Head Teachers to seek guidance.

One Head Teacher introduced the idea of having a 'pebble pond' in the entrance hallway of his school. Gradually it became a way of life at school that if a child experienced a death that they would be encouraged to go to his office and explain what had happened. Many children simply wanted to talk through the meaning of their loss, 'Willow was my first pet and she slept at the bottom of my bed each night.'

Mr Coleman was open to hearing their stories, embracing their sadness as well as their humour. Pupils were then given the opportunity to select a pebble, write the name of the person or pet to be remembered and the date they died. This was then placed in the pebble fountain. If the death was a close family member, Mr Coleman also took the opportunity to discuss how, or indeed if, the child might like this to be shared with his or her classmates.

Their responses naturally varied. Some wanted to be very private; others felt it would be helpful if they could be helped to tell their friends and fellow classmates. The Head was keen that the child had a sense of control while enabling them also to have the opportunity of support from people they valued. He would then offer options for how such delicate issues could be managed to avoid any awkwardness. Children particularly welcomed ideas outlined on the Childhood Bereavement Network's postcards that were specifically designed for use in schools (http://www.childhoodbereavementnetwork.org.uk). Later in the year, the school council voted that the pebble pond be used for other losses, such as parents who had separated or divorced or when relatives were seriously ill. One of the key success factors involves having a shared language around serious illness and death and an appreciation of the natural grief responses following a bereavement. These children and staff were evolving their own special shared language to deal with very important issues.

Memory and resilience

A greater understanding of memory processes will certainly assist us in explaining why some bereaved children show greater resilience than others (Stokes 2004, pp. 69–73).

Maintaining secure attachments and having positive stories to share is a key variable in bereaved children who are perceived as resilient. While the current literature testifies vehemently to the importance of 'continuing bonds', it remains virtually silent as to the particulars of the memory process itself. We need to develop a clearer understanding of the factors that help a child to maintain attachment to a dead parent in childhood (Lohnes 1994). In order to offer services that promote resilience there needs to be a clear theoretical underpinning relating to memory. 'When does the child want to avoid reminiscing?', 'Which of their memories fade?', 'How do different deaths affect a child's capacity to remember?', 'What do they do to retain secure memories?', 'Which memories feel safe to rehearse and with which people?', and so on. Of course all the above questions will be influenced by developmental factors, with a very young child requiring significant prompts to create a narrative around their relationship with a dead parent.

Lohnes' (1994) study supports clinical observations that resilience is associated with positive and humorous memories. Children invest heavily in objects that reduce separation anxiety and prompt story telling. Maintaining an emotional investment in the dead parent permits children to maintain and continue normal developmental processes. However, the nourishing of this bond also requires that children must repeatedly struggle with this loss and feelings of sadness, guilt, anxiety, shame, and rejection, which can run alongside. Child bereavement services need to ensure there is a range of services that help children (and their surviving parent) achieve a balance of holding on, while also letting go, in order to rebuild a different family experience without the person who has died.

The theoretical framework of the Dual Process Model incorporating an understanding of how attachment styles impact on grieving have been core to these developments (Stroebe 2002). In accordance with the Dual Process Model, adults clearly need to be able to tolerate a child's need to jump in and out of grief. It is sometimes a way spontaneously to regulate feeling overwhelmed, and does not mean they are unaffected by the loss. *'I was 6 when my father came down and gently explained that mum had died moments earlier in their bedroom. To my eternal regret I then asked him for a Kit Kat.'*

Younger children are more likely to reminisce with their surviving parent than older children. They are less private and more emotionally dependant on the surviving parent than are older children. Because of the important developmental differences in children it is crucial to design both group and individual interventions that meets the needs of children at different stages of their lives (Silverman 2000).

> There's a land of the living and a land of the dead and the bridge is love, the only survival, the only meaning.
>
> Thornton Wilder (1967)

The following case study demonstrates how memory work can be used to build this bridge, not just of 'love' but also of resilience.

Becky

When Becky was 4 her mother was given a diagnosis of incurable illness. Two years later she died. During that time Becky's mother travelled a parallel path of maintaining 'hope' that she would live, but she also wanted to prepare a memory box for Becky 'just in case' the doctors were right. The memory box contained a variety of objects, each one reflecting a story that would give Becky a sense of being special and loved, and remind her of early childhood memories that may be lost if not rehearsed. The box also contained a bottle of her mum's perfume that was sprayed on a soft scarf, which became a night-time comforter. Some of the items in the box (e.g. letters) were prepared for later in Becky's life when the meaning would be more significant as she approached her teenage years.

Becky took great pride in her memory box, which she chose to keep in her bedroom, underneath her bed. In the early months after her mum died she needed to look through it almost every night with her dad. As time moved on she used it more sparingly and only showed it to those she really trusted. As she got older she knew it would remind her of her mum in a way that was both painful and comforting. Becky was slowly developing her own mechanism for holding on while letting go. Memories reaffirmed her sense of self, allowing Becky to build a resilient mind-set as she encountered future changes, e.g. a new school, dad's new partner and step-siblings. Later, as she moved into adult life, a positive mind-set helped her to make effective personal relationships and good friends, and to feel confident in her own capacity to be a mother.

Conclusions

The death of a parent is one of the most significant losses a child will ever have to face.

Worden (1996)

It is not the fact that a parent dies that matters most; it is the child's attitude to it that will ultimately make the most difference. After the death of a parent or sibling, a child's 'life journey' is forever changed—they can never simply bounce back unchanged. However, a child can be helped to construct a meaning for themselves in relation to the bereavement that will allow the child and others to view them as resilient. It is our job as practitioners in the palliative care and specialist child bereavement field to ensure a child's resilience 'toolkit' is packed full of resources so they do not need to embark on this journey feeling helpless, isolated and stigmatized.

The study of resilience as an outcome for bereaved children gathers vital knowledge that will help us to shape community services. It also serves to shape the attitude of adults who can make a positive difference. Multiple barriers to policy change exist. However, every bereaved child matters and it matters most that we continue to demonstrate that a modest investment in the first year after a death (and in some situations leading up to the death) can mean major financial and emotional savings in future years. As the comprehensive Joseph Rowntree Foundation Report (Ribbens McCarthy (with Jessop) 2005) concludes, research on interventions to promote resilience is just beginning. Only by identifying the multifaceted processes underlying successful adaptation in adverse conditions will we find ways to intervene successfully in the lives of those who remain vulnerable.

Newman (2002) has identified 'a worrying situation where children are seemingly being affected by an absolute increase in many serious problem areas, accompanied by an apparent weakening in their capacity for natural resilience'.

The promotion of resilience-enhancing, child-centred services for the issue children themselves rate as their greatest fear may be one important strategy to reverse this trend. Open access bereavement services that promote well-being, rather than services that simply focus on the identification and elimination of risk, are key to the success of the 'Every Child Matters' agenda in the UK (Rayner and Montague 2000).

Resilience is a concept rather than a theory. Although concepts, by their nature, are not true or false, they can be evaluated with regard to their usefulness. We are slowly beginning to see the emergence of a resilience framework for practice and policy (Newman 2002); however, its active application to child bereavement work currently remains limited.

An understanding and response to the needs of bereaved children could contribute greatly to the quality of life of thousands of families both now and in the future and, indeed, as a result of this, to society as a whole. Bereavement needs to be recognized as having a place on the childhood mental health agenda alongside more familiar subjects such as bullying, drug misuse, and youth offending. Perhaps when it is, we may see fewer bereaved children being bullied or relying on drugs and alcohol to tranquillize their grief before venting their anger in antisocial ways.

This chapter has outlined how parents, schools, and child bereavement services and the wider community can actively seek to promote resilience in bereaved children. A resilient mind-set paves the way forward so that a bereaved child can grow into adulthood, empowered with choices, opportunities, and personal resources that enable them to live a satisfying and successful life in which they have realized their full potential.

Acknowledgements

Thanks to families for sharing their experiences and to Di Stubbs and Danny Nugus for their editorial contribution to this chapter.

References

Allilovic K (2004) Beyond the Rough Rock: offering a specialist group for families bereaved by suicide. In: *Then, Now and Always … Supporting Children as they Journey Through Grief* (ed. Stokes JA). Cheltenham: Winston's Wish.

Aspinwall LG (2001) Dealing with adversity: self regulation, coping, adaptation and health. In: *Blackwell Handbook of Social Psychology: Intra individual processes*, pp 91–614 (eds Tesser, A, Schwazt N). Malden MA: Blackwell.

Bowlby J (1980) *Attachment and Loss: Loss*. Vol 3: *Loss, Sadness and Depression*. New York: Basic Books.

Brooks R, Goldstein S (2001) *Raising a Resilient Child: Fostering strength, hope and optimism in our children*. New York: Contemporary Books.

Brooks R, Goldstein S (2002) *Nurturing resilience in our children: Answers to the most important parenting questions*. New York: Contemporary Books.

Christ GH (2005) Interventions with bereaved children. In: *Loss, Change and Bereavement in Palliative Care* (eds Firth P, Luff G, Oliviere D). Facing Death Series. Maidenhead: Open University Press.

Dfes (2004) *Every Child Matters: Change for children*. www.everychildmatters.gov.uk.

Dowdney L (2000) Childhood bereavement following parental death. *Journal of Child Psychology and Psychiatry and Allied Disciplines* **41**, 819–830.

Dyregrov A, Mitchell JT (1992) Work with traumatised children: psychological effects and coping strategies. *Journal of Traumatic Stress* **5**, 5–17.

Eddershaw R (2006) *Childhood Bereavement Network:* Bulletin Issue 10 October 2006 www.childhoodbereavementnetwork.org.uk.

Freeman J, Epston D, Lobovits D (1997) *Playful Approaches to Serious Problems: Narrative therapy with children and their families*. New York: W. W. Norton and Co.

Furman E (1974) *A Child's Parent Dies: studies in childhood bereavement*. New Haven CT: Yale University Press.

Goldstein S, Brooks R (eds) (2005) *Handbook of Resilience on Children*. New York: Springer Science and Business Media Inc.

Green H, McGinnity A, Mecezer H, Goodman R (2004) Mental Health of Children and young people in Great Britain. London Office for National Statistics.

Grotberg E (1997) *A Guide to Promoting Resilience in Children: strengthening the human spirit*. The Hague: Bernard Van Leer Foundation.

Hughes DA (1997) *Facilitating Developmental Attachment*. Aronson. Lanham MD.

Jordan JV (1989) *Relational Development. Therapeutic implication of empathy and shame*. Work in Progress No. 39. Stone Center Working Paper series. Wellesley, MA.

Jordan JV (2005) Relational resilience in girls. In: *Handbook of Resilience in Children* (eds Goldstein S, Brooks R). New York: Springer Science and Business Media Inc.

Kissane DW, Bloch S, McKenzie M, McDowell AC, Nitzan R (1998) Family grief therapy: a preliminary account of a new model to promote healthy family functioning during palliative care and bereavement. *Psycho oncology* **6**, 197–204.

Lichter I, Mooney J, Boyd M (1993) Biography as therapy. *Palliative Medicine* **7**, 133–137.

Liddle and Solanki (2000) *Missed Opportunities: Key Findings and Implications from Analysis of the Backgrounds and Life Experiences of a Sample of Persistent Youth Offenders in Redbridge*. London: Nacro.

Lohnes K (1994) *Maintaining Attachment to a Dead Parent in Childhood: A developmental perspective*. Unpublished doctoral thesis. The University of Michigan.

Longfield A (2006) A real chance to keep children out of care. *Children Now* 18–24 October.

Love H (2006) *Suicide Bereaved Children and Young-People's Experience of a Specialist Group Intervention; An Interpretative Phenomenological Analysis:* Dissertation submitted to University of Exeter.

Lucinda N (2007) About Our Boys: A practical guide to bringing out the best in boys. lulu.com.uk.

Luks A (1992) *The Healing Power of Doing Good*. New York: Faucett Columbine.

Lyon E (2000) *Welfare, Poverty, and Abused Women: new research and its implications.* Harrisburg PA: National Resource Center on Domestic Violence.

Masten AS (2001) Ordinary magic: resilient processes in development. *American Psychologist* **56**(3): 227–238.

McIntyre B, Hogwood J (2006) Play, stop and eject–creating film strip stories with bereaved young people. *Bereavement Care* **25**(3).

McLaren J (2005) The death of a child. In: *Loss, Change and Bereavement in Palliative Care* (2002), pp 80–95 (eds Firth P, Luff G, Oliviere D). Maidenhead: Open University Press.

Miller JB (1985) *The Construction of Anger in Women and Men.* Work in Progress No. 4. Stone Center Working Paper Series. Wellesley, MA.

Monroe B, Kraus F (2005) *Brief Interventions with Bereaved Children.* Oxford: Oxford University Press.

Newman T (2002) *Promoting Resilience: A Review of Effective Strategies for Child Care Services.* University of Exeter: Centre for Evidence Based Social Sciences: www.exeter.ac.uk/cebss.

Nugus D (2006) *'I Can!': Evaluation Report of the Outward Bound Weekend for Bereaved Teenagers* (In Press) dnugus@winstonswish.org.uk.

Penny A (2007) Grief Matters for Children: Published by the National Children's Bureau.

Pollack WS (1998) *Real Boys: rescuing our sons from the myths of boyhood.* New York: Random House.

Pollack WS (2000) *Real Boys' Voices.* New York: Random House.

Pollack WS (2004) *Creating Genuine Resilience in Boys and Young Males*, pp. 65–77. Cited in Goldstein S and Brooks R (Eds) (2005) *Handbook of Resilience on Children.* New York: Springer Science and Business Media Inc.

Pynoos R, Nader K (1990) Children's exposure to violence and traumatic death. *Psychiatric Annals* **20**: 334–344.

Rayner M, Montague M (2000). *Resilient Children and Young People.* Melbourne: Victoria Deakin University, Policy and Practice Unit.

Resnick MD, Bearman PS, Blum RW, Bauman KE, Harris KM, Jones J et al. (1997). Protecting adolescents from harm. *Journal of the American Medical Association* **278**(10), 823–832.

Ribbens McCarthy J with Jessop, J (2005) *Young People, Bereavement and Loss: Disruptive Transitions.* London: Published for the Joseph Rowntree Foundation by National Children's Bureau.

Roberts JM, Masten AS (2004) *Resilience in context.* Cited in Peters RD, McMahon R, Leadbeater B (eds). *Resilience in Children, Families, Communities: Linking context to practice and policy*, pp 13–25. New York: Kluwer Academic/Plenum.

Rowling L (2003) *Grief in School Communities: Effective Support Strategies.* Bucks: Open University Press.

Sandler I, Ayers T, Wolchik S et al. (2003) The Family Bereavement Program: Efficacy evaluation of a theory based prevention program for parentally bereaved children and adolescents. *Journal of Consulting and Clinical Psychology* **71**, 587–600.

Sergeant H (2006) *Handle with Care–An investigation into the care system.* London: Centre for Young Policy Studies.

Silverman PR (2000) *Never Too Young to Know: Death in Children's Lives.* Oxford University Press. New York.

Stand By Me (1986) Columbia Pictures. Based on the novel *The Body* by Stephen King.

Stokes JA (2004) *Then, Now and Always… Supporting Children as they journey through grief.* Cheltenham: Winston's Wish.

Stroebe M (2002) Paving the way from early attachment theory to contemporary bereavement research. *Mortality* **7**(2), 127–138.

Stroebe M, Schut H (1999). The dual process model of coping with bereavement: rationale and description. *Death Studies* **23**, 197–224.

Stroebe M, Hansson R, Stroebe W, Schut H (2001). *Handbook of Bereavement Research–consequences, coping and care.* Washington DC: American Psychological Association.

Stubbs D (2004) Whispering into someone's ear: providing guidance, information and support over the phone. In: Stokes JA (2004) *Then, Now and Always… Supporting Children as they journey through grief*, pp 152–207. Cheltenham: Winston's Wish.

Thomas G, Hocking G (2003) *Other People's Children–Why their quality of life is our concern.* New York: Demos.

White M, Epston D (1990) *Narrative Means to Therapeutic Ends.* London: Norton.

Wilder TN (1967) *The Bridge of St Luis Rey*, p. 148. London: Penguin Books.

Wood L (2003) *Adolescents' Experiences of a Residential Weekend for bereaved families: An Interpretative Phenomenological Analysis.* For the degree of MSc Health Psychology of the University of Bath.

Worden JW (1996) *Children and Grief—When a Parent Dies.* New York: The Guildford Press.

Resilient families

Talia Zaider and David Kissane

The family is a crucial resource for patients facing life-threatening illness. Family members often serve as primary caretakers; they guide the provision of support for loved ones during their final days of life, actively participate in decision-making processes and serve as liaisons and proxy informants to healthcare practitioners. The journey of illness is thus a shared one, resonating powerfully across the family group. As a result, practitioners and researchers alike have taken an interest in understanding how the family accommodates the strain of serious illness, and in identifying ways to ensure their optimal functioning.

The increased attention given to the needs of families in palliative care has evolved alongside a parallel shift in the field of family therapy toward strength-based models of intervention. This movement, also referred to as the family resilience approach, was intended to counterbalance the prevailing tendency in the mental health field to characterize families on the basis of deficit and pathology. Rather than focusing exclusively on the family's deficiencies, proponents of the family resilience approach feel it is as important to draw attention to the family's skills, existing resources and capacities for growth. In working with families facing severe stress or crisis, this translates into efforts to harness areas of competence rather than simply minimize the 'damage' done by adverse attributes.

The concept of resilience has particular relevance for families in palliative care, who must weather major disruptions to family life, and contend with the real and anticipated losses accompanying these changes. Viewing the palliative care family through the lens of a resilience-based model makes it possible to humanize their experience and to find hope for mastery and reintegration at a time when families may feel challenged and potentially overwhelmed. From a research perspective, this model suggests the need to learn about what factors promote positive outcomes among families facing illness, in addition to investigating predictors of negative outcomes (e.g. distress, impairment).

In this chapter, we examine this model of family resilience as it applies to the setting of palliative care. We begin by addressing the question, what does resilience look like in families? This task is made challenging by the multifaceted and dynamic nature of the family as a unit of study. However, we are guided by existing theoretical models on resilience among families facing adversity. Although not specific to families in palliative care, these models provide a conceptual map with which to recognize key processes implicated in the adaptation of families in crisis. After outlining a general framework for resilience in families, we present a recently developed model for understanding families in palliative care, and an accompanying intervention programme known as Family Focused Grief Therapy (Kissane 2000). This intervention draws heavily from the resilience-based approach through affirming the well functioning family's ability to mutually support each other, or providing specialized support to families considered at some risk during palliative care or bereavement.

Defining family resilience

The concept of resilience first emerged as part of an attempt to explain why some children appeared to fare well in the context of significant adversity, while many others suffered poor outcomes. Generally speaking, the term resilience refers to better-than-expected functioning following exposure to high-risk circumstances. In their extensive review of this literature, Luthar *et al.* (2000) define resilience as a 'dynamic process encompassing positive adaptation within the context of significant adversity' (p. 543). Although the study of resilience has predominantly focused on the individual, the notion proves useful in the family domain as well. Like the individual, the family is an organized, functioning system that responds to major stressors by either marshalling resources adaptively, or suffering distress and upheaval with a potentially adverse outcome (Kissane *et al.* 1994a).

How do we know whether a family under stress is functioning 'better-than-expected'? Drawing from the work of Masten and Coatsworth (1998) on resilience in children, Patterson (2002a) describes three conditions that must be present in order to recognize resilience in families. The first is that there is evidence of competence in key areas of family functioning. The second condition is that there is a level of risk or disruption to the family's life that would ordinarily be expected to yield poor outcomes. Thirdly, there must be evidence of some adaptive mechanism or process operating in the family that prevents the expected poor outcome from occurring. Patterson (2002b) delineates the core functions that families can be expected to serve, to the benefit of both its individual members and the community in which it resides. The implication is that resilience is evident insofar as the family-as-a-whole is able to fulfil and even strengthen these functions during times of stress or crisis. These core family functions include: (1) cohesion, membership, and family formation (e.g. Is the family able to maintain a sense of belonging, and personal and social identity for its members?); (2) economic support (e.g. Is the family able to provide for basic needs of food, shelter and health resources?); (3) nurturance, education, and socialization (e.g. Is the family able to affirm social values, and foster productivity and compatibility with community norms?); and (4) protection of vulnerable members (e.g. Is the family able to protect members who are young, ill, or disabled?). For instance, in the case of chronic illness, this latter function is successfully fulfilled when the family is able to reorganize its roles, rules, and interaction patterns to ensure adequate care and protection of an ill member. Nevertheless, difficulties may arise if, over time, the family continues to channel resources toward this function at the expense of all others.

Despite a growing literature on this topic, efforts to converge on a single definition of family resilience have been prevented by a number of conceptual issues. For example, is resilience best viewed as a family 'trait' (i.e. a stable attribute possessed by some families and not others) or a family 'process' (i.e. a capacity possessed by all families that is activated in some and lies dormant in others) (Luthar *et al.* 2000)? Is it a reflection of successful continuity in functioning, adaptive change in functioning, or both? Is resilience only activated under terrible adversity, or is it evident during the families' adaptation to normative developmental challenges as well (e.g. birth of a child, moving to a new country)?

The questions raised above reflect a central concept in family resilience, which is that the pathway toward resilience is complex and multifaceted (Bonanno 2004). Whereas early empirical work on resilience was devoted to describing the distinguishing traits of resilient individuals (e.g. Masten and Garmezy 1985), recent efforts have focused on understanding the process of resilience, that is, describing the various trajectories that lead to positive outcomes. Bonnano (2004) argues that when we look at endpoints of positive adaptation, we should distinguish between those who reach that outcome by returning to healthy functioning after a period of high distress and destabilization from those who have maintained a stable equilibrium of healthy functioning throughout the course of the stressful event. He recommends that the term 'resilient' be reserved for the latter group, who show an ability to sustain their well-being during a period of hardship. Clearly, psychiatric morbidity emerges for a time in the former setting. Bonanno goes on to argue that the failure to distinguish between these trajectories can lead to missed opportunities for clinical interventions, as one group may benefit from more support than the other, despite similar eventual outcomes. In a slightly different take on this theme of multiple pathways to resilience, Richardson *et al.* (1990) recognized that every family whose life course is disrupted by a major stressor embarks on a process of adaptation and reintegration. They distinguish between resilient reintegration (experiencing growth and gaining strength in response to disruption), reintegration back to homeostasis (recovering from, or simply 'getting past', the disruption in the hope of maintaining previous functioning), reintegration with loss (responding to a disruption but with clear deficits, loss of hope, motivation, or drive), and dysfunctional reintegration (managing disruptions by resorting to maladaptive coping strategies, e.g. substance use). Without the demands of disruptive life events, whether planned (e.g. birth of a child) or unplanned (e.g. accident or illness), there would be no opportunities to exercise the capacity for resilience that otherwise exists as a universal potential.

Definitions of family resilience highlight both the typology of resilient families, and the processes by which they achieve beneficial outcomes. McCubbin *et al.* (1997) define family resilience as a measure of 'elasticity' and 'buoyancy'. In their model, elasticity refers to the degree to which the family maintains its functioning when disrupted by a stressor such as illness. Buoyancy is the degree to which the family can recover from a stressor by adapting to change. According to these authors, a resilient family is one that both maintains its integrity during the crisis, and 'bounces back' through successful adaptation. They identify a number of 'common denominator' factors that contribute to these processes (e.g. communication, flexibility, hardiness, consistency in family routines). McCubbin *et al.* argue that resilience is not simply the absence of pathology, but also the presence of assets empowering growth and transformation. Acknowledging that families are sometimes unable to recover their prior state of functioning, Walsh (2003) uses buoyancy as 'bouncing forward' instead of 'bouncing back'. She defines family resilience as the ability to both '*withstand* and *rebound from* disruptive life challenges … to struggle well, surmount obstacles and go on to live and love fully' (p. 1). As we will see below, the distinguishing characteristic of resilience in families is that it is essentially a relational event, in which acts of connection and collaboration take centre stage.

General frameworks of family resilience

In an attempt to extend the work on individual resilience to families, Joan Patterson and Froma Walsh, among others, developed working models of family resilience. These models provide a conceptual map and ultimately guide clinical practice. Although each author reaches similar conclusions regarding the key processes implicated in family resilience, they do so from different theoretical frameworks.

In her family resilience model, Walsh draws from ecological and developmental perspectives, taking into account the family life-cycle stage as a key contextual variable that influences the family's response to stress. Rolland's (1987) description of centripetal versus centrifugal phases of family life illustrates this developmental influence. According to this model of chronic illness and the life cycle, illness generally has a centripetal effect on the family, drawing family members inward toward increased closeness and teamwork. If the family or its members are in a centrifugal life cycle phase (e.g. young adults leaving home), then an illness can clash with the family's natural momentum toward disengagement and autonomy. Alternatively, if illness coincides with a centripetal phase of family life (e.g. during early child rearing when members are focused inward), the illness may prolong or magnify this phase of the life cycle, and the family may have greater difficulty moving forward when needed. The fit, or lack thereof, between the developmental tasks of the family and the demands of the illness can thus shape the family's adaptation and subsequent developmental course. Positive adaptation thus involves managing the demands of illness without significantly compromising developmental needs. Walsh asserts that no single model of family health can fit all, and that family functioning cannot be assessed meaningfully without placing the family within this temporal context.

Key influences on family resilience occur within three overarching domains: (1) family belief systems; (2) organization patterns; and (3) communication processes (Walsh 2003). Family belief systems refer to the shared explanations and meaning that families ascribe to their hardships. Resilience is a likely outcome for those families who believe that strength is derived from teamwork, and who perceive adversity as a shared challenge to be overcome together. This can require a departure from a culturally endorsed emphasis on self-sufficiency and 'rugged individualism'. Resilient families normalize the distress they experience, view stress as a natural part of life's passage, and avoid responses of blame, shame or pathologizing. Walsh points to attitudes of optimism, hopefulness, and spirituality as noteworthy contributors to resilience.

The way a family organizes itself around an illness influences its potential for resilience. Flexibility is a key component here, as families may need to negotiate role transitions and revise their perceptions of what 'normal life' looks like. The ability to co-ordinate, mutually support one another and pull together cohesively eases the difficulties posed by these transitions. Understandably, the potential for resilience can be severely undermined without adequate financial security and support from social institutions. Finally, communication is the conduit through which all of the above processes operate. Effective communication among family members occurs when members elicit and share accurate and clear information about the source of difficulty, tolerate and encourage open emotional expression and engage in proactive and collaborative problem solving.

Patterson (2002a) draws from family stress and coping theory to specify a somewhat different model of resilience in families. The central premise here is that adaptation to any stressor is contingent on the balance between demands and resources. A family experiences crisis when the demands imposed persistently exceed the family's ability to manage. This disequilibrium prompts a turning point in the family's trajectory. Families that restore the balance and move forward with improved functioning are described as 'resilient'. Meaning plays a prominent role in this model of family adaptation, influencing how families perceive the demands they face as well as the sufficiency of their resources. The resilient family accepts or minimizes the level of threat, makes sense of the information given to them and forms a belief in their ability to respond.

In Patterson's model of family resilience, cohesiveness, flexibility and communication are once again cited as the central processes through which resilience is facilitated. However, rather than assuming that 'more is better', Patterson recognizes that the family's task is to strike a balance within each of these domains of functioning that best suits the needs of its members. Hence, cohesiveness requires an optimal balance between closeness and distance; flexibility reflects a balance between stability and transformation. This balancing act, implicit in Walsh's model as well, suggests that the absolute degree of flexibility or cohesiveness is less important than the family's ability to reach a consensus about the configuration that works well for them.

The theoretical models presented above offer practitioners conceptual approaches to guide the assessment of families under severe stress. An implicit assumption is that if we understand what helps families adapt and thrive under stress, we can cultivate these processes in less resilient families and help them to generate adaptive responses.

Families in palliative care

Families are not always forthcoming about their need for psychosocial support in palliative care, presenting a challenge for healthcare professionals to know which families should be targeted for clinical interventions. Although the models presented above describe processes that are highly relevant to palliative care families, they do not necessarily provide a means of predicting longer-term psychosocial outcomes. In order to efficiently deliver family-centred care to patients with advanced stage illness, it is helpful to have some criteria by which healthcare professionals can recognize which families are in most need of support. These criteria also enable the development and delivery of prophylactic interventions aimed at strengthening families early in their trajectory, thus preventing morbidity. Previous attempts by Rolland to establish such criteria involved the classification of families based on the course (e.g. progressive, constant, episodic) and time phase (e.g. crisis, chronic, terminal) of illness (Rolland 1987). The palliative care phase is characterized by concerns about separation and grief, increased familial involvement in patient care and thoughts about the anticipated death.

Kissane *et al.* (1994a) embarked on a series of observational studies aimed at discerning the specific needs of palliative care families and deriving a predictive model of family functioning in this setting. The substantial distress that reverberates across the members of palliative care families highlights the need for family-centred care. Up to one-half of patients and one-third of their family members exceed clinical thresholds on distress questionnaires (Kissane *et al.* 1994b). Moreover, longitudinal studies indicate that distress can persist for up to 18 months (Ell *et al.* 1988; Northouse 1989). The adult offspring of patients, an often overlooked group, were also identified as vulnerable (Kissane *et al.* 1994b). In a cohort of patients with a life expectancy of less than 1 year, over one-quarter of adult offspring scored above a clinical threshold on the Beck Depression Inventory (Kissane *et al.* 1994b). Moreover, offspring carried significantly higher levels of anger than patients and spouses, and held divergent views on family functioning, perceiving less cohesion and greater conflict. For all family members, hostility was strongly associated with poor family functioning, accounting for 13% of the variance in perceived family conflict (Kissane *et al.* 1994a). While distress is certainly inevitable when a loved one is dying, these findings underscored the need for healthcare practitioners to consider the impact of illness on family as a whole. Family functioning is of considerable relevance to the psychosocial status of each individual family member.

Which palliative care families carry the most vulnerability and distress? Can families be distinguished based on patterns of interaction during palliative care? The high levels of anger reported by the children of palliative care patients led Kissane *et al.* (1994a) to take a closer look at how the family relates and organizes itself during this phase. Family members' perceptions of family life were assessed using two well-validated measures, the Family Relationships Index (FRI) of the Family Environment Scale (FES) (Moos and Moos 1981) and the Family Adaptability and Cohesion Evaluation Scales (FACES-III) (Olson *et al.* 1985). A cluster analysis performed on 102 palliative care families generated five types of family functioning. The same clustering emerged in a second cohort comprised of 115 families in bereavement, who were assessed at various points during the first 13 months after the death of a parent (Kissane *et al.* 1996a) and was replicated in a third cohort who were at baseline for an intervention study (Kissane *et al.* 2003). Thus, this classification is both consistent and predictive of psychosocial morbidity, making it a clinically useful model to guide the delivery of support.

The key parameters that distinguished degrees of family competence in these samples were cohesiveness, conflict, and expressiveness, but not flexibility. Cohesiveness emerged as the hallmark of the well-adapted family, signifying the family's ability to work together as a team, their inclination to spend time together and to provide each other with mutual support. Families with a high cohesiveness feature a kind of instrumental and emotional 'togetherness' that pervades all areas of family life. Conflict management emerged as another key dimension of family functioning, reflected in family members' endorsement of such statements as 'we fight a lot in our family', or 'family members sometimes get so angry they throw things'. As will become evident below, the presence of conflict *per se* is not necessarily a marker of dysfunction, and its impact appears to be mitigated when there is sufficient cohesiveness. Finally, families who score highly on expressiveness readily share feelings and thoughts, endorsing such items as 'we say anything we want to around the home' or 'we tell each other about our personal problems'.

These three parameters that discriminated palliative care families are consistent with those cited by Walsh and Patterson (see discussion above) as central to family resilience and adjustment. The only exception to this was the construct of family adaptability, the family's capacity to revise existing roles, rules and structure to accommodate the demands of illness. Scores on a measure of family adaptability played no empirical role in statistically discriminating family patterns. This could be partly explained by the nature of the subscale used to assess this construct (Green *et al.* 1991), but flexibility appears less important than cohesion, communication, and conflict resolution in determining the clinical outcome for the family.

The family focused grief therapy model

The five patterns of family functioning that emerged from these early studies were named according to their most salient features (Kissane *et al.* 1994a, 1996a, 2003). Two of these are well functioning and resilient, namely *Supportive* and *Conflict Resolving*. Supportive families, comprising approximately one-third, described family life as intimate and mutually supportive, with open and honest communication among its members, tolerance of emotional expression, and little to no escalation in conflict. Family members who perceived their families as such reported low distress and good social functioning, an observation that lends further support to the notion that cohesiveness and communication within the family serve to protect the personal well-being of family members during times of stress (Kissane *et al.* 1994b). During bereavement, supportive families share grief openly and intensely, but with no accompanying morbidity among its individual members. This is attributed to the protective elements of such resilient functioning (Kissane *et al.* 1996a). These families are not likely to need specialized psychosocial support. Healthcare practitioners serve these families best by affirming their strengths and reinforcing their successful teamwork. We now know that the strengths exhibited by these families predict a course of adaptive functioning over time, even beyond the palliative care phase.

The families referred to as conflict-resolving also featured high cohesiveness and above-average expressiveness, but differed from supportive families in their endorsement of moderate conflict. This class was named 'conflict-resolving' because the presence of conflict with little accompanying distress suggested good conflict management and a tendency to both voice and reconcile differences between family members. Like supportive families, those classified as conflict-resolvers (approximately one-fifth in palliative care) carried minimal psychosocial morbidity. Moreover, relative to all other classes, the intensity of grief at 6 and 13 months post-death was lowest and members featured the lowest scores on a measure of depression (Kissane *et al.* 1996b). Levels of hostility were reduced by half over the 13 months following the patient's death. The adaptive functioning and low morbidity observed among family members in this class reminds us that the pathway to resilience is varied and that the presence of certain key processes (i.e. cohesiveness, expressiveness) may both protect against the erosive influence of conflict, and/or facilitate its resolution.

Unlike the families described above, there were two classes of families who appeared to be at risk for poor outcomes during stages of palliative care and bereavement. One such family type, referred to as *Hostile*, presented with low cohesiveness, low expressiveness and high conflict. Family members in this class (approximately 6% during palliative care and 12% in early bereavement) described family life as fraught with frequent arguing, little teamwork or felt closeness among members, and minimal communication. A closer look revealed that these family characteristics were perceived most often by the adult offspring of palliative care patients. Lacking the groundwork needed to cultivate resilience, members of these families carried more depression, hostility, interpersonal sensitivity, anxiety and poorer social and occupational functioning than those in any other group. During bereavement, hostile families were least likely to engage in adaptive coping strategies, such as seeking social or spiritual support, or making use of community resources. To the palliative care practitioner, such families are likely to require a great deal of assistance, although they may not readily seek out support. A family that is fractured, distressed, and has difficulty working together will need considerable help from the palliative care team in planning the patient's care and preparing for the likelihood of his or her death.

The class of families named *Sullen* also featured reduced cohesiveness and expressiveness, but only mild to moderate conflict. Whereas almost half of the Hostile class families had members who met clinical caseness for depression, approximately 35% of Sullen family members reached these levels of depression (Kissane *et al.* 2003). However, up to 13 months after the patient's death, Sullen family members had the highest depression scores relative to other family classes, suggesting that they remain vulnerable to distress long after the palliative care phase. Reports of overt hostility were low in this group, suggesting that anger is muted, with depression gaining more prominence as the anger is directed inwards. Unlike the Hostile class, family members with the Sullen pattern of functioning reported active support-seeking during bereavement and good use of social and community resources. These families appear receptive to and accepting of an intervention providing specialized psychosocial support.

Finally, a fifth class of families was termed *Intermediate* because of its position between the two sets of groups described above. Despite moderate cohesiveness, family members in this group (approximately one-third of families) reported high rates of anxiety and depression and some difficulty functioning socially. These families carry potential for resilience but do tend to deteriorate during early bereavement. They may benefit most from intervention during palliative care to strengthen their existing resources, and may readily engage in a programme of support offered to them by staff.

Importantly, the classes presented above are not intended to be reified as diagnostic categories, as this would be uninformative and misleading in a model intended to be preventive. Rather, the classification offers some organization and meaning to the heterogeneity observed in this population, and ultimately helps the clinician to differentiate the resilient from families at greater risk of morbid psychosocial outcome. The family classes presented above are not presumed to be perfectly stable or mutually exclusive, nor are the patterns described within each class uniformly endorsed by all members of a single family. In addition to alerting us to families at risk, the research informs us that there are strengths and resources among these same families that may not otherwise be apparent (e.g. the positive outcomes reached by conflict-resolving families; the adaptive coping strategies used by sullen families).

A model for assessing family competence: the family meeting in palliative care

Guided by the classification presented above, Kissane and his research group have designed and implemented a model for assessing family functioning and optimizing adaptation in the setting of palliative care. This model includes two tiers of intervention, the first of which is a brief and focused single family meeting held by the palliative care team, in which the key dimensions of competence described above are assessed and affirmed. Table 4.1 presents guidelines to this basic family meeting in palliative care. As is often the case, the assessment of the family during this meeting is itself a form of intervention, as family members are invited to take notice of, and make explicit, their ways relating with each other and with the illness. While the meeting serves certain

Table 4.1 Guideline to a basic family meeting in palliative care

1. Round of introductions and welcome
2. State goal of meeting together

   To review the status of the patient's illness

   To consider the family's needs in providing care

   To complete questionnaire giving information about family

   To aim at optimizing the journey ahead
3. Check for any other agenda that the family might have
4. Clarify the family's understanding of the seriousness of illness
5. Clarify the family's understanding of the current goals of medical care

   Are there key symptoms that are a concern to the patient or family?

   Any medication or treatment concerns?

   Any hygiene issues?

   Any concerns about walking, moving, transferring?

   Any concerns about nursing or hospice visits?

   Any concerns about accessing palliative care resources?

   Any needs for respite?
6. Clarify the patient's and family's view of what the future holds:

   Has the place of death been discussed?

   If at home, who from the family will be providing care?

   If in hospital, who will accompany? Help? Support?
7. Give out the FRI screening to explore family functioning: communication, cohesiveness, conflict resolution.
8. Clarify how family members are managing emotionally: Is anyone a concern or do you expect family members to manage satisfactorily? Is there anything we can do to help?
9. Affirm family strengths: commitment, willingness, caring and concern for one another.
10. If concerns exist and are agreed to, discuss referral for ongoing family therapy.
11. Offer written material in accordance with institutional norms or issues raised at the meeting.
12. 'Before concluding, are there any questions that you have as a family?'

general purposes that are undoubtedly part of routine practice in palliative care services (e.g. introducing the patient and family to the palliative care team, reviewing the goals of care and engaging caretakers in helping deliver this), additional strategies are introduced to aid in planning for the care of the family as a whole.

One such strategy involves the use of routine screening as a tool to gauge the predominant 'family environment', and determine the level of risk facing each family (Kissane and Bloch 2002). The Family Relationships Index (FRI) (Moos 1990) has proven to be a reliable and informative screening device that is minimally intrusive and can be easily administered to patients and their relatives in the clinical setting. Its sensitivity and specificity in detecting families at risk have been confirmed by other groups (Edwards and Clarke 2005). Anecdotally, we have found the FRI to be a feasible and acceptable method of screening across a variety of palliative care settings, although some training and facilitation is needed to help integrate screening into existing practices in each setting (Kissane *et al.* 2006).

The scale is best used on admission to the service, when family members are likely to be accompanying the patient. Each family member completes the scale independently and without consulting with one another in order to ensure honest and confidential responses. Because the scale inquires about aspects of family life that may not seem directly relevant to the patient's care, the administrator of the questionnaire is proactive in highlighting its utility in helping the medical team understand the family's needs. Additionally, a comment to normalize the divergence in views among members of the same family may help clarify the importance of obtaining each member's perspective. The FRI can be used to derive scores on three key dimensions of family competence, namely cohesiveness, communication and conflict resolution. Families are considered to be at risk if one or more respondents score 9 or less out of 12 on the FRI, or less than 4 on cohesiveness, a particularly sensitive predictor of family outcomes (Kissane and Bloch 2002). In our most recent sample of palliative care families, the FRI was found to be extremely sensitive to detecting maladaptive family patterns (86% sensitivity), although some risk for false positives was evident (Kissane *et al.* 2003). Families in which at least one member indicates difficulties in family functioning are offered the option of additional family meetings as part of an ongoing programme of support. The following is a sample script used by the practitioner in this scenario:

> We notice in your questionnaire responses that some of you feel that an aspect of family life—communication, teamwork, or conflict—can be a challenge at times. We'd like to tell you about some options for services that try to help families as they strive to support a sick relative. These services use ongoing meetings like this to support the family …

The screening should supplement, but not replace, a broader discussion with the family that aims to elicit family members' perceptions of family functioning and coping. The family meeting is an opportunity for the healthcare team to gain information from the family, but also for the family to openly acknowledge how they interact and communicate with one another, what values are prioritized, and which members, if any, are suffering significant distress. In this way, the meeting itself models and fosters the very processes that contribute to resilience. Should maladaptive patterns (e.g. high conflict, fractured relationships) emerge during this discussion or from the FRI, the task of the palliative care team is not to solve these problems there and then, but rather to help synthesize the information for the family in such a way that a plan for further support can be established.

For all families, regardless of how well they are functioning, a critical component of this meeting is the affirmation of family strengths and resources. The healthcare team can use this time to reassure well-functioning families that their teamwork, communication, and good conflict resolution will prove to be a great source of support to the patient and to each other. Likewise, families who struggle to cope with the illness and have greater difficulty working together may be reminded of aspects of family life that are valued, unique and genuinely positive (e.g. caring concern for each other, commitment to the patient). Written material can be offered to summarize issues raised during this meeting.

Family-focused grief therapy: a model for preventive intervention

For those families requiring more extensive support, Kissane *et al.* designed a time-limited and focused intervention whose objective is to improve family functioning through the enhancement of cohesiveness, conflict resolution and expression of thoughts and feelings. The premise for this intervention is that families who fall within the Sullen, Hostile, and Intermediate classes of functioning are likely to carry substantial psychological distress and tend to deteriorate under the strain of death and bereavement. For a detailed description of the intervention, with case examples, the reader is referred to *Family Focused Grief Therapy* by Kissane and Bloch (2002).

The intervention begins with an assessment phase (1–2 weekly sessions) in which the story of the patient's illness is elicited, a family genogram is used to understand trans-generational patterns of relating and dealing with loss, and a focus for continued work is agreed upon collaboratively. The intervention phase (typically 2–6 sessions) involves a focus on the agreed-upon agenda, and the termination phase (1–2 sessions) is used to consolidate gains, reaffirm family strengths and bring closure to the work.

In the simple act of bringing the family together for routine meetings (no small feat), the intervention activates a kind of teamwork from the start that can be later summoned to handle illness-related challenges. By inviting the family to share their story and reconstruct their history, the intervention encourages an appreciation for the family's unique identity and the contribution of trans-generational influences. Thematically guided questioning is used throughout sessions to help family members reveal expectations, voice their fears, wishes and express grief, thus facilitating open communication and making way for the family's natural capacities to comfort and soothe each other.

A randomized controlled trial of family-focused grief therapy has confirmed its ability to reduce distress in high-risk families during palliative care and bereavement (Kissane *et al.* 2006). Indeed, reduced depression and distress in individual members with the highest baseline scores points to its protectiveness against pathological grief. A dose–response study, sponsored by the National Cancer Institute, is now underway at Memorial Sloan–Kettering Cancer Center in New York to better understand the mediators and moderators of outcome.

Conclusions

Family resilience is a vital concept for palliative care. The developmental life cycle of the family and its functioning as a group are key parameters in our conceptualization of this resilience. The meeting with the family is clinically crucial as a means to affirm the family's robustness when present, or to offer a preventive approach to bolstering this—family-focused grief therapy—when the family is thought to be at risk. Family strengths prove invaluable to understand and affirm as a path to nurturing greater resilience.

References

Bonanno GA (2004) Loss, trauma, and human resilience: have we underestimated the human capacity to thrive after extremely aversive events? *American Psychologist* **59**, 20–28.

Edwards B, Clarke V (2005) The validity of the family relationships index as a screening tool for psychological risk in families of cancer patients. *Psychooncology* **14**, 546–554.

Ell K, Nishimoto R, Mantell J, Hamovitch M (1988) Longitudinal analysis of psychological adaptation among family members of patients with cancer. *Journal of Psychosomatic Research* **32**, 429–438.

Green RG, Harris RN, Forte JA, Robinson M (1991) Evaluating FACES III and the circumplex model: 2440 families. *Family Process* **30**, 55–73.

Kissane DW (2000) Family grief therapy: a model for working with families during palliative care and bereavement. In: *Cancer and the Family*, 2nd edn (eds Baider L, Cooper CL, Kaplan De-Nour A). Chichester: Wiley and Sons.

Kissane DW, Bloch S (2002) *Family Focused Grief Therapy. A model of family-centred care during palliative care and bereavement.* Buckingham: Open University Press.

Kissane DW, Bloch S, Burns WI, Patrick JD, Wallace CS, McKenzie DP (1994a) Perceptions of family functioning and cancer. *Psychooncology* 3, 259–269.

Kissane DW, Bloch S, Burns WI, Mckenzie DP, Posterino M (1994b) Psychological morbidity in the families of patients with cancer. *Psychooncology* 3, 47–56.

Kissane DW, Bloch S, Dowe DL, Snyder RD, Onghena P, McKenzie DP, Wallace CS (1996a) The Melbourne family grief study, I: perceptions of family functioning in bereavement. *American Journal of Psychiatry* 153, 650–658.

Kissane DW, Bloch S, Onghena P, McKenzie DP, Snyder RD, Dowe DL (1996b) The Melbourne family grief study II: psychosocial morbidity and grief in bereaved families. *American Journal of Psychiatry* 153, 659–666.

Kissane DW, McKenzie M, McKenzie DP, Forbes A, O'Neill I, Bloch S (2003) Psychosocial morbidity associated with patterns of family functioning in palliative care: baseline data from the Family Focused Grief Therapy controlled trial. *Palliative Medicine* 17, 527–537.

Kissane DW, McKenzie M, Bloch S, Moskowitz C, McKenzie DP, O'Neill I (2006) Family focused grief therapy: a randomized, controlled trial in palliative care and bereavement. *American Journal of Psychiatry* 163, 1208–1218.

Luthar SS, Cicchetti D, Becker B (2000) The construct of resilience: a critical evaluation and guidelines for future work. *Child Development* 71, 543–562.

Masten AS, Coatsworth JD (1998) The development of competence in favorable and unfavorable environments. Lessons from research on successful children. *American Psychologist* 53, 205–220.

Masten AS, Garmezy N (1985) Risk, vulnerability and protective factors in developmental psychopathology. In: *Advances in Clinical Child Psychology* (eds Lahey BB, Kazdin AE). New York: Plenum Press.

McCubbin HI, McCubbin MA, Thompson AI, Han SY, Allen CT (1997) Families under stress: What makes them resilient? American Association of Family and Consumer Sciences Commemorative Lecture. Washington DC.

Moos RH (1990) Conceptual and empirical approaches to developing family-based assessment procedures: resolving the case of the Family Environment Scale. *Family Process* 29, 199–208.

Moos RH, Moos BS (1981) *Family Environment Scale Manual*. Stanford, CA: Consulting Psychologists Press.

Northouse L (1989) A longitudinal study of the adjustment of patients and husbands to breast cancer. *Oncology Nursing Forum* 16, 511–516.

Olson DH, Portner J, Lavee Y (1985) *FACES III Manual*. Minnesota: Family Social Science.

Patterson JM (2002a) Integrating family resilience and family stress theory. *Journal of Marriage and Family* 64, 349–360.

Patterson JM (2002b) Understanding family resilience. *Journal of Clinical Psychology* 58, 233–246.

Richardson GE, Neiger B, Jensen S, Kumpfer K (1990) The resiliency model. *Health Education* 21, 33–39.

Rolland J (1987) Chronic illness and the life cycle: a conceptual framework. *Family Process* 26, 203–221.

Walsh F (2003) Family resilience: a framework for clinical practice. *Family Process* 42, 1–18.

Resilient carers and caregivers

Sheila Payne

Caring for a dying family member is unpredictable and uncertain in duration and nature; it is simultaneously challenging and fulfilling. This chapter is presented from the stance that engaging in this type of care can have both positive and negative consequences for carers. Most academic accounts of caring emphasize the work involved in providing physical nursing, housekeeping, financial management, and social surveillance of the ill person (Payne 2004). There is also attention to the psychological demands. It is no accident that this type of psychological support may be described as emotional labour. These ways to construe caregiving appear to be effortful and instrumental. An alternative more nuanced account is revealed in the written and verbal accounts of carers (Clark *et al.* 2005). These accounts tend to present caring as a multidimensional social role rather than a job, that builds upon previous roles and relationships. Moreover it is enacted in different ways throughout the person's illness, when demands fluctuate and resources vary. These roles need to be understood in the context of individual and family circumstances, social position, expectations, and environmental possibilities. The paradox in this role is that while people may engage with many of the tasks and responsibilities of caring, some strongly resist the label of 'carer'. It is therefore largely an ascribed role, placed on family members and less frequently upon friends, by health and social care workers.

This chapter will draw upon theoretical concepts of resilience, both psychological (such as personality traits of hardiness, mastery and perceived self-efficacy) and social concepts of perceived social support, social network and the evidence for their effects upon 'buffering' stress upon the role of carers. The chapter starts by discussing definitions of family and caregivers. It reviews the evidence on the impact of caring on caregivers, drawing both on the available research and also the accounts of caregivers to provide a nuanced and critical account of how caregiving has become constructed as 'burdensome'. The chapter highlights the discrepancies between how caregiving is construed by health and social care practitioners and the representation of the lived experience of caring reported by family members and others. This chapter will focus on the factors influencing carers (see Table 5.1) and suggests how resilience can be enhanced and promoted through self-care and through supportive interventions (see Table 5.2). The chapter then suggests new ways of conceptualizing and responding to carers' needs by enhancing well-being and promoting partnership.

Carers and families: definitions

Carers, who may or may not be family members, are lay people in a close supportive role who share in the illness experience of the patient and who undertake vital care work and emotion management

National Institute of Clinical Excellence (2004, p. 155)

The terminology of caregiving is potentially confusing with a number of terms being used in various situations, countries, and in the research literature (Payne 2004). The following terms are widely used to describe people who provide unpaid care in existing relationships including: carer, caregiver, informal carer, caretaker, relative, family, companion, and significant other. In this chapter the term 'carer' will be used. This marks these people out from paid workers and volunteers who generally have no previous relationship to the cared for person. Carers are crucially important in the lives of those facing the end of life. The presence of capable and willing carers makes possible a range of options and choices such as being cared for and dying at home. A systematic review of the literature indicated that two strong determinants influencing death at home for cancer patients, were living with relatives and having extended family support (Gomes and Higginson 2006). There was also evidence that the preferences of family members to facilitate death at home was important in helping patients achieve this goal. The lack of available or willing carers limits the possibilities for end of life care options and choices and may contribute to a greater number of institutional deaths. This is most marked in older people, especially for women, where evidence suggests that those dying in late old age are more likely to die in care homes or hospitals than at home or in hospices (Seymour *et al.* 2005).

The rhetoric of palliative care claims that the patient and family is the 'unit of care'. Yet it is only relatively recently that carers have attracted attention in their own right (Payne *et al.* 1999; Harding and Higginson 2003; Hudson 2003). Families tend to be construed as readily available and willing to provide care for dying members. In many societies there are strong social norms that mean that caregiving within kinship networks are expected obligations that most people fulfil out of duty, filial piety, and reciprocal altruism. Family is a contested notion, and may comprise anything from a dyad (for example, a mother and child) to an extended multigenerational network. In many families there is a network of support and care from people who may or may not be co-located. NICE (2004) offered the following definition of family: 'those related through committed heterosexual or same sex partnerships, birth and adoption, and others who have strong emotional and social bonds with a patient' (p. 155).

Complex webs of social change impact on family structures, economic viability, and sense of cohesion. Patterns of family life have changed markedly in many developed countries during the last 50 years, with high rates of divorce, marital separation, serial marriage, step-parenting, single parenting and co-habitation becoming commonplace. Increased longevity may result in greater numbers of people enjoying being grandparents or great grandparents but also increasing the possibility of experiencing the loss of, or distancing from, younger family members in late old age. In many developed and some developing countries such as China, there are strong social pressures or government policies to promote smaller family size and fewer children. This reduces the potential number of people related by kinship who may be available to offer care near the end of life. This, combined with changing patterns of employment with more families dependent upon two incomes, increased female employment outside the home, greater geographical mobility, greater job insecurity, more part-time and casual working, means that fewer people are available to offer informal care. For some, technological developments such as the mobile telephone and email, have offered new ways to maintain family relationships and support even when geographically apart. Same sex partnerships are now formally recognized in many countries, giving people the same rights and obligations to provide care, along with or instead of, other biological family members. In parts of Africa, the devastating HIV/AIDS epidemic has impacted on traditional family structures with large numbers of children being raised by siblings, grandparents, or more distant kin (Kwaka 2006). While families may be sources of support, comfort, attachment, care and love, they can also be conflict ridden, abusive, and exploitative of their members.

Arguably, families are influential in determining the possibilities and options available to people facing advanced disease. Family systems theory proposes that families can be understood as dynamic and reciprocal organizations. In dealing with the fluctuations, stresses, and deterioration accompanying terminal illness, families often respond by negotiating and distributing roles and responsibilities for various aspects of care and support throughout their members. These mutually supportive roles belie the simple categorization of a nominated person as the 'main carer'. Health professionals may make assumptions that the 'main' carer is the only person to whom they should direct communication, instructions, and advice. This may be problematic in fractured or disrupted families where communication channels are limited by old or current disputes. However, most families are remarkably adaptive and resilient. They work hard to support all members in systems of interdependence. This is equally true of patients who may seek to protect and support other family members. In older couples, it may be difficult to distinguish caregiving roles, as patterns of mutual dependence overlap and fluctuate as frailty and ill-health take their toll. For example, in a study of patients with heart failure (Gott *et al.* in press), one patient reported: 'He's supposed to be my main carer but at the moment I think it's me looking after him more than the other way round.' (female patient, aged 71, carer is spouse, aged 79).

How are carers construed in the literature?

The early literature tended to construe care provision in largely instrumental terms as a series of (physical) tasks such a nursing care, assistance with activities of daily living, personal and intimate care, and domestic tasks. These tended to be enumerated in measures such as the Carer Strain Index (Robinson 1983) and other measures that itemized tasks and recorded them as hours of labour. Indeed, the number of hours spent on these tasks was used as a criterion to allocate resources and benefits. It is hardly surprising then that caregiving became seen as burdensome and demanding. Within palliative care many families provide supportive care throughout the illness trajectory and only gradually become engaged in direct personal physical care during the dying phase. Therefore, it is argued that this model of care tends to fail to recognize the contribution of families throughout the illness.

Latterly this construction of caring has been challenged by a number of authors including Thomas *et al.* (2002), Hudson (2003), and Nolan *et al.* (2001). Drawing upon a large study of carers of cancer patients (Thomas *et al.* 2002) argued that caring is often seen as a natural extension of existing relationships. Over a lifetime, mutual support in changing circumstances is often faced with courage and achievement provides a sense of pride. In some cultures the privacy and independence of the family are highly valued. For example, in a study of older people living in rural communities in England, there was strong resistance to seeking additional statutory benefits (Scharf and Bartlam 2006) and the opening up to scrutiny of personal and financial affairs that this involved. There was a strong preference for managing even on very limited incomes and being self-reliant.

Drawing upon psychological models of stress and coping and particularly the transactional model of coping (Lazarus and Folkman 1984), Hudson argues that the diversity of responses from caregivers can be understood in relation to their cognitive appraisals of their caring roles. If their current caring activities exceed their capacity to cope, they will be perceived as stressful. He argues that caregiving should not be seen as inherently stressful but depends upon individual internal coping resources such as feelings of mastery and competence, and external resources such as supportive neighbours or sufficient income to purchase additional help. This model celebrates the capacities and skills which people bring to caregiving. It recognizes that people differ in their personal coping styles (such as being optimistic or pessimistic) and personality traits such as hardiness and resilience. Appraisals of caregiving that find meaning in the caring relationship that enhances self-esteem such as feelings of love, duty, moral obligation and social approval are more likely to be sustaining. In addition, if the carer has a sense of mastery, self-efficacy, perceived competence, and perceived control in their role, they are more likely to derive benefits from the role. This may come from previous life experiences such as being a carer of other dependants or from professional backgrounds in social work or nursing for example.

Drawing upon extensive research with carers of frail older people, Nolan *et al.* (2001) have argued that carers should be seen as experts in the care of their family member. For example, they may understand facial expressions of pain or discomfort in confused patients without language. Health professionals should therefore acknowledge carers' 'insider knowledge' and seek to work together with them, rather than taking over or de-skilling them. Nolan *et al.* (2001) also highlight the neglected positive elements of caring that are under-represented in conventional assessments of caring roles. He and his colleagues have developed models of care that move beyond patient-centred care to relationship-centred care (Nolan *et al.* 2003). These have not yet been tested in palliative care contexts but are potentially applicable.

What factors influence the resilience of carers?

The following section examines the factors that are likely to influence the capacity of families to manage the final stage of a person's life (see Table 5.1).

Personal characteristics of carers

While there are no reliable international data, it has been estimated by the charity Help the Hospices that at any one time there are approximately 500 000 people providing care to people with terminal illness in the UK. The personal characteristics of the carer such as their age, gender, health, education, life experience, and their relationship with the patient, are all likely to impact on the performance of caring and how it is construed by them. Within palliative care

Table 5.1 Factors influencing carers

Socio-demographic characteristics
- gender
- age
- relationship to cared for person

Personal and family resources
- mastery
- meaning
- self-concept
- resilience
- health and fitness
- supportive family or kinship networks

Material and social resources
- income
- education
- culture
- housing
- community

Circumstances of care
- type of disease or condition
- nature and pattern of dying trajectory
- timeliness and expectedness of dying
- nature of relationship with cared for person
- information and communication
- access to health and social care services
- nature of health and social care services
- adverse events and concurrent stressors.

contexts, most carers are spouses rather than adult children of the cared for person. In the UK, most patients who access specialist palliative care services have cancer and therefore are in middle or later life. This means that many carers are themselves older people who may be experiencing health problems and other impairments. Differential life expectancy means that many older carers are women. However, each life stage brings challenges as caregiving in mid-life may limit opportunities for employment and social relationships; in young adulthood it may be performed concurrently with other family demands such as childrearing and it is often unrecognized that children may also be care providers (Segal and Simkins 1993). The nature and expectations of spousal and other family relationships may be influential in how willingly people take on caring roles. Certain relationships such as parental carers of adolescents and young people with cancer may require complex negotiations and mutual understanding (Grinyer 2002). Overall, despite the absence of definitive data, it is likely that in palliative care situations most carers are women, spouses of the patient, and are themselves in later life.

Personal and social resources

The psychological characteristics of carers have tended to be researched with a 'deficit' model in mind. Researchers have tended to measure and report the presence of 'problems' and 'needs' including depression, psychological distress and failure to cope (Harding and Higginson 2003). While it is important to recognize those people who experience problems, the remarkable thing is that most carers appear to manage well in difficult circumstances. Bonanno (2004) has argued that resilience in the face of loss and aversive events is perhaps more common than normally acknowledged. Drawing upon a longitudinal study of older adults who were contacted before and after spousal loss, it has been demonstrated that psychological traits such as hardiness, self-enhancement, repressive coping, positive emotion, and laughter are all factors that predict better outcomes (Bonanno 2004). Psychological research indicates that mastery, self-efficacy, and self-concept can also be crucial determinants of those who show resilience in the face of adversity. Maintaining general health and fitness, including the ability to manage stress are important attributes for carers. Those with a greater range of coping repertoires are known to do better because they are adaptable and are able to seek help when necessary. Education and an ability to elicit information and communicate effectively are helpful. Carers who have the skills to elicit the support and information they require, manage better. However, many carers are reluctant to draw attention to their own concerns and tend to prioritize the needs of the dying person. Health professionals may inadvertently assume that carers are managing well because their concerns are not voiced spontaneously.

Some of the most important resources carers have are other family members, extended family and friendship networks. There is evidence that perceived social support 'buffers' stress and that those with larger social networks tend to do better because there are more people to contribute. When family size is small there are greater demands on fewer people and the potential to become overwhelmed is increased. However, while families may be supportive, they also have the propensity to be challenging, conflicted, and stressful to members (Kissane and Bloch 2002).

Material and social resources

People take up caring responsibilities with different material and social resources. It might be assumed that those with access to greater financial resources including higher incomes, savings, and material support from extended family members will be more resilient. The costs of providing medical care, medications, transportation to hospital appointments, additional equipment or home adaptations, laundry, heating, clothing, and special food are rarely acknowledged. A review of the effects of poverty on access to palliative care services and other services in the USA, indicate that poor people and their families do less well (Hughes 2005). Evidence from the USA indicates that patients with advanced illness and their families often have to use all or most of their savings to purchase medical treatment and care (Teno *et al.* 2001). Even in countries with statutory health and social care services, some carers experience significant financial impact. Research on older people in rural areas in England (Scharf and Bartlam 2006) suggest that many live in relative poverty but over a lifetime have adapted to managing on low incomes and have limited expectations. The additional financial demands of caring placed on those already living in marginal conditions may precipitate a crisis but this may paradoxically leverage additional state benefits.

During advanced illness families are likely to be faced with reduced income because either the ill person is the main wage earner or the carer has to cease or reduce employment. Caregivers may be faced with difficult choices about ceasing employment, with short-term loss of income but long-term consequences for career progression, pensions, and social contact. In a comprehensive review of the literature on carer employment in palliative care, only eight research studies were identified (Smith *et al.* 2006). The authors concluded that strategies including flexible working practices, extended leave arrangements, and back to work training after bereavement may be helpful. Caregivers from poorer backgrounds, doing low paid and manual work were most adversely affected as they had few reserves to call on. Other types of income support may be required for those who leave employment such as the 6 weeks 'Eternity Leave' provided in Canada. Expectations about caregiving being largely a female role are most likely to limit opportunities for men for more flexible working (Lee and Owens 2002).

Home ownership and housing tenure are all factors in this equation. A current UK end of life care initiative (DoH 2006), which aims to promote patient choice and facilitate more dying at home, may have inadvertently increased the hidden costs of caring and shifted costs from NHS services on to carers. The nature of the home, the number of people occupying it, sanitary arrangements and willingness and resources to make adaptations to the dwelling such as bringing a bed downstairs all influence the acceptability and comfort for dying at home. For example, in Hong Kong high density living in tiny apartments and with very limited community nursing services, effectively means that it is impractical to die at home (Wee 1997). While family members are often willing to make remarkable changes to their living arrangements, they will continue to inhabit that space once the patient has died and permanent changes may impact on the value of their home. Concerns about this and fears about having to manage alone or the burden placed upon their spouse, may mean that some older people prefer not to die at home (Seymour *et al.* 2005) and in some cultures death may be construed as 'contaminating' the home (Payne *et al.* 2005). The material circumstances of the wider social neighbourhood are rarely acknowledged such as the perceived safety, infrastructure of services and social cohesion, but this may determine if it is safe for community nurses to visit out-of-hours or even if neighbours know each other.

The circumstances where caring is enacted

Caring in advanced illness has some features that are common to all facing the end of life, including the fact that there is no second chance to get things right, while other features are unique to that particular family. The circumstances of care are enacted against a backdrop of complex and interacting personal and social factors, including the disease, access to suitable and affordable services, and other concurrent life events. The nature of the disease and pattern of symptoms in the terminal trajectory has been categorized into four hypothesized patterns (Lunney *et al.* 2003). For example, the prolonged slow trajectory of dying found in late old age has been compared with the more precipitous decline in function of those with cancer and the unpredictable fluctuations of those with end-stage organ failure. There is not yet good empirical evidence to determine if these patterns may be used to allocate services (Gott *et al.* in press). In the UK, specialist palliative care has largely concentrated services upon those with cancer but carers are equally important whatever disease the person is dying with. Family carers may be highly influenced by factors such as duration of dying, level of dependency in the cared for person, presence of complex and difficult symptom clusters such as breathlessness, confusion, or incontinence. A further consideration is the extent to which symptoms may or may not be amenable to medical interventions and of course, the resources available to purchase necessary medication or services. Vicarious suffering by families, who witness intractable pain or distressing breathlessness, may influence feeling of mastery and their feeling of helplessness may precipitate hospital or hospice admissions (Hinton 1994). Beliefs about the timeliness of dying are likely to be related to the age of the person. For example, dying is both anticipated and perceived to be acceptable in late old age but not in young adulthood where it is generally regarded as a tragedy. From a US perspective, Lofland (1985) has argued that most people view all deaths, except those of the very old, as personal tragedies. She suggests that this view of death, combined with relatively few but intense personal relationships, means that caring for a dying spouse is often highly emotional and distressing.

Carers require access to suitable health and social care services for their own needs as well as for the cared for person. Access to specialists palliative care services in the UK is known to be inequitable (Ahmed *et al.* 2004). Most patients and carers have little realistic choice because few options exist or because they fail to understand that they can express preferences. Seymour *et al.* (2005) have highlighted the difficult circumstances many people dying in old age find themselves in. Research has also demonstrated that patients and families with end-stage heart failure found it difficult to access appropriate social care services, with fewer than 25% of a sample of 542 patients receiving these services in their last 2 years of life (Barnes *et al.* 2006). Even for those patients and carers who received services, most found that the services were limited, unsuitable or that they did not qualify because they did not have terminal cancer. Some people who had previously applied for means tested grants and been rejected (when their condition was less severe) were reluctant to apply again.

Caring for a dying family member may take place in the context of wider family and social disruption such as in refugees or asylum seekers or those living in regions where there is social unrest, famine, or war. In these circumstances normal kinship obligations and patterns of support may not be possible. For example, support from extended family members may not be available because they remain in the place of origin or are displaced by social changes. In these families, concurrent stressors may be overwhelming and prevent engaging with caring. For example, in Sierra Leone palliative care services largely deal with patients dying from HIV/AIDS and their model of care has to take account of orphaned and vulnerable children whose parents die in the hospice (Kwaka 2006).

What are the interventions that promote and enhance resilience in carers?

A systematic review of the literature has demonstrated that there is limited evidence for the efficacy of interventions designed to support carers in palliative care situations (Harding and Higginson 2003). A major review of the general caregiving literature (Nolan *et al.* 2002) has identified several unresolved issues in relation to carer support, including:

◆ *When* is support best provided?
◆ *How* is support best provided?
◆ *What* are the intended aims of support?
◆ *Who* is the perceived beneficiary?

Many interventions have been based on the 'deficit' model of carer burden, the most common being respite services that seek to remove the cared for person to give the carer a 'rest'. However, a review of the literature on palliative care respite failed to demonstrate strong evidence of its efficacy for carers

(Ingleton *et al.* 2003). A probable cause of the problem lies in the fact that services are often inflexible and fail to provide care and support that carers see as being of sufficient quality. Many carers are also reluctant to leave their family member when they fear they may die soon (Skilbeck *et al.* 2005). Other interventions have attempted to provide information or education to carers to enhance their skills and better prepare them for their role (Harding and Higginson 2003). Some interventions have sought to address psychological concerns by reducing depression, or offering psychological support, or family problem solving (Kissane and Bloch 2002). A recent project has offered carers of lung cancer patients access to social workers who delivered individual assessment, practical advice, and support with accessing financial benefits (Hardy 2006). This intervention was highly rated by carers who appreciated having their own needs addressed and having a contact person readily available outside normal cancer care services.

All too often the outcomes of interventions are not those that carers see as important (Qureshi *et al.* 2000), and there is a general failure to engage fully with carers as co-experts in care delivery (Nolan *et al.* 2003). Consequently, services are often viewed as obstructing or inhibiting carers' goals, rather than facilitating them (Nolan *et al.* 2003). Another challenge has been to deliver services to carers that they feel able to take up, as most of their attention and energies are devoted to the dying person. Table 5.2 suggests a range of interventions for carers that are based on the principle that carers should be encouraged to enhance their coping skills.

The start of a new way forward

It is a paradox that in an attempt to improve current UK end of life care for patients by prioritizing choice about location of death, with the assumption that most patients prefer to die at home, the one person who lacks any choice will be the carer. The shift of dying patients from hospital to home may well prove to be cheaper for healthcare services, although if comprehensive home support such as 'hospice-at-home' schemes are put in place, this might not be so. The hidden costs for carers are largely unrecognized and unreported. Moreover, the current imperatives to enable people to die at home may place undue moral pressure on families to provide this care whatever the cost. Instead, there needs to be new principles that shift from patient-focused care to relationship-focused care, as has been advocated by Nolan *et al.* (2003) in the context of care for frail older people. In my view this would require:

- Rethinking what end of life care services might look like if they were based on the hopes and aspirations of all family members, rather than the patient.

Table 5.2 Promoting and enhancing resilience in carers

Physical resilience—aims to maintain and improve physical health
- moving and handling training
- exercise programmes such as walking for health or swimming
- self-care such as healthy eating, responsible drinking of alcohol
- opportunities to attend health screening and dental checks
- preventive medicine such as influenza immunization

Mental resilience—aims to maintain and improve emotional and cognitive state
- mastery
- perceived control
- self-efficacy
- optimism

Social resilience—aims to maintain and improve social situation and relationships
- social network
- perceived social support
- engagement with desired leisure activities
- opportunities for intellectual stimulation and education

Financial resilience—aims to maintain and improve social situation and relationships
- financial management
- access to benefits and social welfare
- employment
- pensions

Spiritual/existential resilience—aims to provide meaning in caring role
- finding meaning and purpose in life
- for some people engagement with religion or faith
- anticipatory grief and acknowledging loss

- Establishing a partnership working relationship between family carers and health and social care workers, based on mutual respect and sharing of knowledge.

- Developing a shared understanding of the important relationships within each family and how they impact on the dying person.

- Regarding carers and patients as citizens with rights and responsibilities, rather than vulnerable and needy, or merely as 'users'.

- Highlighting policy and practice developments that promote carers well-being, choice, control and resilience and ensure there is sufficient investment to support them.

Conclusions

In summary, current health service provision for carers of people nearing the end of life is based principally on a deficit model, with variable and generally sparse provision for support. The evidence suggests that alternative perspectives that view carers as resilient, resourceful, adaptable, and capable may more accurately reflect the position of most people. In highlighting this, it should be remembered that additional support that enhances coping, shares skills and knowledge may be more welcome than models of care that seek to remove (temporarily) the burden as with respite services. The chapter has discussed the physical, psychological, social, existential, and financial consequences of caring and described a range of strategies to support care. It ends with suggestions for a reformulation of services to take account of the important relationships that serve to sustain families and in which the dying person is embedded.

References

Ahmed N, Bestall J, Ahmedzai S, Payne S, Clark D, Noble B (2004). Systematic review of the problems and issues of accessing specialist palliative care by patients, carers and health and social care professionals. *Palliative Medicine* 18(6), 525–542.

Barnes S, Gott M, Payne S, Parker C, Seamark D, Gariballa S, Small N (2006). Death and the bereavement period: Family carers' views of end of life care for older people with heart failure living in the community. Summary of methods and findings. *International Journal of Palliative Nursing* 12(8), 380–389.

Bonanno GA (2004) Loss, trauma and human resilience: have we underestimated the human capacity to thrive after extremely aversive events? *American Psychologist* 59, 20–28.

Clark D, Thomas C, Lynch T, Bingley A (2005) What are the views of people affected by cancer and other illnesses about end of life issues? *Carer Perspectives*. Lancaster: International Observatory on End of Life Care, Lancaster University.

Department of Health (2006) NHS End of Life Care Programme Progress Report March 2006. Leicester: Department of Health.

Gomes B, Higginson IJ (2006) Factors influencing death at home in terminally ill patients with cancer: systematic review. *British Journal of Medicine* 332, 515–521.

Gott M, Barnes S, Payne S, Parker C, Seamark D, Gariballa S, Small N (in press) Patient views of Social Services provision for older people with advanced heart failure. *Health and Social Care in the Community*.

Gott M, Barnes S, Payne S, Seamark D, Parker C, Gariballa S, Small N (in press) Dying trajectories in heart failure. *Palliative Medicine*.

Grinyer AE (2002) *Cancer in Young Adults: through parent's eyes*. Buckingham: Open University Press.

Harding R, Higginson I (2003) What is the best way to help caregivers in cancer and palliative care? A systematic literature review of interventions and their effectiveness. *Palliative Medicine* 17, 63–74.

Hardy E (2006) *Macmillan Carers Project*. Bath: University of Bath.

Hinton J (1994) Which patients with terminal cancer are admitted from home care? *Palliative Medicine* 8, 197–210.

Hudson P (2003) A conceptual model and key variables for guiding supportive interventions for family caregivers of people receiving palliative care. *Palliative and Supportive Care* 1(4), 353–365.

Hughes A (2005) Poverty and palliative care in the US: issues facing the urban poor. *International Journal of Palliative Nursing* 11, 6–13.

Ingleton C, Payne S, Nolan M, Carey I (2003) Respite in palliative care: a review and discussion of the literature. *Palliative Medicine* 17(7), 567–575.

Kissane DW, Bloch S (2002) *Family Focused Grief Therapy. A model of family-centred care during palliative care and bereavement.* Buckingham: Open University Press.

Kwaka J (2006) The hospice model in Sierra Leone. *International Journal of Palliative Nursing* 12(4), 157.

Lazarus RS, Folkman S (1984) *Stress, Appraisal and Coping.* New York: Springer-Verlag.

Lee C, Owens G (2002) *The Psychology of Men's Health.* Buckingham: Open University Press.

Lofland LH (1985) The social shaping of emotion: a case of grief. *Symbolic Interaction* 8(2), 171–190.

Lunney JR, Lynn J, Foley DJ, Lipson S, Guralnik JM (2003) Patterns of functional decline at the end of life. *Journal of the American Medical Association* 289(18), 2387–2392.

National Institute for Clinical Excellence (2004) *Improving Supportive and Palliative Care for Adults with Cancer.* The Manual. London: National Institute for Clinical Excellence.

Nolan MR, Davies S, Grant G (2001) (eds) *Working With Older People and Their Families: Key issues in policy and practice.* Buckingham: Open University Press.

Nolan MR, Ryan T, Enderby P, Reid D (2002) Towards a more inclusive vision of dementia care practice and research. *Dementia: The International Journal of Social Research and Practice* 1(2), 193–211.

Nolan MR, Lundh U, Grant G, Keady J (eds) (2003) *Partnerships in Family Care.* Maidenhead: Open University Press.

Payne S (2004) Carers and caregivers. In: *Death, Dying and Social Differences*, pp. 181–198 (eds Oliviere D, Monroe M). Oxford: Oxford University Press.

Payne S, Smith P, Dean S (1999) Identifying the concerns of informal carers in palliative care. *Palliative Medicine* 13, 37–44.

Payne S, Chapman A, Holloway M, Seymour J, Chau R (2005) Chinese community views: promoting cultural competence in palliative care, *Journal of Palliative Care* 21(2), 111–116.

Qureshi H, Bamford C, Nicholas E, Patmore C, Harris JC (2000) *Outcomes in Social Care Practice: Developing an Outcome Focus in Care Management and Use Surveys.* York: Social Policy Research Unit, University of York.

Robinson BC (1983) Validation of a Caregiver Strain Index. *Journal of Gerontology* 38(3), 344–348.

Scharf T, Bartlam B (2006) *Rural Disadvantage: Quality of life and disadvantage amongst older people—a pilot study.* Keele: Commission for Rural Communities, Centre for Social Gerontology, Keele University.

Segal J, Simkins J (1993) *My Mum Needs Me: Helping children with ill or disabled parents.* London: Penguin Books.

Seymour J, Witherspoon R, Gott M, Ross H, Payne S (2005) *Dying in Older Age: End-of-Life Care.* Bristol: Policy Press.

Skilbeck JK, Payne SA, Ingleton MC, Nolan M, Carey I, Hanson A (2005) An exploration of family carers' experience of respite services in one specialist palliative care unit. *Palliative Medicine* 19, 610–618.

Smith P, Payne S, Ramcharan P, Chapman A, Patterson M (2006) *Carers of the Terminally Ill and Employment Issues: a Comprehensive Literature Review*. Report to Help the Hospices. Sheffield: University of Sheffield.

Teno JM, Field MJ, Byock I (2001) The road taken to be traveled in improving end of life care. *Journal of Pain and Symptom Management* **22**(3), 714.

Thomas C, Morris SM, Harman JC (2002) Companions through cancer: the care given by informal carers in cancer contexts. *Social Science and Medicine* **54**(4), 529–544.

Wee B (1997) Palliative care in Hong Kong. *European Journal of Palliative Care* **4**(6), 216–218.

Resilience and paediatric palliative care

Joan Marston

Children and adolescents with life-limiting conditions have very specific palliative care needs which are often different to those of adults. If these children's and adolescents' physical, emotional, social, spiritual and developmental needs are to be met, the caregivers require special knowledge and skill. We ask that the voice of these children and adolescents is heard, respected and acknowledged as part of the expression of hospice and palliative care world-wide.

Korea Statement on Hospice and Palliative Care for Children, The International Children's Palliative Care Network, Seoul (2005)

Introduction

Children live in a world of constant change and surprises. Resilient children have the capacity to learn, adapt, and develop, through interaction with the changed environment, especially when supported by at least one caring adult (Barnard *et al.* 1999). Children are the heroes of their own stories, and the narratives of their lives contain their own unique personhood, the history of their journey, and the different circumstances and environments that they experience. It is the complex interaction of all these that affects whether a child will be the victor or the victim (Bernard 1995).

Children facing life-threatening illness, whether in themselves or a close family member, and children experiencing loss, are made especially vulnerable by external factors and situations over which they have little or no control.

Poverty, illness, the impact on society of HIV and AIDS, orphanhood, and the breakdown of traditional family and community support systems in the developing world, further affect the child's ability to cope with emotional trauma and to adapt to a changed life situation. Despite all these factors, many children show a remarkable ability to affirm the meaning of their lives, to remain an active, contributing part of their family, peer group and community and to experience warmth and humour in situations of illness, deprivation, and trauma.

Good palliative care for children, which is described by the World Health Organization (Sepulveda *et al.* 2002) as 'the active, total care of the child's body, mind and spirit, and also involves giving support to the family, which continues into the bereavement period', promotes resilience by enhancing the child's support systems and providing a safe and structured environment of care for the child and family, whether in the child's home, in a hospital or within a children's' inpatient unit.

Certain core interventions associated with the provision of paediatric palliative care are also interventions that support a child's ability to cope with adversity.

Palliative care is patient and family centred; is based on comprehensive and holistic assessment and ongoing reassessment of the child and family; involves a multidisciplinary approach to ensure care of the body, mind, and spirit; provides good pain and symptom control; is culturally acceptable; and provides psychosocial, emotional, and spiritual support for the child and family, throughout the illness and into the bereavement period. Palliative care promotes the best possible quality of life for each child.

Through support to the child's family, support to the child is strengthened. Palliative care identifies the child and family as the unit of care, and all planning and interventions are directed to improving the quality of life of this unit. Family is not necessarily biological family nor a mother and father, but those closely involved in the primary care of the child. In Sub-Saharan Africa, where millions of children have been orphaned by AIDS, the primary caregiver is often an elderly family member, usually the granny or 'Gogo'; a caring community member; or an older sibling within a child-headed household. Legal guardianship is often difficult to identify especially in families where multiple deaths have occurred, or when the surviving family members are too old or too poor to provide safe care for surviving children. Resilience in children is a combination of inner and outer resources and is enhanced by the presence of at least one caring and constant adult in the child's situation (Mallman 2003). The constant adult may be a teacher, a hospice nurse, or caregiver, or an adult outside of the family unit.

Each child is unique with his or her own strengths and lives within his or her own social environment. Children's responses are different to those of adults, and are affected by age, social competence, and culture. While respecting their individuality within the context of childhood, interventions can be implemented that enhance the child's resilience and response to adverse situations (Barnard *et al.* 1999).

Care of the child's physical body through good nutrition, treatment of acute conditions such as opportunistic infections, and promotion of health, enhances psychological and behavioural interventions (HIV Clinical Resource 2001).

Play is the child's method of communication and learning, and interventions using play techniques strengthen the child's capacity to cope with trauma and stress. The use of transitional objects in play, such as toy animals or dolls, can stimulate communication with ill or bereaved children (Sourkes 1999). Sourkes tells of a child asserting that 'Food, toys and love are all we need to live:' Perhaps this is the basis of all resilience in children?

Research carried out for Save the Children UK in South Africa, to identify the needs of children infected and affected by HIV and AIDS, compared the issues identified by the children with issues identified by their primary caregivers, many of whom lived in rural areas in great poverty. Both groups identified food as the primary need of the child. Children then identified play as their second most important need, but the caregiver group did not identify this at all as essential to their child, focusing rather on material needs and safety. Both groups took for granted the need for a caring adult in the child's life and did not see the need to identify this specifically (Marston and Sephiri 1999).

This difference in the perceived needs of the child may be a risk factor in the development of resilience, especially when the children cannot negotiate their needs with their primary caregiver (Marston and Sephiri 1999).

The International Resilience Project has undertaken research into resilience in children experiencing different types of trauma in a number of countries, and agreed upon the following definition: 'Resilience is a universal capacity which allows a person, group or community to prevent, minimize or overcome the damaging effects of adversity' (Grotberg 1995).

The resilient child

A resilient child exhibits positive adaptation in a situation where one would expect significant degradation in coping skills to take place

Newman (2003)

The impact of paediatric palliative care on childhood resilience will be discussed by examining a number of case studies of children suffering from life-limiting conditions.

Emma's resilience

Emma's mother died of AIDS when she was 3 months old, and Emma is HIV positive. She spent her first 5 years in a crowded and under-resourced children's Place of Safety in South Africa, and was frequently hospitalized for opportunistic infections. Emma was referred to a children's hospice and attended the community palliative day care centre from the age of 6 months, with admissions to the inpatient unit from time to time when she required symptom management. At the age of 6 Emma was placed in foster care by the department of social welfare and was removed 2 months later because of sexual abuse. A new foster placement with a nurse and her family was initially successful but once again Emma had to be removed from the family after sexual abuse by older children. Despite all these traumas in her life, Emma is a delightful, happy and energetic 8-year-old child. Although late starting school because of frequent illness, and dyslexia, she enjoys school and has close friendships there. Emma is described by her teacher as a friendly and hard-working child who is confident enough to participate during lessons, and join in school and class activities. She is warm and responsive to caring adults and has a strong relationship with her weekend parents who fetch her every weekend from the children's home where she now lives in a small family-type unit.

Now on highly active antiretroviral therapy (HAART), her physical health has improved, she has gained weight and seldom suffers from infections.

Geoffrey's resilience

Geoffrey was 12 years old when he died of heart failure. His parents and grandmother had died and he had been sent from one set of family members to another, with his schooling disrupted with each placement, and a consequent loss of friends and a stable environment. His family members all lived in great poverty and none could take responsibility for him for more than 4 months. He was receiving palliative care from a home care team, with admissions to a district-level hospital or a children's hospice when he was ill. His paediatrician referred him for inpatient care to the children's hospice when his oxygen needs increased or whenever the family could not cope with caring for him. With a natural artistic talent, and a love of bright colours, especially red, Geoffrey filled his time drawing and painting and looking after the smaller children in the hospice 'family', despite being on almost continuous oxygen.

Singing was another favourite activity and his sweet voice was often heard singing his favourite song 'I want to pray before I die'. He understood the words of the song and felt this expressed his own feelings. Geoffrey was aware of his prognosis and had experienced the deaths of family and friends. He had a loving relationship with the hospice chaplain and was not averse to discussing death and an afterlife with him in a very matter-of-fact manner. Geoffrey had good communication skills in three languages and through art. Despite little formal schooling he delighted in sending frequent mobile phone text messages asking 'Please bring me Coke and chips' and often including an 'I love you!' at the beginning.

A month before his death, which he told the doctor and staff was imminent (and they did not believe), he gave his nurse a picture that expressed his feelings and uncertainties about death; his love for his young best friend who had just died; and that the children's hospice, painted red in the picture, was his favourite place to be.

Thabo's resilience

Abandoned at birth, Thabo's family was unknown. The only information that could be deduced about his mother was that she was HIV positive, as Thabo also displayed symptoms from a very young age, with a diagnosis of AIDS given when he was just 4 years old. Despite frequent severe infections, including tuberculosis twice, Thabo continued to survive and thrive as an active and friendly child. Although sent to school at the correct age by the children's home where he lived, he never learned to read or write but could express himself verbally in two languages. He attended the children's community palliative day care programme for 3 years, and was often admitted to the children's hospice inpatient unit for short-term care. There he went about setting up a 'family' for himself, with a favourite registered nurse as his 'mother'; the hospice driver as his 'father'; a volunteer fundraiser as his 'granny or gogo' and the maintenance officer as his 'grandfather'. During the last year of his life he also adopted a special teenage patient as his 'big brother'. He enjoyed any machine on wheels, from riding in his mother's car to sitting on the lap of his big brother who was in a wheelchair.

Factors that promote resilience

When looking at Garmezy (1985) and Grotberg's (1995) descriptions of factors that promote resilience, and evaluating Emma, Geoffrey, and Thabo's short lives against them, we can see that they had certain personality factors as well as access to a number of external support systems that enhanced their own strengths.

In 1985 Garmezy identified three protective factors in resilience:

- personality features such as self-esteem
- family cohesion and the absence of discord
- the availability of external support.

Grotberg (1995) also described three similar but slightly different protective factors, which she named the 'I AM; I HAVE; and I CAN' factors. Not all of these factors need to be present for the child to be resilient, but the child needs more than one of these factors.

I AM refers to internal personality features such as self-esteem, which cannot be created but can be strengthened. The child knows that 'I am loveable, have self-esteem and am someone worth knowing and caring about.' The child also recognizes that he or she is competent and has the confidence to carry out certain roles and activities. Peer support groups can play an important part in bolstering self-esteem during times of crisis, and enhance and rebuild self-confidence, while also developing social and communication skills in the child. Support groups should be supervised by a competent, trained adult, to ensure they work towards set objectives, and that each child has the opportunity to participate actively.

'I HAVE' refers to an external support system, whether in the form of a biological family that nurtures the child, or caring adults who provide constancy and structure in the child's life. The system can be present in a school, faith group, sports team, or social activity group. Where a palliative care team is involved in care and support, this often becomes an external support system for the child.

The African proverb, 'It takes a village to grow a child' points to the support that communities can or should provide for children. In a number of African communities any child born becomes the child of that community, and when parents die the community takes over responsibilities of care. Sadly with the increasing breakdown of traditional communities and movement to towns and cities to seek employment and healthcare, this safety net for children is now frequently absent.

Children learn ethical and acceptable behaviour from role models and those who care enough to teach and guide, and to set boundaries for them. Spiritual support, often provided through formal religious structures, provides a system of values and beliefs, and enhances a child's sense of justice. Within countries ravaged by HIV and AIDS, where children experience death on a regular basis, a spiritual belief system helps them to find meaning in their own and others' lives, and in death (Mallman 2003).

'I CAN' features refer to the child's interpersonal skills and social competence and affect the way the child deals with problems, interacts with others, expresses feelings and identifies the right person with whom to share emotions.

- **I am** features cannot be created but can be strengthened by external supports
- **I have** features can be strengthened and also can be provided
- **I can** features can be taught, and must be learned by the child.

Although the concept is complex with a multitude of interacting factors, it is suggested that a resilient child will have at least two of these features in their lives and will be actively involved in developing their own resilience. Caring adults and a concerned community, whether in the family, school, faith system, or peer group are the ideal people to help strengthen the child's resilient response. In some traditional African cultures, the Tribal Leaders would lead the community response to children.

Personality features

Emma has always had a definite sense of her own worth and she was a natural leader among her friends and playmates, even after the two traumatic periods in foster care, after which she regressed to short periods of thumb-sucking and bed-wetting. She received counselling immediately after removal from her foster families, and participated in play therapy. Her art showed the chaos and the anger in her mind at first, emphasized by the use of dark colours in her drawings. However, within 6 weeks, her pictures were once again full of bright colours, friends, and flowers.

The 'I am' personality feature was a primary reason for Emma's resilience after the failed foster placements, and this had been enhanced throughout her life while attending the palliative day care centre each day, and when admitted to the children's hospice.

Geoffrey was always confident in himself as a leader and 'big brother' to the smaller children in the children's hospice, and took delight in his talent for art and singing. Despite little formal education he could express himself clearly in three languages and through his art. He also expressed his faith in going to Heaven after he died, in discussions with the chaplain.

He felt safe in the children's hospice and requested to spend his final illness there, secure in the knowledge that he was cared for and loved.

Thabo was able to define his place in life through appointing a family unit for himself and identifying the family members' possessions as his own. He was confident that the children's hospice was his personal space in life and that there he could be completely himself. Without the ability to draw properly, he expressed himself through play and singing.

Family cohesion and the absence of discord

On both occasions of abuse **Emma** was wisely, and at her own request, returned to the children's hospice, where she was with staff and volunteers whom she knew and who had known and loved her for many years. This provided a safe, welcoming and well-known environment where she could receive care and support from a multidisciplinary team, and known therapists. The 'I can' features included her communication and interactions within this supportive environment, and also her loving weekend family who have given her life structure and meaning and a sense of identity apart from the institutions where most of her life has been spent. The children's hospice staff, multidisciplinary team, and her weekend family worked closely together to ensure Emma felt safe and loved, and that she received the best possible holistic palliative care to support the antiretroviral therapy that was initiated.

Geoffrey was aware that he had family members who could not care for him, and had memories of a loving Gogo. The hospice staff were extra caring people in his life, and he constantly thanked them with his drawings. The younger children became his special charge and could often be found around his bed. Geoffrey was the one who made sure each received a fair share of any items given to the children. He was part of the development of his own supportive and harmonious environment that enhanced his natural communication and interactive skills with others to strengthen his 'I can' factors.

As **Thabo** had created a selected family for himself he was supremely secure and contented within this unit, and within the security of the hospice environment. Palliative care could not at that time include HAART, as it was not available in South Africa in public health facilities, but good healthcare, treatment of tuberculosis and opportunistic infections, a well-balanced diet, spiritual support, and ongoing emotional support all enhanced his ability to explore and interact within his created environment and contributed to an exceptional enjoyment of life. Again, like Geoffrey, Thabo had been part of ensuring 'I can' features to give his life meaning. The children's Place of Safety and the children's hospice worked together with the hospice multidisciplinary team and decided that the best quality of life could be achieved within the hospice environment, with frequent visits from the caring staff of the government institution.

The availability of external support

Apart from the hospice personnel a new support system came into **Emma's** life when a board member of the hospice decided to become her weekend mother, taking her home to her family each week from Friday to Monday, providing her with her own room as personal space, decorated as she wished, and with her own clothes and toys. After the second readmission, Emma was initiated on HAART and her physical health improved rapidly, with a reduction in the periods of ill-health she had experienced all her life.

Now living in a children's home she has been able to organize her life into its different compartments—children's home, hospice, weekend home, school—and function effectively within each area.

Geoffrey had good memories of all the people who had been part of his life, from a remembrance of his mother and Gogo, to fond recollections of various aunts and uncles. At the end of his life he chose to be readmitted to the children's hospice for palliative care from known and supportive staff. While remaining the patient, he made sure that he controlled his treatment, from his use of oxygen to the food he ate, and would not hesitate to call on visitors to assist with extra treats such as cool drinks and chips.

Thabo had been involved with the children's hospice through day care and admissions, from the age of 4 until he died at age 11. He enjoyed playing with his friends but his happiest times were when he was receiving one-on-one attention from his 'family members', especially his 'mother' and 'big brother'. The staff of the children's home were also very caring and concerned about his progress, working closely with the children's hospice staff to provide the best possible quality of life for Thabo.

Spiritual support was given through gentle discussions with the children's chaplain, learning to pray, and involvement in church activities and services.

Thabo was sent to school when he was 7 years old. After 6 months of little progress he became withdrawn and insecure. During the school holidays he insisted on attending the hospice palliative day care where within days he was back to his happy and active self. At school he could not master reading and writing and could not participate in all the class activities, thus his self-esteem was damaged. Back at the day care, he knew that he could play all the games and participate competently in activities, and his self-esteem 'bounced back'. Participation provides opportunities for coping with different situations, and coping enhances self-esteem (Barnard *et al.* 1999).

Protective factors in palliative care

Four processes that protect people against the psychosocial risks associated with adversity were described by Rutter (1987, 1999) as:

1. Reduction of the impact of the risk
2. Reduction of negative chain-reactions
3. Establishment and maintenance of self-esteem and self-efficacy
4. Opening up of opportunities.

Palliative care for children helps to reduce the impact of risk as it provides a protective framework through careful assessment of each child within their own family unit, and holistic child-centred care. Regular assessment and reassessment that leads to adaptations in treatment and care, helps to identify risk factors and either minimize or prevent risks and break negative chain reactions. Care and treatment by skilled practitioners promotes good physical, emotional and spiritual health that promotes participation in activities within and outside the family, and enables the child to take advantage of new opportunities.

Sally was dying from a brain tumour. As a 16 year old, despite weight gain associated with taking cortisone, blindness from the tumour and increasing weakness, she still took great delight in remaining involved in school activities.

The palliative care team worked together with Sally and her parents to enable her to join in as many activities as possible. On hearing of a school dance, Sally insisted on attending. Although her family and the palliative care team realized that she would tire very quickly, they supported her wish, and the hospice community nurse took her shopping for a new outfit, carefully explaining what each dress looked like and allowing Sally to feel the material and imagine her appearance in the dress.

On the night, Sally insisted on wearing a multicoloured wig as she had lost most of her hair, and gaily went off to the dance with her very supportive school friends. Asked to dance by the most popular young man from a local school, she re-lived that evening many times, when she was unable to leave her bed.

Peer support throughout the illness enhances resilience and is often more acceptable than adult support, as the peer group have more sensitivity to the child's needs, so like their own. On Sally's last Christmas Day the hospice nurse and her daughter, also a friend of Sally, went to the family home to look after Sally while the parents spent a few hours with friends. Sally's mother had left a plate of soft vegetables for her daughter, who by this time was having difficulty swallowing. With one look at this, her friend said, 'This is Christmas. It needs junk food!' and fetched ice-cream and a cool drink, which she slowly fed to a delighted and giggling Sally. Afterwards the two girls lay together on the bed, talking quietly, and Sally opened up to her friend about her emotions about dying, something she had been reluctant to speak of to her parents, priest, or hospice staff.

Peer group members also require information and support throughout the illness of their friend or fellow pupil, and the palliative care team will frequently go to the child's school or meet with the child's friends to listen to, provide explanations, and support the other children. While in most communities, peer group members will not have experienced life-limiting illness, in sub-Saharan Africa, where so many children are either infected with HIV or have lost family members to AIDS, a child newly orphaned or diagnosed with HIV will soon find peers who are experiencing similar situations. In certain areas, almost whole classrooms are filled with HIV-infected and affected children, taught by infected and affected teachers. Thus natural support groups are formed as these children share experiences and understand each others' problems.

Promoting self-esteem

Involving the child in decisions concerning care enables them to experience mastery over their illness and external conditions, thus promoting self-esteem.

Jenny was almost 3 and nearing the end of a 1-year battle with cancer. Supported by wise and loving parents and two older sisters, she asked to stay at home within her family unit. As her pain increased she was initiated on Tilidine, an opioid analgesic, for pain control, which was effective, but Jenny decided she did not like the taste. The doctor changed her prescription to morphine syrup, which was also effective, but, once again, found to 'taste nasty'. Instead of trying a different medication or route, the palliative care nurse put the Tilidine in a teaspoon and the morphine syrup into a syringe, explained which was which, and gave Jenny the choice of drugs. After a few moments hesitation, Jenny grasped the syringe, swallowed the morphine syrup, and continued to take the syrup for pain without ever again complaining of the taste. Despite her young age, she was given control over this decision and took responsibility for her choice.

Sitembi was dying of AIDS and severe heart failure. Although 4 years old, he had never learned to walk, and spoke very few words. Despite lack of verbal skills he had mastered the art of non-verbal communication, using his face, his eyes, and arms very effectively. He was orphaned and his only remaining family member was a young and loving uncle who visited him regularly. As he was dying, Sitembi indicated to the hospice nurse that he wanted to go outside, ride in his favourite car, visit much-loved staff members and volunteers, and see his special places again. For 2 days he organized his farewells, and then died peacefully in his uncle's arms. His mastery of non-verbal communication had allowed him to control his last few days and achieve completion and peace before his death.

Play as a vehicle for resilience

Play helps build resilience and is used in paediatric palliative care (Kernberg 2004):

- to enhance communication skills, both verbal and non-verbal
- to promote self-confidence through the development and mastery of skills

- to enable the child to experience control over situations and enhance self-esteem
- to facilitate the expression of emotions related to illness and bereavement
- to provide a safe environment for the discussion of fears and feelings
- to learn more of the illness and procedures related to diagnosis and treatment
- to provide enjoyment and relaxation.

Gloria was so withdrawn when admitted to the children's hospice programme that the staff believed her to be severely mentally and physically challenged. At 3 years of age she neither walked nor talked, and would not play with other children nor with the hospice staff. Nothing made her smile and no one could remember hearing her laugh. Gloria had lived with her ill mother in a shack, with no other family or friends, and only the hospice nurses visiting the patient and child. Once her mother died, Gloria was placed in a children's home among many other children, and taken to day care once a week. It appeared that all she could do was to eat and drink. One of the palliative care nurses caught Gloria walking to fetch a biscuit one day when she thought no one was watching her. After discussion with the multidisciplinary team, an intensive programme of play therapy was initiated, at first with absolutely no response from Gloria.

In the end, persistence paid off, and a simple ball game led to Gloria slowly beginning to participate, then to enjoy and laugh during the play sessions, until finally she initiated play with the therapist and then with the other children. She died a few months later, but enjoyed these last few months, actively interacting with others, and taking delight in being with other children and playing her favourite games.

Play enables children to express emotions and to feel in control of their activities (Kernberg 2004). Mastery of any activity enhances self-esteem and builds internal resilience. Most children will enjoy creating something through art or other activities, such as sand bottles or a mandala, which encourages the external expression of inner emotions and allows the child to live safely in the present while describing past and present experiences.

The role of the family or primary caregiver

The family will usually wish to provide the best possible care and support for a child requiring palliative care, but the family members' own situation of living with the illness and the feelings of grief and loss associated with this, may hamper the factors that promote a child's resilience. A desire to protect the child from difficult decisions and situations may prevent the child from developing coping strategies and building confidence in themselves, which encourages them to make sense of their illness and manage their responses (Newman 2003). It can be very difficult for a caring parent or primary caregiver to allow a child to experience the emotional, spiritual, and social pain of a life-limiting illness, and not try to protect them from this. At times, the palliative care practitioner may also do his best to provide (or become!) the cotton wool of caring that shuts out reality (Marta 2004). Through education of the family or primary caregiver, and involvement in both multidisciplinary team discussions and planning of care, an enabling environment can be established to promote resilience. Discussions with a psychologist to identify the child's and their own personal qualities that can be strengthened, promote coping by the whole family unit.

Sister Silke-Andrea Mallmann worked in Namibia with children infected and orphaned by HIV and AIDS and often either living on their own in child-headed households, or with elderly relatives. She examined the reasons many children cope with seemingly overwhelming adversity coupled with extreme poverty. She recognized that children and their families coped better when they have three capabilities:

- the capability to understand an adverse event
- the capability to believe that they can cope with a crisis because they know they have some control over what happens
- the capability to give deeper meaning to an adverse event.

And that these required both inner and external resources (Mallmann 2003).

When the family unit understands and identifies these resources, they can participate in strengthening them. The palliative care practitioner can also assist the child and family's capacity to reframe adversities so that the beneficial effects are recognized (Newman 2003).

Promoting resilience through paediatric palliative care

The aim of paediatric palliative are is to promote the best possible quality of life for the child and family, through skilled and compassionate holistic care, involving a multidisciplinary approach. Paediatric palliative care practitioners seldom have the enhancement of the child's resilience to enable them to cope with illness or bereavement as a primary objective of care. However, the presence of the practitioner as a caring and constant adult may be one of the most important factors in the development of resilience in a child, especially within a child-headed household, or where the primary caregiver is too ill, too poor or too old to provide simple care to meet the child's basic needs, let alone meet the emotional, developmental, spiritual, and social needs of a child facing life-limiting illness or loss (Marston and Sephiri 2000).

Support from others, and structures within their own and the greater community may be both formal and informal. Where unemployment is common, the availability of a grant to provide food, clothing, and shelter, and enable the older child to possess the necessary materials to attend school, is seldom available in the developing world. Aid agencies and international donors are often the only source of school materials, clothing and food support for an increasing number of children in poorer areas of the world. Palliative care programmes may be seen as channels for aid donations, and the true purpose of the home visit obscured by the expectation of material assistance, and disappointment when this is not available. The impact on resilience of a culture of external dependency, needs further research.

Resilience is enhanced where children enjoy school as a positive experience; where teachers treat them with respect, and where they have good interpersonal relationships with staff and other pupils (Newman 2003). Palliative care programmes often establish open communication with the child's teacher and school and include teachers as part of the multidisciplinary team (Yule and Gold 1993).

Respect at all times for the child and family, including children in decisions, where the child is old enough and competent enough to participate, and accepting that the child and family know what is needed, and know what is best for the child, are all part of family-centred care. Paediatric palliative care can do much to enhance resilience in children by providing a safe and caring system to support the child's inherent personality factors, in an holistic, respectful and culturally-sensitive manner. In paediatric palliative care the voice of the child *is* heard, respected, and acknowledged.

References

American Psychological Association Help Centre (2001) Resilience Guide for Parents and Teachers.

Barnard P, Morland I, Nagey J (1999) *Children, Bereavement and Trauma. Nurturing Resilience*. London: Jessica Kingsley Publishers.

Bernard B (1995) *Fostering Resilience in Children*. Education Resource Information Centre (ERIC) Digest. Chicago: University of Illinois.

Garmezy N (1985) Stress resilient children: the search for protective factors. In: *Recent Research in Developmental Psychopathology* (ed. Stevenson J). Oxford: Pergamon Press.

Grotberg E (1995) *A Guide to Promoting Resilience in Children. Strengthening the Human Spirit*. Early Childhood Development. Practical Reflections Series. Bernard van Leer Foundation The Hague: International Resilience Project.

HIV Clinical Resource (March 2001) Department of Health AIDS Institute. New York State.

Kernberg P (2001) Resilience of children in the face of trauma. *Psychiatric Times* **XV111**(4).

Mallman S (2003) *Building Resilience in Children Affected by HIV/AIDS*. Cape Town: Maskew Miller Longman.

Marston J, Sephiri K (1999) *Identifying Children in Distress*. Unpublished research for Save the Children (UK).

Marta S (2004) *Healing the Hurt. Restoring the Hope*. London: Rodale Ltd.

Monroe B, Kraus F (2004) *Brief Interventions with Bereaved Children*. Oxford: Oxford University Press.

Newman T, Blackburn S (1978) *Transitions in the Lives of Children and Young People: Resilience Factors*. Ilford: Barnardo's Policy, Research and Influencing Unit.

Rutter M (1987) Psychosocial resilience and protective mechanisms. *American Journal of Orthopsychiatry* **57**(3), 316–331.

Rutter M (1999) Resilience concepts and findings: implications for family therapy. *Journal of Family Therapy* **21**(2), 119–144.

Smith S (1999) *The Forgotten Mourners. Guidelines for Working with Bereaved Children*. London: Jessica Kingsley Publishers.

Sepulveda C, Marlin A, Yoshida T, Ullrich A (2002) Palliative care: the World Health Organisation's global perspective. *Journal of Pain and Symptom Management* **24**(2), 91–96.

Sourkes B (1995) *Armfuls of Time. The Psychological Experience of the Child with a Life-Threatening Illness*. Pittsburgh: University of Pittsburgh Press.

Yule W, Gold A (1993) *Coping with Crises in Schools—Wise Before the Event*. London: Calouste Gulbenkian Foundation.

Resilience and spirituality

Stefan Vanistendael

Introduction

Resilience (Manciaux 2001; Theis 2001) and even more so spirituality (Watson *et al*. 2005) are human realities that seem to be hard to define and to grasp adequately. Yet most people, if not all, are sooner or later in life confronted with both. This specific discrepancy goes beyond the gap between what we have to face in life and what we do know, because it also raises questions about what we can know, and how (Schweizer *et al*. 2001).

Because of such complexity the exploration of resilience and spirituality in relation with palliative care requires us to draw on a variety of sources of learning ranging from scientific research to ongoing practical experience or even artistic expression. Wolfgang Edelstein from the Max Planck Institute in Berlin has formulated this challenge for the field of resilience in a private conversation in Potsdam in 1994: 'In order to explore a subject like resilience we must gradually build up a form of wisdom which integrates science'. Manciaux (2003) and Cyrulnik (1999) confirm this orientation. The same can be applied to the wider exploration of the relations between resilience and spirituality and their relevance for palliative care. This may not respond to strict canons of science, but in a sense it increases the complexity and difficulty of learning and of building up knowledge. Ideas emerging from such an exploration may inspire practice but they should always be used with great care and remain open to correction. In spite of this added complexity resilience (Wortman *et al*. 2002) and spirituality (Koenig *et al*. 2002) remain relevant for people involved in palliative care: professionals, volunteers as well as patients with their families and friends.

The present chapter first gives a pragmatic clarification of the concepts of resilience and spirituality, followed by the presentation of a resilience model for practical use, with special emphasis on the importance of meaning, as a key element of spirituality. This exploration suggests all along the way some practical implications for palliative care.

Resilience

Resilience is the capacity of an individual person or a social system to grow and to develop in the face of very difficult circumstances (Vanistendael 2002). This pragmatic definition allows us to point out the reality we are referring to while making a clear distinction with resilience as known in physics and engineering, the latter not being a growth process. This definition has evolved over the years, from the consultation of scientific literature on resilience (Werner and Smith 1992; Rutter, 1994; Opp *et al.* 1999; Lecomte 2002; Suárez Ojeda 2002; Titus 2002; Gilligan 2005; Theis 2006), and others, but even more so from discussions with participants in over 100 resilience presentations—workshops or conferences—in over 15 countries in four continents, between 1994 and now. Such presentations have responded to requests from the field, they are not part of a systematic research design. They have brought together a wide variety of fieldworkers, such as doctors, nurses, psychotherapists, teachers, social workers, street workers, specialized educators, prison chaplains, hospital chaplains, as well as a variety of volunteers, covering a wide range of languages, cultures, and concerns.

Beyond a pragmatic definition, discussions about what resilience exactly is can become quite confusing. It is somewhat comparable with efforts of defining time or love. It is therefore helpful to remind us how resilience is rooted in human reality. An Argentinean psychologist, Ramon Lascano, working in the province of Jujuy, has formulated this approach in a resilience workshop in Buenos Aires in 2003: 'What is the starting point of resilience? We observe the fact that some persons or some families do very well in difficult situations, whereas other comparable persons or families have great trouble in similar situations. We then ask: what can we learn from the first group that could be useful for other persons or families not doing so well?' This observation and questioning could also apply to various processes in palliative care. Such 'rooting' of the concept of resilience in real life may be more important for practice than an artificially clear definition.

The process of discovery of and exploration of resilience allows us to specify a series of nuances that have gradually emerged from science as well as from the experience of fieldworkers in diverse countries, cultures, and professions. It is the convergence of experience in contrasting contexts that gives strength to such nuances. That is part of the 'rooting' of the concept in life. All nuances mentioned below may be relevant for palliative care, but they cannot be applied in a mechanical way; they are more like signposts suggesting a path:

1. Resilience is never absolute (Rutter 1993).
2. Resilience is variable in time and in space (Poletti and Dobbs 2001; Lecomte 2002).

3. Resilience consists of two dimensions: resistance and construction. The latter implies a capacity to project oneself into the future (Vanistendael 1998, 2002).

4. In certain cases resilience becomes the capacity to transform a negative event into an element of growth (Lecomte 2004). This is particularly relevant in palliative care, for example when a person dies in a very dignified way, which is even inspiring for relations and staff, or when a grieving process develops into a new start in life.

5. Resilience is built in a life-long process of interaction between the person (group) and its environment (Silva Pañez 1997; Brissiaud 2001; Lecomte 2002).

6. Resilience contains a strong ethical dimension. For example: what does 'positive' mean in positive growth? What is being 'well adjusted' to an impossible and unacceptable situation? (Manciaux 1998; Fuchs 2001). This will sound familiar in palliative care, probably more so than in less extreme situations. For example, what is understood by 'a good death' (Chochinov 2006)?

Fieldworkers often discover in their own context such nuances from experience well before scientific researchers do, but whatever the way of discovery we must remain prudent with generalizations. Two more nuances come even more specifically from discussions with fieldworkers:

7. Often resilience is referred to as positive adaptation or growth in spite of adverse circumstances. Yet on several occasions, the first time in Buenos Aires in 1996, professional fieldworkers have pointed out to the author that the problems to be overcome may open up access to some hitherto hidden inner resources in a person, and trigger off a growth process. If certain problems turn out to be positive challenges stimulating growth, others will be destructive. So, in a difficult situation, growth will sometimes happen in spite of problems, sometimes thanks to them, and in many situations it will be a mixture of both.

8. Resilience is not limited to victims and patients, but also to their families and friends, and to the professional staff and volunteers active in care. This may be particularly relevant in palliative care.

Spirituality

Spirituality and the related concept of religion also raise problems of definition, of what we can know, and how (Watson *et al.* 2005; Chochinov 2006; Echard 2006; Raffin *et al.* 2006). Spirituality is based on the conviction that there is more to life than what we can observe materially (Echard 2006), and yet this 'more' seems to be related to the material world as we know it. For example, a person can be overwhelmed by the beauty of a masterpiece in painting; however, the description and explanation of such beauty and its effect on the person, uniquely in terms of the chemistry and physics of the paint and its support, combined with some neurological processes in the brain of the spectator, may meet certain scientific standards, but it does not seem to do justice to the experience. It is like trying to see a magnificent landscape through a tiny crack rather than a proper window. Spirituality is the exploration of this world beyond what is immediately visible, as well as its connections to life as we know it. As spirituality is less tangible than resilience, it may be even more difficult to grasp.

Spirituality, so broadly defined, is not identical with religion, although there may be overlaps (Watson *et al.* 2005). One can gradually 'funnel' this broad concept of spirituality by accumulating specifications (Vanistendael 2002), which allows for a wide range of applications.

1. A number of people believe in a positive core reality behind the visible world, and some of them will call this 'God' (Armstrong 1993).

2. Some people will develop a personal relation with 'God'.

3. Some communities try to express such beliefs in more concrete and systematic ways: in rituals, celebrations, symbols, art, holy texts, doctrine, rules of conduct.

4. Some communities organize such beliefs and their expressions more formally and that may lead into religion; religions vary a lot according to culture and according to their founders' intuitions (Raffin *et al.* 2006).

5. Christians believe that God made himself present in Jesus, about 2000 years ago, in a way that was radically new and has not been equalled since.

It is not easy to define a common ground in the wide variety of concrete expressions of spirituality. In the frame of a pilot project of Zürich University on spirituality in a home for the elderly, Anemone Eglin describes spirituality as a relation to an ultimate reality. She specifies that from such a relation a human being gains meaning and force for shaping everyday life. She defines three existential questions that show the relevance of spirituality for anybody towards the end of life, independently of his or her religious convictions (Vögeli 2005; Zentrum für Gerontologie 2006):

◆ What meaning does my life have?

◆ What does it mean for me that at one point I shall have to let everything go?

◆ What holds and supports me at this time in life when everything is slipping out of my hands?

Such questions have the advantage of cutting across cultures and personal convictions, without being a sort of uninspiring biggest common denominator. First experiences in this pilot project suggest that some form of spiritual support to the elderly often gives them a profound sense of peace and well-being, beyond the status of their physical health. Spiritual support requires special attention from the staff, so as to see the person in care and his or her situation and history as a whole, beyond the immediate physical needs (Vögeli 2005). This is coherent with the broader principles of palliative care (Watson *et al.* 2005).

A pragmatic synthesis of some factors contributing to resilience: the 'casita'

The concept of resilience has to be interpreted and made more practical for palliative care. The model presented below may be helpful in such exercise without any claims of being the only possible way.

Many factors can intervene in the promotion of resilience. Different presentations and syntheses of such factors are possible (Benard 1991; Goldstein and Brooks 2001; Gilligan 2005). The model presented here first was a communication tool for presenting factors of resilience in a workshop for psychologists, street workers, and social workers in Chili (Vanistendael and Lecomte 2000). However, spontaneously and gradually it has developed into a working tool for people wanting to inspire their action by resilience. This has been very explicit in a few Dutch schools (Broers 2005), but without any exclusivity. The synthesis is based on the scheme of a house. In most places it has kept its original Spanish name, 'casita', little house, for reasons of convenience in pronunciation across languages. Every room of the house represents a major potential factor of resilience: basic physical health; fundamental acceptance of the person as a person, which mostly happens in informal social networks of family and friends; sense and meaning (Vanistendael and Lecomte 2003); self-esteem; competences; humour; and others (open model). The rooms form like a succinct guide for possible fields of action for those who are seeking to operationalize resilience thinking. In practice one has to see in a given situation, what concretely and specifically can be done in each room of that 'casita'. All the rooms can relate to a variety of situations and people, also in palliative care.

The search for positives

How the 'casita' model can function exactly in a given situation has to be worked out by staff and others involved, on a case to case basis, gradually learning from experience.

Yet there is a general underlying orientation: while recognizing the need for dealing with problems and negative situations, particularly in palliative care, resilience requires us to look for positive elements to (re)build life (Fozzard 2002). Such elements may be small, apparently insignificant, relevant to this

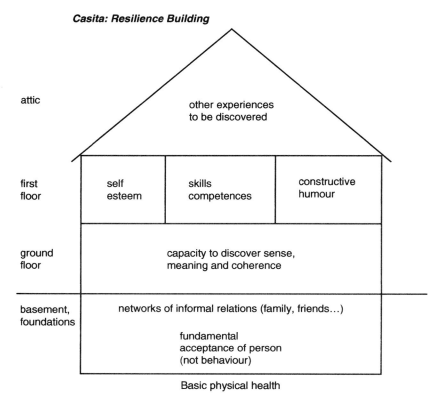

Figure 7.1 (Stefan Vanistendael, BICE, Geneva, 1998).

individual person only, or even hidden behind negative behaviour, and by no means they have to be 'perfect' (Vanistendael 2001). The list of examples can be endless, from an inspiring poem to a cherished photograph, from the favourite cuddly toy to the peaceful smile of a person, from a little encouraging success to an approving and welcoming look, from a favourite piece of music to a much appreciated flower, from a certain type of humour to a silent and welcoming presence, etc.

The search for positives is not a denial of what goes wrong, but a more inclusive and realistic view of the situation, not exclusively determined by problems. It also recognizes that in the end we cannot build with negatives as such, but that we need some positive elements, or some negative experience, which is not exclusively seen as problematic. This may happen, for example, when a severe illness can be recognized and dealt with as a factor of human growth (Büchi 2005), but such processes are often more clearly perceived with hindsight.

We also must avoid the other extreme, the exclusive insistence on positive elements or worse, the denial of the problem. Resilience is not a panacea neither a miracle solution. Resilience does not allow, for example, taking shortcuts in a grieving process: the loss, the pain, and the bereavement have to be fully admitted (Hanus 2001) for sustainable positive growth to be possible in and beyond the grief.

Friedrich Lösel confirmed, when asked in a discussion in 1993 in New York what resilience brings to our activities: 'Resilience gives us back a sense of realistic hope'. Resilience offers a framework where those two elements can be held together. It is interesting that we find 'fostering realistic hope' mentioned among the principles of spiritual care in the palliative sector (Watson *et al.* 2005).

This search of positives does not always come naturally in certain professions, to the extent that their agenda is set exclusively by the response to problems, which can lead to reducing people to a set of problems to be dealt with. That risk is very real in medical care: after all, the patient comes to the doctor because of a problem. However, that should not prevent from opening up other horizons so as to include positive elements and resources. Otherwise some real chances for growth may be missed. One practical challenge could be how to adapt certain assessment or diagnostic instruments so as to include explicitly relevant resources of the patient and his or her environment.

The 'casita' model may be helpful for such a review. It also helps to give shape to a process of continuous learning about resilience. In that epistemological sense, it is close to science, while remaining close to real life. If science is seen in a stricter, more controlled and exclusively quantitative way, the model is not scientific.

The use of the 'casita' model

The 'casita' can be used essentially for structuring experience and discussion related to resilience, with individuals or groups or even institutions.

The model has a number of advantages:

1. It is simple to understand intellectually, while allowing to take into account a fair amount of real life complexity;

2. It is holistic;

3. Given normal care and prudence, it can be used in a variety of situations with or by different sorts of people such as professionals, volunteers, patients, friends, family;

4. It is adaptable to culture;

5. It is flexible and open enough to remain close to the evolving experience of life and of resilience; people can (re)design their 'casita's' according to their experience of resilience; the attic of the house is a free space providing an openness to new experiences not anticipated by the model;

6. It can be used with individuals, groups or even institutions;

7. For many people the image of the house or home allows to establish a strong positive emotional bond with the model; caution may be needed in some delicate situations, such as with some refugees or people who realize that they will never see their home again; although such problems have not been reported yet, it does not imply that they cannot exist;

8. It articulates two opposite dynamics many fieldworkers have to face: on the one hand the search for factors that can be generalized (the rooms of the house); on the other hand the need to contextualize and specify interventions, even individually; following the imagery of the model such specification would be like furnishing the rooms; this may consist of a listing of positive resources and ways how to mobilize them, specified for each room in the house;

9. For those interested in the relation between qualitative and quantitative thinking, the 'casita' is a qualitative model that seems to reflect the basic levels of a mathematical function; the general structure of the house would correspond to the structure of a function, the rooms to the parameters in a function, the furnishing of the rooms to the variables.

Building resilience: physical health or comfort, and feeling accepted as a person

For palliative care the importance of the physical well being or comfort of patients is obvious in many ways, while at the same time being relative: the appropriate response to disease, the care for physical comfort, pain control, they are all important, but in very different ways, according to the evolving condition of the patient. This may be valid not just for the patients but for everybody dealing with the demands of care, from staff to family and relations.

The foundation of the 'casita' is the fundamental acceptance of the other as a person, not necessarily the person's behaviour. Originally the expression 'unconditional acceptance' was used (Werner 1989), but field workers have often found this expression exaggerated. Still it refers to the fact that people grow in stable and profound relations with others, or at least in profoundly positive encounters. This is an old psychological insight, confirmed from a different angle by the research on the foundations of resilience. As Werner pointed out early on, people in informal networks of families and friends around a person are often in a better position for offering such acceptance than professionals dealing with the obligations and constraints of their professional status. She concludes that part of a professional intervention could consist of tapping such informal resources and organize them around a person in need (Werner 1989). Werner's research dealt with children in distress, but her conclusions seem to be coherent with a concept of comprehensive palliative care in general, without diminishing in any way the importance of staff empathy. In practice it is important to remember that acceptance is not a one-way process. A minimum of acceptance has to go two ways in order to work well.

The previous point also clarifies the great positive potential volunteers may have, provided volunteer work is set up carefully. Volunteers, not the least volunteer visitors, can play a role complementary to professionals, because they can focus more on the quality of the relation to the patient (or relatives) as such. They can contribute to the vital informal support networks Werner (1989) mentioned. This is even more important in the case of lonely patients.

In German there is a substantive, 'Geborgenheit', with its derivatives, that expresses very well what is so important for the foundations of resilience. Its meaning integrates elements of feeling respected, protected and secure, feeling accepted and welcomed, a degree of intimacy and of peace, a feeling of being truly held in life.

Meaning is considered to be so important in relation to spirituality, to resilience and to palliative care, that it is discussed separately in the following section of this chapter. The other elements of this resilience model will be mentioned only briefly, because they are often less foundational for resilience.

Building resilience: self-esteem, competences, humour

Self-esteem is typically built in two ways:

- the ordinary words and deeds of everyday life can reinforce or diminish self-esteem; at times this can be a very slow and hardly perceptible process;
- successfully confronting difficult but not ultimately overwhelming challenges.

Even in an individual patient's history the practical implementation of both points may change considerably over time. The respect of self-esteem is closely related to the autonomy and dignity of the patient, two major themes in palliative care (Vinant 2006).

Competences, socially or otherwise, are considered to be important for resilience. They are often 'hands on' and can be learnt (Goldstein and Brooks 2001). For that reason they can be practically important, even if they may be less profound than the discovery of meaning or the feeling of being accepted as a person. A concrete learning experience can help a person to find meaning and it may boast self-esteem, while increasing competences. This applies to many fields, from everyday life to arts. But the continuous adaptation of a patient in palliative care to his or her changing health is a peculiar sort of ongoing learning experience in extreme circumstances, with its own successes and potential for nurturing self-esteem. In a different way this is also true for the accompanying family and relations.

Humour can be a major component of resilience and of spirituality, if it is constructive humour, which keeps us smiling in the face of adversity (Nussenbaum 1995; Schreiner 2003). In its strongest form such humour is not imaginary, but on the contrary, it reveals in a difficult situation a very real positive point that was overlooked or forgotten. Humour may not solve a problem but it can offer some precious breathing space for life to go on, it can restore confidence and a taste for life (Escarpit 1981). It has also its downsides, particularly when it is perverted into sarcasm and irony, or when it functions as a screen that blocks communication (Vanistendael 2003). The latter may occur in palliative care. The relaxing and easing of tension through humour can be positive, but if it makes more serious and essential communication impossible, humour is problematic, particularly when faced with limited time towards the end of life.

Humour can be a great resource for all involved in palliative care, provided it is used prudently. Its positive influence on health has been studied, particularly for reducing stress (Svebak 1987). The full explanation of the links between humour, resilience, and spirituality is beyond the scope of the present text, but the following points may be helpful:

◆ constructive humour requires a climate of confidence; in the absence of confidence humour is easily perceived as aggressive and demeaning (Bariaud 1995);

◆ humour needs boundaries; they can be very different according to cultures, particularly in delicate situations; at least avoid laughing at people (Soebstad 1995);

The attic of the 'casita' is deliberately free for other experiences to be discovered, which have not been anticipated by the model. This reflects the conviction that a resilience model needs to be close to life and open to new elements in order to be workable.

Meaning

Meaning is a key element of both spirituality and resilience, valid both in a religious or non-religious context. It is also a key element of psychological well-being. The logotherapy, developed by the Austrian psychiatrist Viktor Frankl, has its roots in the rediscovery of meaning in life, even in extreme circumstances (Frankl 1963). Frankl articulates three ways for assuming responsibility for life and hence discovering meaning: creative action, experience, or love, of which the latter is the most important (Frankl 1982).

The reflection here comes close to the ideas of Frankl, but in a very pragmatic way. The direct question 'What is the meaning of life?' is avoided, because it would probably lead into an infinite discussion with not much practical relevance. Instead another question is explored in the context of palliative care: 'What does connect a person positively to broader life?' The underlying hypothesis is that such positive connections to life around us give us the feeling that our life has meaning, even without us reflecting upon it, even unconsciously.

This hypothesis has one immediate practical consequence: if the positive connection to life is so important, more than how good or pleasant life is as such, people can in principle discover meaning in very difficult situations, to the extent that they can build such positive connections. For example, a person with serious problems in his private life, volunteers as a visitor for a terminally ill patient in hospital; the two may have a positive relation, which they both see as meaningful. Nevertheless both face serious problems in their respective lives, each one in a different way.

The latter example could happen in palliative care. But there are many other ways in which people connect positively to broader life: relations, projects, responsibilities big and small, special objects, rituals, non-sectarian religion or philosophy. Beauty deserves special attention here. Experienced alone, or shared with others who can appreciate the same beauty, it can be a powerful means of discovering meaning, and yet relatively simple to put into practice. The underlying reason is perhaps that beauty is a strong affirmation of value even in the absence of utility, and even when life becomes fragile.

All these suggestions open up possibilities for the exploration of meaning in a person's life, while avoiding manipulation. In that hypothesis the discovery of meaning is the result of a balance between active inquiry and letting life come. Meaning is not a pure construct, it has to be discovered.

Sects are an example of how the search for meaning can be perverted. They give a false security by not respecting the freedom of conscience and they can easily turn against life itself and become destructive. Yet their promise of security can make them attractive to vulnerable people.

We can now clarify a specific strength of constructive humour that is often overlooked. To the extent humour makes us see a positive point in life, where we had seen problems only, it also establishes a positive connection between us and broader life surrounding us. In that sense constructive humour reveals meaning, in a modest way in comparison with philosophical discussion, and often unintentionally, but no less true, close to life, precisely when things go wrong.

Rituals are often a codified 'hold' offered by a group, a community or society in order to sustain life in a challenging situation, such as entering life, entering adult life, commitment to a partner, commitment to a vocation, forgiveness, sickness, and death. In the last case it helps the survivors to say farewell to the deceased and get on with life. Positive rituals hold life and encourage people in a moment of great fragility (Warner 1997). Negative rituals will sustain people in their aggression against life. It follows that positive rituals can play an important pacifying role in palliative care, both for the patients and their surroundings, probably including some staff. But rituals need to remain convincing for the people involved.

This extends to bedtime rituals (Warner 1997), because falling asleep is a moment of great vulnerability and abandonment (Ekirch 2001), even for the strongest person, and particularly towards the end of life when there is a higher probability of a person not surviving until the next morning. Bedtime rituals are widespread, also with healthy people, in a great variety of forms, such as prayer, a moment of silence, listening to a favourite and pacifying piece of music, reading or listening to a story, all sorts of drinks, from a glass of milk to a whisky. They are easily accessible and understood. But bedtime rituals need to be well adapted to the person concerned, as they are very intimate and touch directly upon our vulnerability.

Meaning in palliative care: the transformation of hope

The ultimate positive connection to life is the belief that life is basically good, has a positive core, in spite of all problems, traumas, death, and grief. In other words: the belief that, after all, we can expect something positive from life. This can be expressed in many ways, for example poetry, as in Bonhoeffer's poem 'Von guten Mächten' (Bonhoeffer 1990). Some people call such a positive core at the heart of life 'God'.

Yet in palliative care this approach to meaning seems to be based on a contradiction: death is a major disconnection from life. How is it possible to expect something positive from life in the face of death? Such questions are relevant for all involved, not just the patient.

In order to search for an answer it is useful to see how the human and spiritual reality of hope can be transformed in palliative care. In fact, what the word 'hope' stands for may change completely in a matter of months, weeks, days, or even hours, while we keep using the same word. This can easily lead to confusion between different people involved in palliative care. It is important to be aware of such potential confusion.

With a view to the future, the positive commitment to life can change, at least in principle, from 'fighting for life' to 'letting go' or even a peaceful farewell and departure.

In that sense the very nature of hope changes (Chochinov 2006; Raffin *et al.* 2006). There can be a shift from hope based on the expectation of obtaining a desired result, such as restoration of health, to hope based on confidence in a future which, in principle, is unknown. The latter can be filled out in different

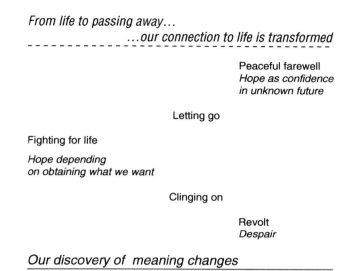

From life to passing away…
*   …our connection to life is transformed*

Peaceful farewell
Hope as confidence
in unknown future

Letting go

Fighting for life

Hope depending
on obtaining what we want

Clinging on

Revolt
Despair

Our discovery of meaning changes

Figure 7.2 (Stefan Vanistendael, BICE, Geneva, 2005).

ways, according to the beliefs of the person concerned: a good afterlife, mere trust, absence of worries and pain, meeting beloved ones who passed away earlier, meeting God, or just a peaceful farewell. It is important to understand that such a transformation of hope is not the same as giving up hope. This new form of hope is in a sense purer, perhaps less vulnerable, because less instrumental, less dependent on control, success, and achievement as we normally understand it. Ideally this gradual transformation of hope can be an expression of the desire for a fulfilled life, of which the farewell is an integral part. Such farewell is very different from a process of losing one battle after another or from merely letting life slip away. This is a specific form of the 'realistic hope' mentioned before and so typical of the resilience processes.

The process of transformation of hope can also be perverted, at least in two ways:

- whatever reality there would be after death is perceived as terrifying, for example as a severe punishment
- the nature of hope does not change, and the fight for recovering health shifts increasingly to clinging on, revolt, bitterness, despair—as reality catches up with false hope.

Spiritual accompaniment can try to help with the positive transformation of hope, but with no guarantee of success.

The patient and a variety of people connected to him or her may all go through such processes but not necessarily in a synchronized way. The patient, family, friends, the professional staff, and the volunteers may all have to deal with such transformation of hope, or the lack of it, in different ways and with different intensities. At any given time they may be at different stages of that process.

Transformation of hope as a way of not losing meaning is closely related to a distinction easily overlooked in a performance-driven society and yet essential for many situations in palliative care, not the least for the staff: success and meaning are to be distinguished. We easily confuse success and meaning. What is successful appears to be meaningful; failure looks meaningless. When confronted with the limits of medicine, with severe disability or with death, such identification of success and meaning can be most disturbing. But although the two often coincide, they do not overlap each other entirely. Certain actions can be 'successful' but with questionable meaning, such as murder. Certain activities are not successful in a narrow sense, but most meaningful. For example, if a suicidal person is well cared for but finally commits suicide, we cannot automatically conclude that the care has been without meaning. For as long as it goes, such care may have established a constructive connection to life, and in that sense meaning, even in a way that would not have been possible otherwise.

Some particular opportunities for spiritual growth in palliative care

The transformation of hope leads us to the opportunities for growth in palliative care. This can be a field full of life's paradoxes. Generally speaking it may appear as a newly gained intimacy and dignity, such as:

◆ a new openness to what is felt to be really important in life

◆ a new awareness of and perspective on vulnerability

◆ forgiveness and its positive mirror-concept of gratitude.

The first point is probably a relatively common experience, although by no means universal: a patient who knows the end is near and who may gain a new perspective on what really matters in life, or at least question what was considered important before. This is an opportunity for growth, not just for the patient, but possibly also for family and friends, sometimes even for staff and volunteers. How this is accompanied will vary according to the situation. Attentive listening, with the occasional question to sustain the process of searching for new perspectives, will probably be more important than long discussions. In principle, all caregivers or relations involved can have a smaller or bigger part in it. In a sense, the patient supports the careful listener inasmuch as the listener supports the patient, because both may be facing together some fundamental questions about life and death. The risk is that such questioning may end in despair, particularly when a person feels life has been wasted in the light of what is considered important in the face of death.

The care of the sick and particularly the end of life confront everybody involved, even the staff, in a radical way with each person's fundamental limits and vulnerability (de Hennezel 2004). Vulnerability is usually not considered to be positive. Yet, at the heart of a really intimate and profound relationship we often find vulnerability rather than performance or success: two people go beyond mutual admiration or given roles, they recognize each other's vulnerability and limits, and they respect that. Sometimes people may be aware of such a subtle balance in a relation. Vulnerability can in that sense become a real test of acceptance: does the other accept me as I am, even when things do not go well, when my limits become so visible? It is then that we have to make a real decision to choose for the other, beyond natural sympathies or mechanical reactions.

At first sight this may seem obvious for the medical staff accepting the sick patient. Yet not the least a vulnerable patient may be very sensitive to the way in which a medical intervention is carried out, with great care and attention for the patient or not. But particularly in palliative care the acceptance of limits and vulnerability also goes the other way. Gradually the patient will be challenged to accept the limits of the medical and other staff, directly as related to his or her deteriorating condition, but also indirectly because of staff tiredness and even irritation caused by the stress of working under extreme conditions. To the extent people are capable of such acceptance, it can have a profound and humanizing influence for all involved. Such mutual acceptance of respective limits and vulnerability is neither an invitation to sloppiness nor a justification of sagging standards, but an ultimate reaction of our humanity when life challenges us where it hurts most. If it succeeds, it is a powerful way of reconnecting to life and to each other, of re-establishing meaning, in the face of life's fragility.

This is a specific application of how suffering and sickness can also become a moment of growth. The hospice movement has contributed to the awareness of such potential (Vranckx 1993). This does not play down pain, illness, and death, because it is not the suffering as such that makes people grow as what people make of suffering (Jollien 2002).

Finally there may be special opportunities for the discovery of meaning opening up through forgiveness. In order to see the connection between forgiveness and meaning, it is helpful to specify what forgiveness is not:

- forgiveness is not denial, because in that case there would be nothing to forgive; it is based on the clear recognition that something evil and hurtful was done;

- in the same sense it is not playing down evil, neither explaining it away and even less so justifying it; explanations about why the bad happened may be useful and can help us draw lessons for the future, but they are no justification;
- forgiveness is not forgetting what has happened;
- it is not necessarily switching to good feelings towards the person that has perpetrated something bad, neither spontaneously nor by a forceful act of will;
- it is not identical with the healing of hurt feelings; such healing may accompany the process of forgiveness or be a consequence of it; it may take a much longer time than forgiveness, or even turn out to be impossible within a lifetime.

Forgiveness recognizes that life has been badly hurt, and that this has damaged or even broken some relations; some lives have been disconnected from each other and in that sense there is loss of meaning. Forgiveness takes one step forward beyond such recognition and gives expression to the will to reconnect with life by granting the perpetrator of something bad that reconnection. It can be as much a liberation for the person forgiving, as for the person being forgiven. Ultimately forgiveness is an act of will, inspired by an intelligence of life. Feelings may follow or may not follow. In some cases forgiveness will be a long process, rather than a single act.

In extreme cases where the perpetrator does not recognize the evil done, forgiveness can even be unilateral. But in such case reconciliation is not possible, because the latter requires a two-way process. Forgiveness is necessary but not sufficient for reconciliation; reconciliation is not necessary for forgiveness (Lecomte 2004). This nuance can be important in extreme situations towards the end of life.

In the interpretation of meaning as presented here, forgiveness is a powerful means of reconnecting to life and hence of searching for meaning where life was terribly hurt.

From a resilience perspective forgiveness plays on several important elements at once: the acceptance of the person to be forgiven, the rediscovery of meaning for both the person forgiving and the person to be forgiven, and in doing so it may also contribute to the self-esteem of both.

It may also be helpful, particularly towards the end of life, to remember with gratitude good things experienced in life. This is somehow the positive mirror image of forgiveness, including the good received as well as the good done, in the hope that this may contribute to a sense of peace and fulfilment. This must be balanced, however, against some risks:

- it may increase the pain of the farewell
- it may increase the sense of meaninglessness, to the extent that not the positive connections with life prevail but the loss of opportunities.

Final reflections: exploring life beyond strict utility

First, palliative care invites us to explore the areas of life that lie between strict utility, as defined by ordinary standards in society, and the ultimate limits of life. Such exploration is only possible if:

1. we recognize that there can be great value in what is not useful;
2. we can fully recognize that life is limited and vulnerable, not only as a general principle but also for everyone, including caregivers, and ourselves.

Both points are coherent with life and death in a very inclusive way, with no shortcuts. They are coherent with the idea of the physically disabled Swiss philosopher, Alexandre Jollien, that it is not worth desiring to control everything because one would lose what is essential (Jollien 2002). In the end it also implies that we accept a sense of failure as a part of life, not to be looked for, but unavoidable and not robbing life from all meaning. Such ideas are at the heart of the dynamics of resilience and of spiritual growth, but they may be uneasy and go against many mainstream opinions in modern Western society.

In her action for the dying poor in India Mother Theresa of Calcutta gave witness of such convictions in a very different culture. Many people across various cultures, countries, and beliefs recognized the greatness of such commitment, but some criticized her work as a waste of resources. However, one can take this respect for the dying even further. The most extreme example the author has come across is a person who attends funerals of people unknown to her, where she knows that nobody will be present, except the obligatory representative of public authority. The reason is that she can simply not accept that somebody's parting from existence is not acknowledged by another human being, beyond pure administrative obligations, and independently of who that person was or what the person did (Lennon 2002).

Second, the challenge of palliative care is to set a sustainable framework that will make a dignified life possible, for the patient and the relatives. This does not imply that everything can or must be planned in detail. Even if such careful planning is necessary for certain sectors of care, it requires an openness that allows positive things to happen, that is attentive to unexpected possibilities for growth, so that positive surprises are not lost in all the suffering and planning for care.

Such a framework must also give ample space to family, friends, relations, or volunteers, because of their closeness to the patient, in a very different way from the professional caregivers. The former have in principle a great potential to contribute to the human and spiritual well-being of the patient, which is truly complementary to professional care.

Such a framework must help all involved, even the medical staff, to help preserve human dignity when life is slipping away. In the end this implies that it must be possible to 'wake', i.e. to be present with great attention, even silently, when nothing can be done.

Third, the exploration of life beyond utilitarian criteria, so fundamental to palliative care, refers us to some other people in society who are in different ways much involved in a similar exploration without being involved in palliative care. Is it too much to say that this exploration creates a sort of unofficial complicity with the contemplatives, men and women, with the artists, the clowns and the little children? The contemplatives because they withdraw from ordinary active life, in order to be more attentively present to life in greater depth, an apparent waste. The artists, because they explore so often life beyond narrow utility, in beauty but also in the expression of immense suffering. The clowns, because they often acknowledge the limits and the tragedy of life, while clearly signalling that life cannot be reduced to its tragedy. Is it a coincidence that they have become active in hospitals? But also the little children, because they have such an uninhibited capacity for exploration of every bit and shred of life, even what the adult sees as unimportant or useless. Would it be possible to find a practical articulation of such complicity between those explorers of life and some or all people involved in palliative care?

Fourth, the same exploration beyond strict utility invites us to keep wondering about three more questions: What is health? What is a fulfilled life? Which leads to the question: What is a human person?

Such questions are perhaps more important as ongoing questions than for the provisional answers they may inspire. The experience of palliative care suggests looking for answers that move us away from strict human perfectionism. Does the greatness of a civilization show—at least to some extent—in its capacity to appreciate vulnerability as an integral part of life?

References

Armstrong K (1993) *A History of God*, pp. 432–457. London: Mandarin.

Bariaud F (1995) Les premiers pas. In: *L'humour. Un état d'esprit*, pp. 39–50 (ed. Cahen G). Autrement, Série Mutations nr 131. Paris.

Benard B (1991) *Fostering Resiliency in Kids: Protective Factors in Family, School, and Community*, pp. 3–20. Portland: Northwest Regional Educational Laboratory.

Bonhoeffer D (1990) *Widerstand und Ergebung*, p. 219. Munich: Kaiser.

Brissiaud P-Y (2001) *Surmonter ses blessures. De la maltraitance à la résilience*, pp. 127–129. Paris: Retz.

Broers A (2005) *Als een huis. Resilience op de basisschool*, pp. 7–12. Bergen op zoom: Akros.

Büchi S, Baumann-Hölzle R (2005) Den Sinn des Leidens ergründen. Fragen zum Gesundheitsverständnis und zu den Zielen der modernen Medizin. *Neue Zürcher Zeitung*, nr 271, 19–20 November, 75.

Chochinov HM (2006) Dying, dignity, and new horizons in palliative end-of-life care. *CA cancer Journal for Clinicians* **56**, 84–103.

Cyrulnik B (1999) *Un merveilleux Malheur*, pp. 10–15. Paris: Odile Jacob.

Echard B (2006) *Souffrance spirituelle du patient en fin de vie. La question dus ses*, pp. 41–62. Ramonville Saint-Agne: Eres.

Ekirch AR (2001) Sleep we have lost: pre-industrial slumber in the British isles. *The American Historical Review* **106**(2), 343–386.

Escarpit R (1981) *L'humour*, p. 72. Series 'Que sais-je?'. Paris: PUF.

Fozzard S (2002) *Surviving Violence. A recovery programme for children and families*, pp. 6–7. Geneva: Bice (International Catholic Child Bureau).

Frankl VE (1963) *Man's Search for Meaning*, pp. 171–176. New York: Simon and Schuster.

Frankl VE (1982) *Der Wille zum Sinn*, pp. 27–34. Bern: Hans Huber.

Fuchs E (2001) L'éthique et la résilience ont-elles partie liée? In: *La résilience: résister et se construire*, pp. 225–227 (ed. Manciaux M). Geneva: Médecine et hygiène.

Gilligan R (2005) Promoting positive outcomes for children in need. In: *The Child's World. Assessing children in need*, pp. 180–193 (ed. Horwath J). London: Jessica Kingsley.

Goldstein S, Brooks R (2001) *Raising Resilient Children*, pp. 295–302. Chicago: Contemporary Books.

Hanus M (2001) *La resilience à quell prix? Survivre et rebondir*, pp. 49–72. Paris: Maloine.

de Hennezel M (2004) *Le souci de l'autre*, pp. 80–94. Paris: Robert Laffont.

Jollien A (2002) *Le métier d'homme*, pp. 26–53. Paris: Seuil.

Koenig MD, Harold G, Cohen AB (2002) Spirituality in palliative care. *Geriatric Times* **3**, www.geriatrictimes.com/g021225.html, consulted on 4 January 2006.

Lecomte J (2002) Qu'est-ce que la résilience ? Question faussement simple. Réponse nécessairement complexe. *Pratiques Psychologiques* **1**, 7–14.

Lecomte J (2004) *Guérir de son enfance*, pp. 82–191. Paris: Odile Jacob.

Lennon P (2002) Friend of the dead. *Guardian weekly*, 27 June–3 July, 21.

Manciaux M (1998) La résilience: mythe ou réalité ? In: *Ces enfants qui tiennent le coup*, pp. 109–120 (ed. Cyrulnik B). Revigny-sur-Orain: Hommes & Perspectives.

Manciaux M (2001) Conclusions et perspectives. In: Fondation pour l'enfance, ed. *La résilience: le réalisme de l'espérance*, pp. 305–315. Ramonville Saint-Agne: Eres.

Manciaux M (2003) La résilience: réalité de vie. *L'enfance majuscule* September-December, 6–9.

Nussenbaum D (1995) L'envers de l'angoisse. In: *L'humour. Un état d'esprit*, pp. 33–35 (ed. Cahen G). Autrment, Série Mutations nr 131, Paris.

Opp G, Fingerle M, Freytag A (1999) Erziehung zwischen Risiko und Resilienz: Neue Perspektiven für die heilpädagogische Forschung und Praxis. In: *Was Kinder stärkt. Erziehung zwischen Risiko und Resilienz*, pp. 9–21 (eds Opp G, Fingerle M, Freytag A). Munich: Reinhardt.

Poletti R, Dobbs B (2001) *La resilience*, p. 80. St Julien-en-Genevois: Jouvence.

Raffin S, Sinclair S, Pereira J (2006) A thematic review of spirituality literature within palliative care. *Journal of Palliative Medicine* **9**(2), 464–479.

Rutter M (1993) Resilience: some conceptual considerations. *Journal of Adolescent Health*, **14**(8), 626–631.

Rutter M (1994) Stress research: Accomplishments and tasks ahead. In: *Stress, Risk and Resilience in Children and Adolescents*, pp. 354–385 (eds Haggerty R, Sherrod L, Garmezy N, Rutter M). Cambridge: Cambridge University Press.

Schreiner J (2003) *Humor bei Kindern und Jugendlichen*, pp. 199–207. Berlin: Verlag für Wissenschaft und Bildung.

Schweizer D, Vanistendael S, Lecomte J, Manciaux M (2001) Conclusions et perspectives. In: *La résilience: résister et se construire*, pp. 214–253 (ed. Manciaux M). Geneva: Médecine et hygiène.

Silva Pañez AG (1997) *Psychische Widerstandsfähigkeit von Kindern, die politisch-motivierte Gewalt ausgesetzt waren*, pp. 15–16. Zürich: Phd university of Zürich, Zentralstelle der Studentenschaft.

Soebstad F (1995) *Humor i pedagogisk arbeid*, p. 106. Otta: Tano.

Suárez Ojeda EN (2002) Una concepción latinoamericana: la resiliencia comunitaria. In: *Resiliencia. Descubriendo las propias fortalezas*, pp. 67–82 (eds Melillo A, Suárez Ojeda EN). Buenos Aires: Paidós.

Svebak S (1987) Humor og helse: et perspektiv paa mestring av stress. In: Senter for barneforskning, ed. *Barn og humor*, pp. 206–227. Trondheim: NAVF's Senter for barneforskning, Universitet Trondheim.

Theis A (2001) La résilience dans la littérature scientifique. In: *La résilience: résister et se construire*, pp. 33–44 (ed. Manciaux M). Geneva: Médecine et Hygiène.

Theis A (2006) *Approche psychodynamique de la résilience. Etude clinique projective comparée d'enfants ayant été victimes de maltraitance familiale et placés en famille d'accueil*, pp. 14–42. Nancy: Phd university of Nancy.

Titus CS (2002) *Resilience and Christian Virtues. What the psychosocial sciences offer for the renewal of Thomas Aquinas' moral theology of fortitude and its related virtues*, pp. 11–22. Fribourg, Switzerland: Phd university of Fribourg.

Vanistendael S (1998) *Growth in the Muddle of Life*, p. 9. Geneva: International Catholic Child Bureau.

Vanistendael S (2001) La résilience au quotidien. In: *La résilience: résister et se construire*, pp. 179–187 (ed. Manciaux M). Geneva: Médecine et hygiène.

Vanistendael S (2002) *Résilience et spiritualité*, p. 10. Geneva: Bice.

Vanistendael S (2003) Humour et résilience: le sourire qui fait vivre. In: *Impasses, ratages, échecs. Sources de créativité pour les pratiques systémiques et travail social*, pp. 75–99 (eds Julier CR, Amiguet O). Geneva: IES.

Vanistendael S, Lecomte J (2000) *Le Bonheur est toujours possible. Construire la résilience*, pp. 205–212. Paris: Bayard.

Vanistendael S, Lecomte J (2003) Découvrir et créer du sens. Une composante essentielle du processus de résilience. *Enfance majuscule*, September–December, 14–17.

Vinant P (2006) Soins palliatifs: quelle autonomie pour le patient? *Laennec* **54**, 39–58.

Vögeli D (2005) Sinn suchen, Sinn geben im Pflegeheim. Das Diakoniewerk Neumünster erprobt Instrumentarium. *Neue Zürcher Zeitung*, nr 286, 7 December, 57.

Vranckx J (1993) *De zinzoekers*, pp. 78–84. Leuven: Davidsfonds.

Warner J (1997) Bedtime rituals of nursing home residents: a study. *Nursing Standard* **11**, 34–38.

Watson M, Lucas C, Hoy A, Back I (2005) *Oxford Handbook of Palliative Care*, pp. 625–629. Oxford: Oxford University Press.

Werner E (1989) Children of the garden island. *Scientific American* **260**, 76–81.

Werner EE, Smith RS (1992) *Overcoming the Odds. High risk children from birth to adulthood*, pp. 189–209. Ithaca, NY: Cornell University Press.

Wortman CB, Tweed R, Sonnega J *et al.* (2000) Resilience to loss and chronic grief: a prospective study from preloss to 18-months postloss. *Journal of Personality and Social Psychology* **83**, 1150–1164.

Zentrum für Gerontologie ZfG (2006) *Spiritualität in der stationären Alterspflege*. Website university Zürich, www.zfg.unizh.ch/projekt/spirit_de.print.html, 8 August.

8

Resilience and rehabilitation

Adrian Tookman

This chapter is written for 'Ray Ray'—extraordinarily resilient and a very special man.

Introduction

Over the last 25 years there have been significant changes in cancer care that have been poorly recognized. Prolonged, increasingly effective, multimodality treatments for cancer are now commonplace and these have led to increasing numbers of cancer survivors who live with cancer. These treatments are often arduous and the survivors are often disabled and in need of physical and emotional support. I have been part of a team that has had a particular interest in this cohort of patients; supporting them through their life-threatening illness and its consequences. Despite over 20 years of experience in this area I have never been able to understand fully how an individual develops the resilience to cope with what must be one of the greatest challenges of their life.

There is also a challenge for palliative care professionals to recognize that there have been significant changes in cancer care and to develop services that can respond to this population of patients and their increasing needs. This may be uncomfortable for some, as it requires a paradigm shift. Palliative care should now actively engage and respond to this growing diversity of need and be resilient enough to care for all patients with advanced progressive illness; no longer can we 'cherry pick' patients who are 'easy' to look after. In the past we have adopted a professional stance that all too often criticizes our colleagues stating that, in some situations, they do not treat patients adequately and humanely. We must recognize that we are now an established and integral part of healthcare and we must engage as such. Palliative care specialists in the statutory and voluntary sector have a responsibility to be a part of their local healthcare environment and demonstrate that they recognize these changing needs and wish to respond to them. This will require a fresh look at the patient population and the development of an approach to service delivery that is proactive rather than reactive. A rehabilitative approach to care will allow us to do this. If palliative care fails to respond to the challenges of modern healthcare there is a real risk of a loss of status and, once again, acquiring the label of being a 'Cinderella specialty'.

Rehabilitation and palliative care may seem to be a contradiction in terms (Tookman 2004), but it can be a practical approach to management that is appropriate for patients with complex, progressive illness. By adopting a rehabilitative approach to care people can reach their maximum capacity, realize their true potential and grow and develop when faced with a difficult situation. The approach can be applied at any stage of the illness—at its core is goal setting.

Rehabilitation in palliative care is different to rehabilitation in general medical care (Nocon and Baldwin 1998). In general medical care rehabilitation is often for a disability that has occurred at one point in time. The aim is to achieve the patient's maximum potential in the hope that further deterioration is unlikely. In palliative care, patients are not only disabled but also have progressive illness (or the threat of progressive illness): consequently a mix of skills is necessary that combines both rehabilitative and palliative expertise. Customarily rehabilitation is the domain of the physiotherapist and the occupational therapist. However, in palliative care it is crucial to engage the whole team to address the multiple needs of patients with advanced, complex, and progressive illness.

Specialist palliative care and hospice care have traditionally been focused on end stage disease, enabling individuals to 'come to terms' with their circumstances. However, there is now a population of patients referred to specialists in palliative care who, because of the trajectory of their illness, have prolonged survival and different requirements for their care. As a consequence this 'passive approach' must now be reviewed. It is important to recognize that some patients now survive with cancer for long periods of time and there are growing numbers of referrals to palliative care of people with progressive non-cancer conditions. Enlightened services now adopt a proactive approach to care that enables patients to manage the concurrent physical and emotional difficulties associated with these progressive illness.

All patients with cancer who are referred to specialist palliative care face a life-threatening illness. This is a huge emotional burden. Dealing with uncertainty is difficult enough, but when one considers the additional physical assault that comes with complicated and often demanding cancer treatments, it is not surprising that patients feel traumatized by their cancer and its management. The need for support and rehabilitation during and after treatment is well recognized (Calman and Hine 1995; Department of Health 2004). However, the resources available to do this are, at best, limited. Therefore a rehabilitative approach to cancer care can be applied at all stages in the illness and the following patients are appropriate:

- **Patients who have undergone treatment and may be cured**: need a range of psychological and physical therapies to enable them to recover, re-socialize and adapt to any disability that may be present. The object is to enable patients to live as normal a life as possible. Setting time frames for recovery is important and the aim is usually a relatively limited intervention.

- **Patients who have had treatment, are in remission and are not cured**: these patients may have disability. They are living with great uncertainty and need help to manage this. They have often had arduous treatments and when their disease recurs can feel disappointed, angry and cheated that the treatment has not worked. They need the full range of rehabilitative resources to reframe their life and maximize their potential.

- **Patients with progressive disease**: often these patients have had multiple courses of treatment and feel defeated by their cancer. They have complex physical and emotional problems and can feel cheated of a healthy future and resentful that things did not progress as anticipated. These patients have a disease trajectory that is often characterized by gradual decline and progressive frailty. As care transfers more into a palliative setting patients can feel abandoned by their oncology teams. Frail patients often 'fail to thrive' and need support from a full range of rehabilitative therapies. Despite frailty much can be done to maximize potential, optimize symptom control and reassure patients that they can have control of their future and will be supported.

- **Patients who are close to death**: ease and solace goals, giving patients a sense of control and negotiating care are important. These goals can be achieved by a rehabilitative approach to care, even at this stage of the illness.

Rehabilitation and the dilemma of diversity

There are changes in the demographics of patients with progressive illnesses. In addition, there are changes in referral patterns to palliative care with earlier referrals, referrals for rehabilitation and for non-cancer conditions. Palliative care is no longer limited to caring for patients solely in the terminal phase of their illness. The dilemma of diversification is real. The best use of specialist palliative care resources is a challenge that clinicians have had to face in the past; it remains an even greater challenge for the future. The changing patient population has greater need for palliative care. This and the growing acceptance that palliative care is now an integral part of medicine, should encourage us to develop strategies that meet the requirements of all patients with palliative care needs. Rehabilitation is one area of care where we must establish our role, define our patient population and empower other teams to assess the rehabilitative needs of patients with advanced illness to ensure appropriate referrals are made.

The changing demographics of cancer patients

As stated previously there are gradual, poorly recognized, changes in the cancer population. People now live for much longer periods of their life with cancer (Scottish Executive 2006). Issues related to survivorship are of growing importance. The reasons for improvement in survival are multifactorial. Cancers can be diagnosed earlier and treatments have undoubtedly improved prognoses. However, the impact of sophisticated imaging techniques cannot be underestimated. The result of improved imaging has led to earlier recognition of progressive and metastatic disease with resultant earlier interventions with more effective cancer treatments. This has resulted in patients who require multiple courses of multimodality therapies, which can be disabling and certainly demanding both emotionally and physically. For many, cancer has undergone a transformation from an acute to a chronic illness (Tritter and Calnan 2002), which has significant implications for designing services. The support of people who are living with cancer and the resultant disabilities requires a fresh approach and new skills; the rehabilitative framework is ideally suitable.

Non-cancer: similarities with cancer

Cancer patients and patients with progressive non-cancer conditions have similar prognoses (Cancer Survival England and Wales 1991–2001; Vestbo *et al.* 1998; Stewart *et al.* 2001) and a similar burden of symptoms (Solano *et al.* 2006). Consequently a rehabilitative approach to the palliative management of patients with progressive non-cancer conditions is entirely appropriate. However, it cannot be assumed that specialist palliative care can meet all the needs of all patients with malignant and non-malignant disease (National Council for Palliative Care 1998). It is therefore vital to ensure that involvement is appropriate to the stage, symptom burden and trajectory of the illness (Lynn and Adamson 2003).

The trajectory of illness for cancer used to be a period of good health followed by a rapid decline (Figure 8.1). This is different to some non-cancer conditions, for example, Chronic Obstructive Pulmonary Disease and Chronic Heart Failure where there is a gradual decline punctuated by periods of extreme poor health from which recovery often takes place. Ultimately patients die, usually during one of these episodes of decline. Overall the prognosis is poor,

A Good Health & Rapid Decline

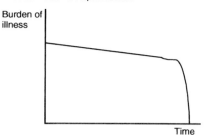

B Gradual Decline with periods of ill health

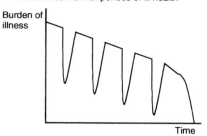

C Gradual Decline with periods of ill health

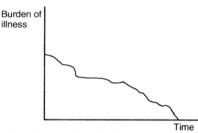

Trajectory	Examples	Rehabilitative interventions	Model of working
Period of relatively good health followed by a rapid decline **A**	Cancer of the lung Many cancers treated in the past Renal failure	Needs brief interventions at beginning and during illness and a large resource during decline	Shared model of care with oncologists (& renal physicians) at beginning of illness
Gradual decline with periods of ill health **B**	Chronic Obstructive Pulmonary Disease Chronic Heart Failure	Needs intermittent rehabilitation throughout illness, especially following acute episodes of illness	Shared model of care with specialist teams (c.f. cancer model) during acute episode
Gradual decline and frailty **C**	Many chronic illnesses and some cancers. Body has limited reserves and in the terminal phase can become rapidly overwhelmed	Needs constant support throughout illness	Palliative approach important with specialist palliative care for complex symptom control

Figure 8.1

but an accurate prediction for an individual patient is extremely difficult. The other and increasingly common trajectory is gradual decline and frailty. This is seen in many chronic conditions and is now the common course for many patients with cancer. Clearly there is much overlap in these trajectories but by understanding them one can design rehabilitative services that are fit for purpose and make the best use of limited resources.

Services must also be developed that allow patients with complex needs to access the support and expertise they rightly require. The model of care that has been developed in cancer, where patients receive oncology expertise from medical and clinical oncology teams in parallel with palliative care, has been highly effective in achieving this in patients with cancer. Similar models of shared care must be developed in non-cancer.

Rehabilitation: levels of intervention

Rehabilitation is an approach to care that can be provided by all professional groups and in all settings. There is a view that rehabilitation is the domain of the physiotherapist and occupational therapist and this is largely supported by National Institute of Clinical Excellence (NICE) Guidance, *Improving Supportive and Palliative Care for Adults with Cancer* (Department of Health 2004). The role of the allied healthcare professionals is of great importance but to deny patients full and ongoing access to the integrated multiprofessional team ignores the attention to detail that is needed to give optimal care to patients with complex needs (Richardson and Tookman 2004). However, the key to delivering rehabilitation is to recognize that there is a need. The NICE guidance recommends four levels of assessment and support and this provides us with a helpful framework. Although the guidance is directed at cancer patients the approach is also applicable for patients with non-cancer conditions.

- ◆ **Level 1:** a rehabilitative approach by all healthcare professionals should be delivered by generalists in all settings (home and hospital). This requires an assessment of rehabilitative needs by all professionals. To ensure that generalists can assess need there has to be local education to raise awareness of the place of rehabilitation and adequate resources must be available to deliver this level of care. The specialist palliative care team will have an important role in education and empowering Primary Care teams and teams in Acute Trusts.

- ◆ **Level 2:** specific generalist interventions for specific common problems and impairments during cancer treatment. An example is postoperative physiotherapy following breast surgery. There should be care pathways and protocols for specific common rehabilitation problems. These interventions are usually delivered in an inpatient environment, commonly post-surgery.

◆ **Level 3:** these are specialized interventions by professionals with extensive experience, training, and education who have worked extensively with cancer patients. This will adopt particular importance in a cancer center, e.g. management of mild, uncomplicated lymphoedema.

◆ **Level 4:** highly specialized interventions by advanced practitioners. This needs a fully integrated multiprofessional approach to holistically manage the complex needs of patients, e.g. patients who have had complex surgical procedures. Palliative care patients often have complex needs and may benefit from a level 4 rehabilitative approach to their management. This will need involvement of a fully integrated, well functioning, informed multidisciplinary team and this approach is most likely to be developed in a hospice setting when there are close links with a cancer centre/unit. There is a description of one such unit below.

Comment on NICE guidance

NICE provides a practical framework to understand the different levels of rehabilitation that are needed to support patients with cancer. Survivorship is an issue that will adopt greater importance in healthcare in the future and will need an approach that embraces all of the skills of the multiprofessional team. In addition to the allied healthcare professional involvement, the role of clinical nurse specialists, physicians, and the psychosocial team in rehabilitation is fundamental to safe, effective, and high-quality care. Structures will need to be developed that ensure all skills are integrated. There are few examples of effective integrated multidisciplinary teamwork in the NICE guidance.

The success of integrated multiprofessional care is hard to measure. There are a range of assessment tools for function and daily living that have been used for specific conditions and by different disciplines (Turner-Stokes 2000). These are generally unhelpful for measuring the outcome of a multiprofessional approach to rehabilitation. However, as no meaningful measurement is available it does not follow that the approach is ineffective. The rehabilitative approach is a complex intervention and should be assessed as such. The trap into which many outcome measures fall is to try and break down complex interventions into their simple component parts and assess each part individually. A complex intervention is not the sum of its parts (Hawe *et al.* 2004). Reducing a complex system to its component parts amounts to 'irretrievable loss of what makes it a system' (Casti 1997). The challenge is to develop and refine this premise so that a highly complex intervention, such as rehabilitation, can be meaningfully assessed.

A level 4 rehabilitation unit in palliative care

At present there are few hospices who have committed significant resource to rehabilitation in either an inpatient or outpatient setting. The model described below is an example of an initiative that has grown over a 15-year period. It was developed within the voluntary sector to respond to a recognized and growing unmet need – often the catalyst for new initiatives. It is interesting to reflect on the development of such a unit, as unmet needs are often recognized by clinicians but they are rarely responded to. The reasons for its growth and success are:

- Senior physician with an interest (Clinical Champion)
- Proximity of cancer centre to Hospice and shared posts with local oncology unit = geographical convenience and shared knowledge (House of Commons Health Committee Report: Palliative Care Fourth Report of Session 2004)
- Recognition of unmet need and enthusiasm to respond. The unmet needs include:
  - recognition of limitations of current services in both statutory and voluntary sectors to support all patients with cancer holistically;
  - growing population of cancer survivors and an inability of the daycare provision to provide a responsive service that meets the needs of these patients;
  - no rehabilitation facility in the NHS—there is an understandable focus in oncology practices on timing and delivery of highly complex multimodality therapies.
- Lack of clarity about which discipline is 'responsible' for delivering the supportive care agenda (including rehabilitation): site-specific clinical nurse specialists, allied healthcare professionals, and specialist palliative care are some of the key stakeholders.
- 'Sign up' by staff.
- 'Sign up' by organization.
- A desire to change the model of daycare from a social/medical model to a therapeutic model.
- Early successes as confirmed by:
  - acceptance of therapeutic model by other units;
  - success of nurse led outpatient clinics;
  - success of physiotherapy, in particular the gym.
- Good feedback from patients.
- Good feedback from professional visitors and at national presentations.

The Day Therapy Unit (DTU) is led by nurses who are the point of contact for both patients and professionals. They have a fundamental role in communication: between patients and professionals; updating teams in the community and acute trusts about their patients; ensuring there is effective interprofessional communication. Referrals are initially triaged by the nursing staff for the first appointment. If the needs are assessed as symptom control then patients are initially seen in a medical clinic. If the needs appear to be predominantly nursing then they are referred to the nurse led clinic. All patients are ultimately seen in a medical clinic for reasons outlined later in this chapter.

The clinical nurse specialist:

- explores the impact of illness on the patient's physical, emotional/psychological and role function and the effects on family members/significant others
- assesses patient awareness of illness and disease progression
- prioritizes patient need
- facilitates goal setting
- discusses strategies to assist with achievement of goals
- assesses the appropriate time and pace of planned intervention
- monitors changes in (and responses to) interventions and treatments.

After the first appointment (medical or nursing) all new patients are discussed in the weekly multidisciplinary meeting (MDM) to determine their programme of care, to set goals and, most importantly, to be given a review date. This ensures that all patients are reviewed on a regular basis. The purpose of regular review is threefold: to acknowledge that the needs of patients change and to ensure the rehabilitation programme remains appropriate to the patients changing needs; to ensure inappropriate patients do not continue in the daycare unit long term; to discharge patients who have achieved their goals and completed their programme.

In addition to reviewing all new patients the weekly MDM allows the team to discuss individual patients who may have specific problems, assesses all patients who have reached their review date and also discusses all patients who have died.

The medical review

The palliative medicine physician plays a key role in the DTU. All patients are ultimately assessed in an outpatient clinic where they are seen by a physician together with one of the DTU nursing staff. There are understandable anxieties about this approach. 'Medicalizing' care can give status to physical symptoms and being unwell. This could potentially delay a patient's readjustment to their disabilities and return to a more 'normal' social environment. However, the benefits of an in-depth medical overview should not be underestimated. The initial consultation is an invaluable opportunity for a patient to give a biographic account of their care. It enables patients to recount their experiences. They are given permission (and time) to discuss anxieties about their diagnosis and treatment, very often for the first time. Uncertainties can be discussed and misperceptions can be corrected.

Furthermore, the medical consultation allows for confirmation of the diagnosis and ensures that all treatment options for symptom control have been fully explored. The assumption that every patient arrives in the DTU with the correct diagnosis and treatments (palliative or otherwise) is naïve and a view that could lead to unnecessary suffering. Good palliative care is underpinned by paying attention to detail (Richardson and Tookman 2004). This approach, when applied in the outpatient setting, will allow an accurate assessment of patients' complex problems and optimal symptom control. Paying attention to detail will often confirm the diagnosis but, in those patients with an incorrect 'label', it is an opportunity to correct it. An incorrect diagnosis is often perpetuated by successive clinicians; one of the consequences of this is inadequate symptom control.

Patients are referred to the unit for many reasons (Tookman 2004):

1. To enable patients to seek advice on pain, symptom control, and end of life issues

This is, perhaps, the traditional role of a hospice and remains an important part of the activities of the unit. The DTU is an excellent opportunity for patients to understand the role of a hospice and introduces the range of services provided by the unit. A rehabilitative approach can also be applied in these settings; however, there is much to commend an outpatient approach to this aspect of care. It enables patients to have exposure to the wider healthcare team and all the services of the unit in one visit. It provides a single point of contact with specialists and, if necessary, enables fast track admission to the inpatient unit. This area of care is often ignored by referring agencies and the clinic can be a safe environment to facilitate these discussions. The regular use of advance statements has been found to be particularly useful; they can act as a vehicle to explore issues that may be too threatening for patients to discuss directly. A rehabilitative approach is taken to these issues, setting realistic goals for symptom control, and an opportunity is provided to proactively explore and discuss end of life decisions.

Palliative care is also accessed outside the hospice—in the community and in the acute trust. This is an example of an 'ambulatory model of care'—an approach that is recommended by the Department of Health to facilitate access and the provision of high-quality of care. In addition, offering outpatient care in a day therapy setting is an economic way of delivering care. There is a considerable time saving when compared with community visiting. Patient preferences are paramount and some will express a desire to have all their treatment at home; however, many patients are happy to come to the DTU, indeed many see attending a healthcare setting as a positive, supportive and beneficial experience.

2. To access support during and following cancer treatments

There is a growing recognition that a patient need support during cancer treatments (both curative and palliative). There is also a growing realization in both the professional and lay press that cancer is, for many, a chronic illness.

In the past there has been some confusion whether specialist palliative care has a role with patients who are receiving active cancer management or not. There is now growing acceptance in the specialist palliative care community that cancer treatment has changed and many patients may be receiving palliative treatments (chemotherapy and/or radiotherapy) even though they may have very advanced disease. To deny these patients access to specialist palliative care would seem inequitable. Whatever view is taken there is little doubt that this group of patients have significant needs and many of these can be addressed in a rehabilitative setting. The DTU has many patients who are concurrently receiving chemotherapy, some of which may be with curative intent. They certainly have physical and emotional needs and benefit from a rehabilitative approach to their management. The DTU can support this group of patients in the outpatient medical and nursing clinics together with the physiotherapy and occupational therapy services and the psychosocial team. The complementary therapists and volunteer services are an essential part of the DTU team and these resources are often seen as a priority for some patients.

The shared care model between palliative care and oncology is well established and it is only by excellent, timely communication that this model can be successfully implemented. Patients often have specific concerns about their cancer therapies many of which need to be addressed by their oncologist. However, the specialist palliative care clinician can empower patients prior to their oncology outpatient appointments by helping them to ask the right questions in the right way. Another role for the palliative care clinician is to acknowledge that both the oncologist and patient often underestimate the time it takes for recovery following cancer treatment. The optimistic perception that recovery from chemotherapy starts immediately when treatment ends and is complete within a few months is unhelpful when realistic goals need to be set for rehabilitation. Setting time frames for recovery that are realistic is fundamental for patients who want to succeed with their rehabilitation programme, and it is the palliative care clinician who is often involved in this dialogue.

A specific area of interest in our unit is the use of exercise. We have espoused the benefits of exercise for some time and have developed a gym and a hydrotherapy pool to enable us to do this. We have gained enormous experience in this area and our exercise programme is one of the great successes of our rehabilitation programme. The benefits of exercising frail people have been well documented (Heath and Stuart 2002). There should be an expectation that there will be improvements in both function and levels of fatigue (Aminoff *et al.* 1996; Allman and Rice 2003). Certainly graduated and targeted exercise should enable an individual to maximize their potential. Exercise optimizes physical fitness and brings considerable emotional and social benefits. When faced with a life-threatening illness attending an exercise programme is seen as a positive approach to care; offering hope that there are real gains to be achieved. Patients need to be carefully assessed by the physician prior to entering the programme to ensure that no harm will be caused and to help the physiotherapy team design the best programme for the individual patient. Careful assessment, including radiographs, may be necessary if there is any anxiety that there is a risk of pathological fracture; however, this risk is largely overestimated. An individual who can carry out their daily activities without pain is unlikely to suffer a pathological fracture.

3. Longer-term disability (cancer)

Many patients now survive with their cancer. Some are in remission, which may be long term, and these patients live with the knowledge that the cancer will almost certainly return. Some patients manage this phase by denying the inevitable recurrence, hoping that they are cured. Others acknowledge the reality but have an ability to live with this, compartmentalizing this information to an area of their mind that is accessed intermittently (often when stressed or when they develop an unanticipated symptom). There are patients who find the uncertainty of their future extremely difficult to come to terms with. They need constant reassurance and regular follow-up for support. The rehabilitation unit is a resource to do this.

There are some patients who attend the unit who should be cured. They usually attend for a time-limited series of interventions, the goal being to 'move them on', perhaps back to their job, perhaps to a gym in the community, perhaps into a day centre for older people.

All these groups of patients are surviving cancer but seldom does anyone survive without any residual disability. Supporting patients to come to terms with their disabilities is an important role of the DTU. It can take many months before patients can acknowledge that they have a disability, sometimes it can be years—this acceptance can be a goal in itself. Often in palliative care we have to make 'quick fixes' to treat difficult symptoms speedily. In patients with long-term disabilities we have to adopt a different approach. We cannot treat their disability, therefore we must have an approach that enables the individual to manage their own disability rather than let the disability manage them. This is a new skill for palliative care clinicians to learn.

Case scenario 1 Mrs X is a 62-year-old married lady with an elderly disabled father to whom she is devoted. She had a lymphoma that required extensive treatment with chemotherapy. More recently she had had a stem cell transplant and had been in remission for 3 years. During this time she developed a lump in the breast that proved to be malignant and was excised. She was referred to the unit with an inability to cope and 'get on with her life' (the words of her general practitioner). The likelihood was that she was cured; however, she was immobilized by her fatigue, despair, and anxieties about her future. She had lost her ability to face the future with any certainty and felt overwhelmed by her circumstances. She had complex physical and emotional symptoms. Untreated pain from abdominal surgery to remove a necrotic mass (thought to be lymphoma) had not been well managed and required analgesia. She attended the nurse-led clinic to oversee her analgesia and to provide ongoing support. She attended the psychosocial team for counselling, accessed complementary therapies and the gym. After 1 year of support she felt much more able to cope and felt that if a rehabilitation programme had been offered earlier in her illness that her recovery would have been much quicker. She has managed to cope with the subsequent death of her father with some further counselling. She is once again painting and feels extremely positive about an art exhibition that she has personally arranged.

4. Longer term disability (non-cancer)

There can be no doubt that patients with advanced progressive non-cancer conditions have a need for palliative care. Patients with many progressive non-cancer illnesses have a similar prognoses (Cancer Survival England and Wales 1991—2001 ONS; Vestbo *et al.* 1998; Stewart *et al.* 2001) to those with cancer and they have similar symptom burdens (Solano *et al.* 2006). The anxiety that services will be overwhelmed (National Council for Palliative Care 2000) by the anticipated extra workload has not yet been realized; however, the fear remains and this has to be acknowledged. Current specialist palliative care provision cannot meet all the needs of patients with progressive non-cancer conditions, especially when one considers the rehabilitation requirements of this group of patients. However, there has to be active involvement with this group to help plan and design future services and to encourage investment.

If the non-cancer population is engaged in a similar way to the cancer population then the workload should be manageable. The model that has been developed in cancer is one where care is shared with the oncologists, often until late in the illness. This way of working has served oncology patients well and makes best use of the skills of specialists in palliative care. The model must be duplicated in non-cancer care.

Palliative care involvement should be determined on the basis of need rather than disease (National Council for Palliative Care 1998). However, accessing specialist palliative care for all appropriate patients remains a challenge both in terms of acquiring adequate resources and appropriate skills. Although specialists in palliative have to remain aware of their limitations they also have to have an understanding that they possess transferable skills appropriate for symptom control in non-cancer patients. The rehabilitative approach to care is another transferable skill.

Finally, there is an assumption made by non-cancer clinicians (and also by some palliative care clinicians) that palliative care will 'take over' the care of patients as soon as a patient is labelled as having far advanced disease and reaching the end of life. To confine palliative care only to this stage of the illness is not in the best interests of any of the clinicians involved. More importantly it is an approach that will lead to inferior care and certainly is not in the best interests of patients or the specialty of palliative care.

Referred with no expectation of service

Some patients are bewildered by their diagnosis, searching for support and looking for help. They have been referred to the unit and have no expectations but hope that, maybe, something can be done to help them or their family. Sometimes these patients need signposting to other services, e.g. information services. Often these patients have enormous needs and will need the support of the full interdisciplinary team.

It is not uncommon that a patient has real needs but has problems conceptualizing this. This is challenging and a strategy needs to be developed to support the patient. To be able to deliver a rehabilitative package of care requires a patient who is both resilient and compliant and has a desire to change. The team needs to understand that a patient can present to the unit with no intention to change or may be contemplating change but is unable to actualize it. Some patients may be ready for change or in the process of changing. The team needs to acknowledge these complexities and to tailor their support to match the different needs of individuals. This flexible approach will lead to a rehabilitative package that is centred on the needs of the individual rather than the needs of the unit. There are various stages a person goes through to actualize change. This has been described by Prochaska and Velicer (1998) (see Table 8.1)—this helpful model helps the team plan, implement and sustain change.

Case scenario 2 Mr Y is a well known actor; he is 72 years old and was still working and travelling until he became suddenly unwell after a collapse at his home. He was found to have renal failure and further investigations revealed multiple myeloma. His former good health has been dramatically affected and he now has to have renal dialysis three times a week and intensive chemotherapy. He is likely to respond to this treatment and survive for several years. He is finding his new status as a 'sick man' extremely difficult to handle: he is weak and fatigued and spends much of his time sitting at home and staring at the wall. He was reluctant to come to the DTU and felt little could be done; however, it was clear that he had significant need for rehabilitation. His wife was keen for him to attend but he was in a 'pre-contemplative' phase. Initial consultations were confined to discussing his illness and helping resolve practical

Table 8.1 Modified from Prochaska's article on the Transtheoretical model of change (Prochaska and Velicer, 1998)

STAGE	Patient's perception and ability to accept change	Objective - Potential for rehabilitation	Member/s of team involved in care and response. (MDM – Multidisciplinary Meeting MDT – Multidisciplinary Team)
Pre-contemplative No intention to change	The patient may not wish to have any involvement with the unit. Options are limited to interventions that are perceived by patient to be relevant and useful.	Objective is to reassure patient that they will not be burdened or forced into treatments. The aim is to gain patient's confidence and 'capture' patient. Intervention may be limited to out patient F/U or the suggestion that re-referral at future date may be most appropriate. Little potential for rehabilitation.	Medical and/or nursing staff is often key worker. MDT involved in a non-rehabilitative capacity. (Good relationships with external health care providers important).

Table 8.1 (continued) Modified from Prochaska's article on the Transtheoretical model of change (Prochaska and Velicer, 1998)

STAGE	Patient's perception and ability to accept change	Objective - Potential for rehabilitation	Member/s of team involved in care and response. (MDM – Multi-disciplinary Meeting MDT – Multi-disciplinary Team)
Contemplative – There is an intention to change	Concepts of new therapies/goals can be discussed. The patient is introduced to the unit.	Objective is to inform patient about the services available in the unit and nudge in right direction. Potential for rehabilitation is good.	Medical and / or nursing staff.
Preparation - Behavior is planned	Care package discussed with patient and team. Team may have useful input at this stage.	Plan package of rehabilitation. At this stage treatment is often confined to limited interventions. For example out patient care alone.	MDT are engaged in planning care. Introduction to members of MDT to discuss potential therapies and interventions.
Action - Plan is operationalised	Therapies are undertaken.	Rehabilitation therapies are organised that are appropriate to the patients needs. Goals are set. Review date is set.	MDT involved in delivering and monitoring care. Referrals to members of MDT as appropriate.
Maintenance - Strategies employed to sustain change	Condition of patient may change. Therapies need monitoring. Package needs reviewing.	The rehabilitation program is underpinned by constant assessment and monitoring on a weekly basis (MDM). Program may need to change if patient's condition changes. This ensures that therapies are appropriate to changing need.	Medical and/or nursing staff. MDT as appropriate.

Table 8.1 (continued) Modified from Prochaska's article on the Transtheoretical model of change (Prochaska and Velicer, 1998)

STAGE	Patient's perception and ability to accept change	Objective - Potential for rehabilitation	Member/s of team involved in care and response. (MDM – Multi-disciplinary Meeting MDT – Multi-disciplinary Team)
Relapse - Return to contemplation or pre-contemplation	Changing physical or emotional needs may make a patient disillusioned and reluctant to continue the rehabilitation program.	Weekly MDM to monitor. Flexibility in program.	Medical and or nursing staff. MDT if appropriate. Good relationships with external health care providers for re-referral if patient unwilling to continue with rehabilitation program.

issues, such as managing his renal diet. Time was spent in the outpatient clinic rehearsing the best way to handle his outpatient appointments and we were able to help co-ordinate his care. With this support he gradually grew more confident in the ability of the unit to help him. He soon accepted the input of the wider team and now regularly attends the unit for the graduated exercise programme and complementary therapies. Although he remains fatigued he now understands his symptoms and is managing them much better. He has improved with regular exercise, his mood has been helped with both counselling and antidepressants, and both he and his wife have learnt to adapt to their new situation. Despite his limited prognosis, he now feels that he can still contribute to the wider world in a meaningful way.

Operational issues in the DTU

The DTU is managed by the nursing team and the senior nurse leads the weekly MDM. Patients can regularly access the medical outpatients, nursing assessments and interventions, physiotherapy, social activities and group psychosocial activities. The weekly MDM is an opportunity for the clinical team to discuss an individual patient's progress and condition. Teamwork is fundamental to an effective service. The team must have a clear and understandable vision of the service and be aware of the ground rules and boundaries. There is an overt understanding that leadership is important and can change. This approach is crucial and facilitates successful teamwork; if it is not understood then the team becomes a group of professionals with no clear direction. The key worker for the patient is generally one of the nursing team. However, it may be a doctor if care is predominantly medical (e.g. outpatient follow-up) or a physiotherapist if the exercise is the key intervention and so on. Other therapies (e.g. art therapy, aromatherapy, reflexology, hydrotherapy, etc.) are arranged for a limited number of sessions. The patient is made aware of this. This ensures that the best use is made of these limited resources.

There is always an anxiety that patients with long-term needs can become dependent on the unit and difficult to discharge. Despite having systems in place to avoid this there continue to be patients who prove difficult to 'move on'. These tend to be highly dependent patients who no longer have rehabilitation needs. An example could be a frail elderly patient who was accepted to the unit with multiple needs. Having done well with the rehabilitation programme the patient has become very dependent on the unit and there may be few resources in the community to take over the care. These complex problems are challenging and require teamwork and collaborative working.

It is noteworthy that there are patients with chronic illness and multiple needs who do not fit into any current support system. This is partly a reflection of the general shift in healthcare away from chronic illness and rehabilitation and towards acute care (Nocon and Baldwin 1998). These patients have complex symptom control needs and often have chronic pain. As a consequence, patients are often on long-term opioids. General practitioners and other healthcare professionals find these a difficult group of patients to manage and will, understandably, refer them to a service that has expertise in managing complex illness and pain. As a consequence a palliative care rehabilitation service that cares for people with chronic problems and chronic illnesses will 'attract' referrals of patients such as these. Whether these patients should access the full range of services that are available in the DTU is debatable as they are a group of patients who are demanding of resources. Therefore, rationing has to be applied to ensure that all patients attending the unit can have appropriate and equitable access to treatment. The way in which these patients are catered for reflects the maturity and resilience of the unit.

Conclusions

This chapter outlines the changing face of cancer management with the consequent increase in survivors. Survivorship has many consequences: physical, social, and emotional and to adapt and cope requires resilience in the patient and their family. Whether the resilience is an 'inner strength' or a primitive part of our response to crises is unknown. It certainly exists.

The concept of a 'rehabilitative approach' is a paradigm shift. It requires the interdisciplinary team to understand that patients, when faced with a life-threatening illness, need support to look at what they can achieve rather than solely on 'coming to terms'.

It is important that patients understand the implications and limitations of serious illness and the resultant disabilities. Setting goals for the future can be challenging especially when intellectual understanding of the illness is not always matched by the emotional capacity to acknowledge the reality. Patients often see themselves as curable (Turton and Cooke 2000), or certainly as long-term survivors, despite having (and understanding that they have) advanced illness. A rehabilitative approach can support patients through this: helping them grow and develop strategies to cope with their disabilities and an uncertain future.

This shift of paradigm requires professionals to move away from their stereotypical roles in hospice care and embrace the changing healthcare environment, developing services that meet an unmet palliative need. No longer can we rest on our past achievements, we must now be an active and integral part of healthcare—indeed this was the original philosophy of the modern hospice movement. To do this we should adapt our current best practice and in addition develop new ways of working. We must persuade our colleagues and our organizations that they should acknowledge the inevitability of change and respond; this takes strength and courage and will require both personal and organizational resilience.

References

Allman BL, Rice CL (2003) Perceived exertion is elevated in old age during an isometric fatigue task. *European Journal of Applied Physiology* **89**(2), 191–197.

Aminoff T, Smolander J, Korhonen O, Louhevaara V (1996) Physical work capacity in dynamic exercise with differing muscle mass in healthy young and older men. *European Journal of Applied Physiology* **73**, 1–2, 180–185.

Calman K, Hine D (1995) *A Policy Framework for Commissioning Cancer Services: A report by the Expert Advisory Group on Cancer to the Chief Medical Officers of England and Wales.* London: Department of Health.

Cancer Survival England and Wales (1991–2001). London: Office of National Statistics.

Casti JL (1997) *Would-be Worlds: How simulation is changing the frontiers of science.* New York: John Wiley & Sons.

Department of Health (2004) *Improving Supportive and Palliative Care for Adults With Cancer.* Cancer Services Guidance. National Institute for Health and Clinical Excellence. London.

Hawe P, Shiell A, Riley T (2004) Complex interventions: how 'out of control' can a randomized controlled trial be? *British Medical Journal* **328**, 1561–1563.

Heath JM, Stuart MR (2002) Prescribing exercise for frail elders. *Journal of the American Board of Family Practitioners* **15**, 218–228.

House of Commons (2004) *Health Committee Report: Palliative Care Fourth Report of Session July*. London: Stationery Office.

Lynn J, Adamson DM (2003) *Living Well at the End of Life. Adapting health care to serious chronic illness in old age*. Washington: Rand Health.

National Council for Palliative Care (1998) *Reaching out: Specialist Palliative Care for Adults with Non-Malignant Diseases*. London: NCPC.

National Council for Palliative Care (2000) *Fulfilling Lives: Rehabilitation in Palliative Care*. London: NCPC.

Nocon A, Baldwin S (1998) *Trends in Rehabilitation Policy. A review of the literature*. London: King's Fund Publishing.

Prochaska JO, Velicer WF (1998) Behavior change: the transtheoretical model of health behavior change. *American Journal of Health Promotion* **12**, 38–48.

Richardson E, Tookman A (2004) Foreword. In: *The Essence of Palliative Care: a Personal Perspective*. London: National Council for Palliative Care.

Scottish Executive (2006) *Cancer in Scotland: Action for change*. Edinburgh: Scottish Executive Health Department.

Solano JP, Gomes B, Higginson I (2006) A comparison of symptom prevalence in far advanced Cancer, AIDS, heart disease, chronic obstructive pulmonary disease (COPD), and renal disease. *Journal of Pain and Symptom Management* **31**, 58–69.

Stewart S, MacIntyre K, Hole DJ, Capewell S, McMurray JJV (2001) More 'malignant' than cancer? 5 year survival following a first admission for heart failure. *European Journal of Heart Failure* **3**(3), 315–322.

Tookman A, Hopkins K, Scharpen-von-Heussen K (2004) Rehabilitation in palliative medicine. In: *Oxford Textbook of Palliative Medicine*, 3rd edn, pp. 1019–1032 (eds Doyle D, Hanks G, Cherny N, Calman K). Oxford: Oxford University Press.

Tritter JQ, Calnan M (2002) Reconsidering categorization and exploring experience. *European Journal of Cancer Care* **11**(3), 161–165.

Turner-Stokes L (2000) *Measurement of Outcome in Rehabilitation—'Basket' of Measures*. London: The British Society of Rehabilitation Medicine, Clinical Guidelines.

Turton P, Cooke H (2000) Meeting the needs of people with cancer for support and self management. *Comp Th Nurs Midwif* Aug 6(3), 130–137.

Vestbo J, Prescott E, Lange P, Schnohr P, Jensen G (1998) Vital prognosis after hospitalization for COPD: a study of a random population sample. *Respiratory Medicine* **92**, 772–776.

Resilience and bereavement: Part 1

Linda Machin

Introduction

Following her study of holocaust survivors Moskovitz asserted that, 'practitioners needed to rethink the idea that adversity inevitably leads to negative outcomes' (1983, p. 201). In the field of bereavement greater recognition is being given to the possibilities for positive adaptation to grief. Estimates vary but there is consensus among researchers that a large proportion of people ultimately recover from grief (McCrae and Costa 1993; Sanders 1993; Raphael *et al.* 2001) and that 'Resilience is an innate self-righting mechanism that assists people in redirecting their lives onto an adaptive path following disadvantageous or stressful circumstances' (Greene 2002, p. 4). Researchers and theorists (Seligman 1998; Grotberg 1999; Greene 2002) have used different ways to define resilience but three common elements can be seen:

- *personal resourcefulness* involving qualities such as flexibility, courage, and perseverance;
- *a positive life perspective* in which there is optimism, hope, a capacity to make sense of experience and motivation in setting personal goals;
- *social embeddedness* in which there is availability of support and a capacity to access it.

As practitioners, how might we recognize these characteristics in the work of bereavement care and how might we promote resilience in those who seek our support?

Recognizing resilience in bereavement

Traditionally practitioner attention has focused upon those people who are thought to be at risk following bereavement. The notion of risk was predicated on the basis of circumstantial factors shown to heighten vulnerability, e.g. age, gender, relationship to the deceased, the nature and the manner of the death, etc. (Parkes and Weiss 1983; Sanders 1993). However, an alternative concept used to appraise the impact of loss and trauma is based upon a theory of stress and coping (Lazarus and Folkman 1984; Folkman 2001; Stroebe *et al.* 2006).

It suggests that the dominant need in a stressful situation, is to decide whether the source of stress is greater than the resourcefulness of the individual, and the extent to which it is putting personal well-being at risk. This perspective provides a different theoretical emphasis where coping capacity is not predictable but has to be understood by looking at individual resources/pressures and strengths/vulnerabilities in a particular context. When viewed from this perspective, individual variations in loss response are enormous and represent a full spectrum of reactions from risk to resilience. Bereavement care needs to engage with this complex blend of intrapersonal and interpersonal factors.

My experiences in counselling and research lead me to observe and identify a range of distinctive responses, which span the spectrum of grief reactions (Machin 1980). The three themes, which emerged were:

+ a state of being deeply sunk in the distress of grief—*overwhelmed*;

+ a dominant need to subdue emotions and maintain a focus on ongoing life demands—*controlled*;

+ a capacity to face the emotional, social, and practical, consequences of loss with equilibrium—*resilience.*

This concept of difference provided a framework—the Range of Response to Loss (RRL) model—through which the varied elements of loss and their manifestation in grief might be understood. It allowed for the identification of both risk and resilience. Without theoretical acknowledgement of the former the latter cannot be fully understood.

The notions contained within the RRL perspective are consistent with other theoretical models. Table 9.1 identifies the conceptual parallels between the

Table 9.1 Theoretical parallels between the RRL framework and other models

Range of Response to Loss (Machin 2001)	Overwhelmed by loss	Resilient in the face of loss	Controlled response to loss
Ainsworth et al 'Attachment' Style (1978)	Anxious/Ambivalent attachment	Secure attachment	Avoidant attachment
Horowitz Stress Theory (1986)	Intrusion		Avoidance
Stroebe + Schut 'Dual Process' Model (1999)	Loss Orientation	◄----------------- oscillation -----------------►	Restoration Orientation
Martin and Doka Personality-related patterns of grief (2000)	Intuitive grief	Blended grief ◄-----------►	Instrumental grief

categories proposed in the RRL framework and other models, which have been highly influential in providing a knowledge base for practitioners working with the dying and the bereaved.

The RRL model proposes that two elements lie at the heart of a grief reaction. The (**overwhelming**) distress generated by the powerlessness of loss and the desire to recover a sense of power (**control**). These two dimensions of grief and the management of their competing forces characterizes the grief dynamic. For some people overwhelmed feelings will dominate—sadness, anger, guilt, etc. The overwhelming nature of grief is likely to be evident in the early days of a loss or bereavement. For other people diversion from feelings and attention to thinking and action will demonstrate a controlled loss response. This response may be characterized by a predominant focus on practical day to day concerns and planning for the future. These two dimensions of loss response may create uncomfortable contradictions between a felt sense of powerlessness and the urge to regain some personal power (see Figure 9.1).

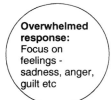
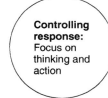

Overwhelmed response:
Focus on feelings - sadness, anger, guilt etc

Controlling response:
Focus on thinking and action

Figure 9.1 Core grief responses.

Set alongside the overwhelming and controlling responses is a **resilient** reaction characterized by an ability to face the feelings of distress, while still being able to distinguish those areas of life where control and active choice are possible. The distress, tension, contradictions, and uncertainties of grief are mediated by an awareness of personal resourcefulness, a capacity to access and use social support and an evolving sense of meaning. Resilience has an executive role in integrating the overwhelming and controlling elements of grief (see Figure 9.2).

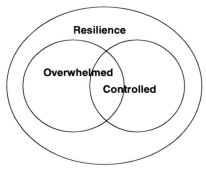

Resilience

Overwhelmed

Controlled

Figure 9.2 Resilient grief response.

The three categories in the RRL model were statistically validated in a sample of bereaved people, using a scale (the Adult Attitude to Grief (AAG) scale) devised to test this proposition of difference in grief reaction (Machin 2001). The AAG scale, as the name of the measure suggests, focuses upon the attitudes people have towards their loss rather than the circumstances, which shape their loss. The AAG scale is made up of nine statements with a self-report response—strongly agree/agree/neither agree nor disagree/disagree/strongly disagree. This revealed the nature of people's perspectives within the overwhelmed, controlled and resilient dimensions of loss.

Table 9.2 Adult Attitude to Grief Scale (Machin 2001)

(Overwhelmed items)
2. For me, it is difficult to switch off thoughts about the person I have lost.
5. I feel that I will always carry the pain of grief with me.
7. Life has less meaning for me after this loss.

(Controlled items)
4. I believe that I must be brave in the face of loss.
6. For me, it is important to keep my grief under control.
8. I think its best just to get on with life after a loss.

(Resilient items)
1. I feel able to face the pain which comes with loss.
3. I feel very aware of my inner strength when faced with grief.
9. It may not always feel like it but I do believe that I will come through this experience of grief.

(Numbers relate to the order of statements on the AAG scale).

What became clear from the 2001 (Machin) study was a fourth dimension, identified as vulnerability. The characteristics of this category were:

♦ an **absence of resilience** (i.e. disagreement with the resilient items on the scale—1, 3, 9).

♦ **tension** between an overwhelming sense of powerlessness and the pull to be in control, when control is central to the person's sense of well-being (i.e. agreement with items in both the overwhelmed and controlled categories).

♦ **overwhelming feelings** and thoughts being especially **powerful and persistent**.

♦ **control** is the normal coping style but the usual strategies **fail to subdue distressing emotions** of grief (see Figure 9.3).

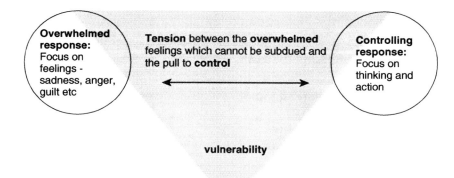

Figure 9.3 Vulnerable grief response.

The fourth category described in the RRL model as vulnerability is consistent with the fourth attachment style identified by Main (1991) as disorganized, in which there is a mix of anxious and avoidant responses.

While the broad categorical differences had been statistically validated (Machin 2001) what became clear in looking in detail at the individual respondents' scores on the AAG scale was the complex blend of perspectives across all of the categories. The scale was providing an individual profile of the biases and blends of overwhelming, controlling, and vulnerability/resilient elements manifest at a particular time by a particular mourner. This capacity to understand the complexities of grief within individuals, suggested that it might be a useful measure in practice settings. The possibility of using the scale in practice was explored in more detail (Machin and Spall 2004) and found to have face validity for practitioners and clients. It was used as a tool of assessment, as a cue for therapeutic dialogue and as a framework for suggesting therapeutic goals, especially that of resilience.

It was also important to address the social context of grief as well as the attitudes expressed through the AAG scale, by exploring the extent to which there was opportunity for comfort and practical support within the social network of the mourner and how far that person was able to access the support (Cleiren 1991). Cultural elements play an important part in the integration of the bereaved and in the social opportunities for meaning making, e.g. through ritual, commonly held beliefs, etc. (Rosenblatt 1993; Schaefer and Moos 2001). Resilience is a capacity to manage external dimensions of stress as well as internal distress (Folkman 2001).

Promoting resilience

If personal resourcefulness, a positive life perspective and social embedded-ness characterize resilience, how can these qualities be promoted in bereave-ment care? To begin it is important to be able to **appraise** the perspectives, which give shape to current grief. The AAG scale can be used quantitatively to assess the relative significance of overwhelming, controlling, and resilient elements of loss response. Used in this way the scale can also help track the changes taking place in the grief over time (Machin—Sage Publications Ltd forthcoming 2008).

In the therapeutic context, qualitative use can be made of the themes prompted by the items on the AAG scale, which provide cues for deeper exploration of atti-tudinal perspectives and provide a structure for the telling of the story of loss (see Table 9.3).

Table 9.3 Qualitative themes prompted by the AAG scale (Machin 2008)

Overwhelmed themes
2. The unwelcome intrusion of grief or chosen rumination about the death and the deceased.
5. The persistence of grief – an incapacity to see beyond the pain.
7. A struggle to find either old or new meanings in life.

Controlled themes
4. Valuing courage and fortitude.
6. Keeping emotions in check to protect self or others.
8. The need to divert and focus on the future.

Resilient themes
1. The ability to confront emotions and the reality of what has been lost.
3. A sense of personal resourcefulness.
9. A positive outlook which can see beyond the present pain.

(Numbers relate to the order of statements on the AAG scale).

1. The goal for building on the initial story of grief is to enhance **personal resourcefulness**. The two objectives for working with the diverse and complex grief perspectives are (a) to facilitate safe exploration of the distress alongside (b) a realistic appraisal of the ways in which it is possible to think and act outside that distress. To work with these two elements may require focus on the area that is outside the usual coping frame of the mourner. For example, a cognitive approach to explore the possibilities for greater control will counter a predominantly emotion focused (overwhelmed), response to loss. Conversely, where control dominates a safe opportunity to examine and understand feelings is necessary.

Schut *et al.* (1997) have observed in their research the usefulness for therapy to provide a compensating approach to the usual coping style of grieving people. This will help achieve some balance between the immobilizing (overwhelming) distress of grief and the desire to have some degree of agency (control). It increases the perception that at a personal level there is a capacity to meet the needs of the situation by making the divergent components of grief more manageable (Antonovsky 1988).

2. A **positive life perspective** will follow more readily when a grieving person has greater engagement with their own resources. It allows for the emergence of a more optimistic perspective. From this may follow a capacity to revisit the story of loss and find alternative ways of understanding events, as thoughts are (re)organized and meanings communicated (McLeod 1997; Neimeyer and Anderson 2002). Frankl, himself a holocaust survivor, asserts that, 'Suffering ceases to be suffering in some way at the moment it finds meaning' (1963, p. 117). For Frankl three important components make up meaning in life:

   ♦ creativity—striving to produce something, setting a personal goal or a cause to follow

   ♦ experiential—experience centred on truth and beauty but most of all found through love

   ♦ attitudinal—a capacity to turn tragedy into triumph, transforming human predicament into achievement.

   Achieving greater comprehensibility and meaningfulness (Antonovsky 1988) requires the therapist to act as a co-constructor in the process of change, by helping the client explore potential routes to a more positive life perspective (Neimeyer and Anderson 2002; Joseph and Linley 2006).

3. While the focus of therapy is the individual, attention should not be confined to the inner processes of grief and its management but should also look to understand the **social embeddedness** (or not) of the client. The grief perspective of clients is likely to reflect attitudes held in a wider social context. Family, religion, and culture may provide a coherent background to beliefs about grief or they may present dissonant voices and variable pressures to react to loss in different ways. The extent to which a person is held within a supportive network of people who are able to offer comfort and assistance will contribute to the level of resilience shown in the face of loss. Therapy needs to address the ways in which a client might access and use the relationships and social resources at their disposal (Schaefer and Moos 2001).

Conclusions

Exploring the full spectrum of loss responses has opened the way for new awareness about the capacity for resilience in the face of grief. The RRL model, through the AAG scale, provides a way of identifying and engaging with this diversity in individual grief reactions—from vulnerability to resilience. Grief is a journey and it is likely to render most people vulnerable for a time. However, for some people the circumstances of their loss and the inadequacy of their resourcefulness will put them at particular risk. For these people and for all who may demonstrate a need for bereavement care, the challenge for the practitioner is to harness the natural mechanisms for recovery from grief. It is an approach that aims not only to restore former equilibrium but strives to nurture the development of new strengths within a joint therapeutic enterprise.

> You shall be free indeed when your days
>
> Are not without a care nor your nights
>
> Without a want and a grief,
>
> But rather when these things girdle your life
>
> And yet you rise above them naked and unbound.
>
> Kahlil Gibran, the Prophet

References

Ainsworth MDS, Blehar MC, Waters E, Wall S (1978) *Patterns of Attachment: A Psychological Study of the Strange Situation*. Hillsdale, NJ: Erlbaum.

Antonovsky A (1988) *Unraveling the Mystery of Health: How People Manage Stress and Stay Well*. San Francisco, CA: Jossey-Bass.

Cleiren M (1991) *Bereavement and Adaptation: A Comparative Study of the Aftermath of Death*. Washington, DC: Hemisphere Publishing.

Folkman S (2001) Revised coping theory and the process of bereavement. In: *Handbook of Bereavement Research*, pp. 563–584 (eds Stroebe MS, Hansson RO, Stroebe W, Schut H). Washington, DC: American Psychological Association.

Frankl V (1963) *Man's Search for Meaning*. London: Rider.

Gibran K (1960) *The Prophet* New York: Knopf.

Greene R (2002) Holocaust survivors: a study in resilience. *Journal of Gerontological Social Work* **37**.

Grotberg EH (1999) Countering depression with the five building blocks of resilience. *Reaching Today's Youth* **4**(1, Fall): 66–72.

Horowitz M (1976/1986) *Stress response syndromes*. Northvale, NJ: Aronson.

Joseph S, Linley PA (2006) *Positive Therapy*. London: Routledge.

Lazarus RS, Folkman S (1984) *Stress, Appraisal and Coping*. New York: Springer.

Machin L (1980) *Living with Loss*. Research Report for the Lichfield Diocesan Board for Social Responsibility.

Machin L (2001) Exploring a framework for understanding the range of response to loss; a study of clients receiving bereavement counselling. Unpublished PhD thesis: Keele University, UK.

Machin L (2008) *Mapping Grief* (forthcoming). London: Sage Publications Ltd.

Machin L, Spall R (2004) Mapping grief: a study in practice using a quantitative and qualitative approach to exploring and addressing the range of response to loss. *Counselling and Psychotherapy Research* **4**, 9–17.

Main M (1991) Metacognitive knowledge, metacognitive monitoring and singular (coherent) vs. multiple (incoherent) model of attachment. In: *Attachment Across the Life Cycle*, pp. 127–159 (eds Parkes CM, Stevenson-Hinde J, Marris P). London: Routledge.

Martin TL, Doka KL (2000) *Men Don't Cry … Women Do*. Philadelphia, PA: Brunner/Mazel.

McCrae RR, Costa PT (1993) Psychological resilience among widowed men and women: a 10-year follow-up of a national sample. In: *Handbook of Bereavement: Theory, Research and Intervention*, pp. 196–207 (eds Stroebe MS, Stroebe W, Hansson RO). Cambridge: Cambridge University Press.

McLeod J (1997) *Narrative and Psychotherapy*. London: Sage.

Moskovitz S (1983) *Love Despite Hate*. New York: W.W. Norton.

Neimeyer R, Anderson A (2002) Meaning reconstruction theory. In: *Loss and Grief*, (ed. Thompson N). Basingstoke: Palgrave.

Parkes CM, Weiss RS (1983) *Recovery from Bereavement*. New York: Basic Books.

Raphael B, Minkov C, Dobson M (2001) Psychotherapeutic and pharmacological interventions for bereaved persons. In: *Handbook of Bereavement Research*, pp. 587–612 (eds Stroebe MS, Hansson RO, Stroebe W, Schut H). Washington, DC: American Psychological Association.

Rosenblatt PC (1993) Grief: The social context of private feelings. In: *Handbook of Bereavement: Theory, Research and Intervention*, pp. 196–207 (eds Stroebe MS, Stroebe W, Hansson RO). Cambridge: Cambridge University Press.

Sanders CM (1993) Risk factors in bereavement outcome. In: *Handbook of Bereavement: Theory, Research and Intervention*, pp. 196–207 (eds Stroebe MS, Stroebe W, Hansson RO). Cambridge: Cambridge University Press.

Schaefer JA, Moos RH (2001) Bereavement experiences and personal growth. In: *Handbook of Bereavement Research*, pp. 145–168 (eds Stroebe MS, Hansson RO, Stroebe W, Schut H). Washington, DC: American Psychological Association.

Schut HAW, Stroebe MS, van den Bout J, de Keijser J (1997). Interventions for the bereaved: Gender differences in the efficacy of two counselling programmes. *British Journal of Clinical Psychology* **36**, 63–72.

Seligman MEP (1998) Building human strength: psychology's forgotten mission. *American Psychological Association Monitor* **29**.

Stroebe M, Schut H (1999) The dual process model of coping with bereavement: rationale and description. *Death Studies* **23**, 197–224.

Stroebe M, Folkman S, Hansson RO, Schut H (2006) The prediction of bereavement outcome: development of an integrative risk factor framework. *Social Science an Medicine* **63**, 2440–2245.

Resilience and bereavement: Part 2

Phyllis R. Silverman

In this chapter I am considering how a public health approach might be adopted in a community based response to the grief people experience after a death of someone important in their lives. I am focusing on what takes place in Western societies. In public health the emphasis is on prevention, taking a population approach to particular illnesses or social conditions. The target population would be those who will be mourners. The goal of this intervention is not only to prevent serious problems from developing, but to enhance people's ability to cope, when someone important in their lives dies. In looking at issues related to grief after a death we are dealing with a universal experience with which, at one time or another, we all have a need to find a way of coping. Death is not an experience that we can realistically prevent. In the end we have very little control over matters of life and death. What we have control over is how we deal with this fact of life and how we find a place for death in the way we live our lives. I am suggesting that as we look at dealing with the fact that we all die and that we are all likely to be mourners at one time or another in our lives, it is not simply a personal issue that rests primarily in our own psyches, it is not something we do alone. We do it in a community of others and these others frame our behaviour, provide us with a vocabulary that directs our actions and what we expect of ourselves and this vocabulary determines what help is available. Given that we cannot prevent death, we can, however, consider how to promote people's ability to deal with their grief in a meaningful and more competent manner; in a way that would help to prevent maladaptive behaviour. Deviating from typical public health language I cannot talk about prevention of the basic cause of any one person's grief as might be done in a more traditional public health approach in which, for example, the water supply is kept clean to prevent gastrointestinal problems. I am instead suggesting promoting competence toward a more comfortable outcome and helping people to be more resilient when faced with this fact of life.

The language of grief

The language we use reflects the attitudes and beliefs about grief that exist is any community. The current vocabulary, used in most Western societies, may not provide the bereaved with an adequate and open vocabulary that reflects the complexity of the bereavement process and identifies the realities of the impact of the death on their lives. I am suggesting that we need to change our vocabulary to help people see the fullness of what grief means in their lives.

I am asking, as a way of promoting people's ability to be resilient, what expectations a particular society has for the way people cope with death? These expectations also affect how non-mourners respond when they are faced with the grief of others.

The vocabulary we use to describe and explain the experience may not be consistent with the experience of the bereaved. We focus on the sadness associated with the loss, the emptiness we may feel, and the emotional pain and stress associated with the loss. We hear from those around us that we are expected to get over it, and to get on with our life, in a relatively short period of time. Mourners are expected to recover, to in some way put the past behind them and go on as before. Grief is often seen as having a clear beginning and a clear ending. This view does not take into consideration the fullness of the impact of death on those who were mourning for: spouses, partners, siblings, parents, children, and friends. For the bereaved this notion that they can recover, as if they have an illness or are infected by a 'virus', often leaves them feeling as if something is wrong with them when they do not 'recover'. It is not unusual to be asked why grieving is taking us so long, as if there is something wrong with us that we are still sad and not able to get back to 'normal' even 1 or 2 months after the death of someone important in our lives. Our personal experience does not always seem to coincide with popular theories of grief that inform our expectations and that influence the community of friends and family around us who may think they are being helpful by sharing what they have learned, for example, from the media or from books they have read. In the words of a young man mourning the death of his friend:

> I always have the feeling I haven't grieved Corey's death. I read Kubler-Ross and I am not following her stages. They don't match my experience and I keep feeling that I am doing something wrong. Yet when I think about it, what I am doing feels right to me. I'll never get over it. It has really changed me in so many ways. When I visit his mother she tells me she has the same feelings.
>
> Silverman (2000, p. 6)

Machin (2003) observed this discrepancy between some of what the bereaved experience and the findings of researchers who maintain that they need a certain objectivity to do good research. As a result of staying outside the experience of those they are studying, she points out that many researchers are not able to hear the fullness of the stories the bereaved tell.

There is also a haste to give labels to human experiences by many professionals. There is a growing movement in the Western world to define some experiences of bereavement as an illness (Parkes 2006, Pettus 2006; Prigerson 2006, Walter 2006). When grief is seen as resting primarily in the inner psyche of the bereaved individual, the mourner is led to believe that with proper treatment this grief can be 'cured'. Thus when someone is grieving, the focus is often on 'fixing it', on ridding ourselves of these feelings. Grieving is seen as time limited and often associated with a formula that should be followed to grieve successfully. Treatment is provided by an 'expert' and the focus is on eliciting these painful feelings and thereby making it possible to recover. In this approach the personal experiences of the bereaved in finding ways of dealing with their loss are often insufficiently valued.

Professional knowledge, rather than experiential knowledge guides the helping process (Horowitz 2006), and for the most part this seems to be adopted in the larger community partly in deference to and out of respect for professionally generated knowledge. The bereaved are not empowered to use their own abilities and experience on their own behalf. People in their own community feel self-conscious about not having professional credentials and knowledge, and are therefore reluctant to try to be helpful (Silverman 2004; Stroebe and Schut 2006). Sometimes the vocabulary of recovery is used to avoid getting close to the pain of the bereaved, suggesting that if they were doing it right they should no longer be in pain or be thinking about the deceased. Amitai Etzioni, a professor of sociology wrote, on the 'op ed' page of the *New York Times* (10 October 2006, p. A27) about being told to mourn in the right way after his wife died more than 20 years earlier. He is being told the same thing today after his son died leaving a pregnant wife and a 2-year-old child:

> 'I presume that many a psychiatrist and New Age minister would point out that by keeping busy we avoid "healthy grieving". To hell with that; the void left by our loss is just too deep. For now focusing on what we do for one another is the only consolation we can find.'

Professional knowledge may not translate well as it moves from the research project to implementation in the community. People struggle to deal with a sense of loss, of something missing, and of slowly becoming aware of the fact that their lives have changed forever. They soon discover that there is no correct way to mourn, that they have to find their own way through it and that grief is an ongoing process of change without necessarily having a clear ending. It also implies recognizing the role of the deceased in this process.

When we talk about putting recovery and the past behind us, these needs are not taken into consideration. A radical change in vocabulary would occur if the word 'recovery' was deleted.

A process of change

Change on many levels is an integral part of the bereavement process. To look for a return to what was once 'normal' is not really possible. We cannot go back to what was. We soon learn that change is an essential part of the process. Our world is changed in ways we could not imagine. This world can feel very different and it may require the development of different ways of living in it. As mourners try to manage this it is important to ask what is lost when someone important in our lives dies? What is lost is a person, a relationship, a way of life and a self in that relationship. Loss is something that we must make sense out of, give meaning to and respond to. The vocabulary that we learn as we deal with this fact of life must include a way of looking at the change as a consequence, that occurs on many levels and that includes a new relationship with ourselves and the world. Each aspect of this process influences the others. Thus, when a person is grieving, change is a constant companion and it can be seen as a new beginning (Silverman 1988, 2000). This aspect of the grieving process needs to be acknowledged and legitimated.

Stroebe and Schut (1999) describe how people can vacillate between their feelings of pain and the sadness that is typically associated with grief and then reach out to find ways of dealing with the world as it is newly constructed. They describe this as a back and forth movement, yet we are never wholly in one place or another. Over time we integrate the sense of loss, how we make meaning out of it and the changes in our lives, so that in a sense this dynamic becomes part of the whole, of the way we accommodate to the loss and all that it brings with it.

One aspect of change is an emerging sense of a new self (Silverman 1988, 2000). A widower describes his experience with a changing sense of self:

> To me there is a death of the self—that's what you have to come to terms with. I have to find a ritual that says the old self is dead because part of the old self was the relationship with my wife and one of the things that I've learned is that change is inevitable. For me part of what I have to do is let go of the old self and not feeling that I am not still connected to my wife but it's not in the old way. Something different is happening to my sense of who I am.

> Silverman (2004, p. 66)

What does the death of the self mean? As noted above the self that existed as part of the relationship with the deceased is lost as well, and so in many ways this involves finding a new self even though it may still hold parts of the old self and other relationships. Mourners find themselves beginning to develop a new perspective on their own behaviour and their relationship to others. They talk of moving from one way of seeing themselves in the world to another more complex vision that gives them greater understanding of themselves and their relationship to others. In the words of one widow:

> 'My friends find it hard to believe how I have changed since my husband died. I expect different things from people. I say things I never said before. I decide what is best for the family. If I was going to survive that is what I had to do.'

> (Silverman 2000, p. 19)

One way of understanding this new sense of self that seems to evolve out of grief is to look at it as a developmental process. The old way no longer is effective. The bereaved are open to the fact that they cannot go back, but they need to know that this dynamic is part of the grieving process. They find themselves relating to the world in a more and more complex manner. I am talking about a cognitive process that is usually reserved to describe the growth in children. Children grow from a place where they are the centre of their world, to a place where they are aware of the needs of others and eventually develop a mutuality and exchange with others with whom they interact. In the face of a changing life situation, if this is understood as part of the process, our ability to observe expands. We begin to see changes not only in the external properties of our world or our experience with it, but also in the properties of our mind that help compose order and make sense of the experience. We also become more sensitive to the needs of others, with a growing awareness of our interdependence. Michael White (1988) describes this as the growing ability to be both performer and audience to our own performance. Regardless of where we have been, facing death and grief creates new opportunities for change. To promote resilience we need to recognize that change continues throughout our life time on many levels, and make these ideas part of the vocabulary of grief. A new scheme for the bereaved dealing with all the changes in their lives, involves a growing sense of self, of personal authority, a new awareness of others and a new sense of mutuality (Silverman 2000). In the words of a widower:

> 'I am a more caring person. Grieving and sharing it with my dear friends and family have made me more open and I deeply appreciate the need to share and to be sensitive to the feelings of others.'

> (Silverman 2004, p. 141)

Role of the deceased

Is there a language for including the dead in how we deal with our grief? How in any given community do we honour the dead? What are the customs, the traditions that are there for us to follow when a death occurs in our family, in our community? Do we really let go? Do we really put the past behind us (Silverman and Klass 1996)? My colleague Stephen Nickman and I (Silverman *et al.* 1992; Silverman and Nickman 1996; Nickman *et al.* 1998) discovered in looking at the data from the Child Bereavement Study (Silverman and Worden 1993) that these bereaved children had not 'read the book', so they did not know they were supposed to 'let go'. We found that there were many ways in which children connect to the deceased. This is not a simple phenomenon and in our limited sample we found that the nature of the connection changed over the 2 years of the study, but it did not end (Normand *et al.* 1996). We recognized the tension created if people tried to live in the past, but if we disconnect from the past then who are we? A good example of this process is found in the following quotation from one of the most famous orphans of this decade:

> You think the dead we love ever truly leave us? You think that we don't recall them more clearly than ever in times of great trouble? Your father is alive in you Harry and shows himself most plainly when you have need of him … Harry in a way you did see your father last night … you found him inside yourself

Rowling (1999, p. 428)

There are many lessons to be learned from the popular series of books about Harry Potter. Harry can be seen from many perspectives but the fact that he is an orphan may be the most important part of his story for us. The essence of the series is about his increasing awareness of the importance of his parents in his life, and his need to find out more and more about them. He slowly begins to recognize that he has a relationship with his mother and father. Since they died shortly after his birth, for this relationship to be sustained requires a good deal of learning on Harry's part.

In the wake of the 9/11 tragedy, those helping the surviving families kept looking for ways to foster and hasten their healing and find closure. As a result, each family received an urn of ashes from the World Trade Center that was intended to 'bring closure.' However, this provided little solace to some mourners (personal communication, 2002). In many ways, these initiatives actually compounded the survivors' pain because as they lived with their grief they began to realize that closure, as such, is unattainable. One kind of closure did come with the confirmation of the death, the other kind of closure that would involve closing the space in their lives was not possible. Mourners learn that relationships must change after a death, but they do not end. Playwright Robert Anderson summarized his experience 15 years after his first wife's death:

> 'I have a new life … Death ends a life but it doesn't end a relationship, which struggles on in the survivor's mind toward some resolution, which it never finds.'

(1974, p. 77)

As much as the bereaved may try, they find that they cannot put the past behind them. They must now deal with a world without the deceased, but they need to find a place in that world for the deceased. As survivors they make their way through their pain and as part of this face the silence of the grave, but the past is still very much a part of who they are. The grave is not totally silent. To carry on with their lives the bereaved soon discover the need to find a way of remembering and honouring the dead, of knowing who they were, and the ways in which they shaped their lives. The deceased are in many ways still part of the conversation.

I see grief as a dynamic process involving the deceased, multiple mourners, those who are part of the mourner's lives, and the cultural traditions and mores that shape people's behaviour and understanding (Klass *et al.* 1996). The past, the present, and the future come together. The language of grief needs to include this perspective.

Grief can be seen as a dynamic process that invariably must connect both to how we understand the experience and to what we do about it. It is not so much what happens to us but what we do about it. We cannot separate the two. When we talk about how we understand what we are experiencing, this gives form to how we cope and towards what end we are working.

The new vocabulary I propose has to come not only from the professionals who study bereavement and grief but from the bereaved themselves. The grief counsellor, the physician, the hospice worker have become the guardians of how we grieve and how we die. The emphasis is on doing it correctly! What we learn from living has not been valued and those of us who want to comfort the bereaved have become very self-conscious about what we have to offer and are often fearful about saying or doing the 'wrong thing'. In the same way we can ask who defines a good death: me or the professional who takes care of me? Are we abdicating the care we can provide to each other to professionals? Caring has become a *commodity* for which we expect to pay. McKnight (1995) reflects on this:

> 'Care is the consenting commitment of citizens to each other ... care cannot be produced, provided, managed, organized, administered or commodified. When care is over professionalized to the extent that provider (professionals deliver services to dependent clients (the rest of us)) ... people begin to doubt their ability to help each other...'
>
> (McKnight, 1995, p. x)

The professional is typically the guardian of how we die. Farber *et al.* (2004) write about a 'respectful death' suggesting that the person who is dying and his or her community take the lead rather than the professional. Is this a subject that should be discussed primarily in my doctor's office or in the privacy of my home? Is the knowledge that comes from living with this fact the province of some professionally trained expert to administer and tell us what to do? What is my part? The burden in this instance is that the family and the dying person need to know what seems most comfortable to them and to be able to articulate what is right for them—it also means those of us who are in the role of professional need to learn to listen. We also need to translate what we learn from research to recognize its limitations and to make room for the experience that people bring to this period in their lives.

When we allow experts to tell us how to live and how to die, we are not prepared for taking charge of the difficult times in our lives. To be partners in the process we need to have confidence in our own ability to take hold as needed. Resilience is fostered when people appreciate their own ability to learn what they may need to know to be effective. Many years ago when I first started working in this field I found this quote from a sociologist that I have carried with me ever since as a guide to help me understand why I am uncomfortable about what I see in the present situation. McKnight's concern about commodifying care is consistent with Friedson's thinking 30 years earlier:

> 'A pathology arises when an outsider may no longer evaluate the work by rules of logic and the knowledge available to all educated men and when the only legitimate spokesman on an issue relevant to all men must be someone who is officially certified.'

> (Friedson 1970)

Considering what Friedson said we need to ask is there a pathology in our society today? In many ways I think there is. I am concerned with the commodification of care and with the place of the citizen/persons defined as consumer because we are all citizens and we are all consumers in this area of living. We should all be expert in issues that concern all of us. In our world generally we no longer respect experiential knowledge. We ask for people's qualifications, where were they trained? How did we get to a place where mourners ask when grieving, 'what is wrong with me'? The parents who participated in the Harvard/MGH Child Bereavement Study (Silverman and Worden 1993) agreed to talk to us if we would tell them whether their child was psychologically okay. How did they get to a place where they considered their child's pain and angst about a parent's death as a sign of something being wrong with them? What do we do when people fail to reach out to the bereaved or the dying because they fear they might say the wrong thing or because they take literally what they learned from popular literature?

We learn by example, from others who have been there before us. Learning is facilitated when we are offered a vocabulary to explain what we are experiencing. The bereaved have to find new meaning in a world where they feel helpless in their ability to control what has happened to them. Resilience comes from being able to take charge, from having an appreciation of our own abilities, and from learning a vocabulary that describes what we are experiencing, that does not disenfranchise us, but gives us room and support to build on our own experiences.

Helping in this context

The implication of what I am saying is that there needs to be an expansion of ways in which we learn about the nature of grief that promotes resilience and competence. There may be many ways to do this, beyond changing vocabulary, that include educating teachers, clergy and healthcare professionals so that they can see the bigger picture and provide appropriate support to those who turn to them for help, without being prescriptive or looking at the pain as something that must be gotten rid of. The bereaved themselves also need to be involved, as experiential knowledge is included in how we understand what is happening. Educating journalists is critical. Judith Foreman (2007), a syndicated writer on issues of health, questioned the value of studying the obvious and giving it a label. She was reacting to a study of people's reactions to being told they have an incurable illness. The study found that half of these people met the criteria for a significant psychiatric disorder. She wondered if it was really news that a serious medical diagnosis could shake a person to the core? She asked of what value is such a label?

I have said that most mourners do not grieve alone. On a more personal level, we all need some help from a friend. I have said that our best teachers are often those who have been through the pain, who understand what we are experiencing and from their own experience provide a listening ear and some ideas about how to cope (Silverman 2004). There seems to be something special about meeting others who are or were in the same situation. Helping and being helped by other people with whom you share a common experience, seems to provide the participants with a special opportunity to feel hope and see the possibilities for the future that they had not seen before. It normalizes our experience.

While it was probably common practice throughout the ages for the bereaved to help each other, formal mutual help programmes for the bereaved, as we have come to know them, were rare and may not have been needed. Help was there in the community and the customs and mores of the society were intact.

A mutual-help exchange, as used here, involves people who share a common problem, a problem that one of the participants has coped with successfully. The helping person has expertise based on personal experience and has learned to solve a particular problem. Borkman (1976, 1999) distinguishes between at least two sources of information, one that comes from formal learning, or what she calls professional knowledge, and the other is experiential knowledge, which is accrued from personal experience. A helper, in the process of helping, may work out some aspect of his or her own difficulty, obtain new perspectives, and get a renewed sense of self-adequacy from discovering the capacity to help someone else. Self-help is a first step; the individual becomes aware of the problem and then tries to do something about it. Once the individual engages someone else in sharing experiences, in an exchange, then it becomes mutual help. A mutual-help organization limits its membership to individuals with a designated common problem and their purpose in coming together is to offer one another help and guidance in solving their common problems or mutual predicaments:

> "You alone can do it, but you cannot do it alone" is an often-quoted saying in the literature on self help and mutual aid … and produces a special form of interdependence in which the individual accepts self-responsibility within a context of mutual aid—that is giving help to others and receiving help from others.'
>
> (Borkman 1999, p. 196)

Informal mutual exchanges go on all the time, as people discover in each other common experiences that until that moment they may have believed were theirs alone. When informal encounters develop into formal clubs or organizations, it may occur because people in the group sense they have a mission to extend their discovery to others like them. The literature on mutual help and bereavement tells us more about the formal encounters. However, as we talk of promoting competence in many ways it is the informal encounters that need to be encouraged and that are the major influence on the way a community responds to grief and is helpful to the bereaved.

When a group becomes formalized, in order to maintain its character as a mutual-help organization, it must develop a sustainable organizational structure, with officers, a governing body and procedures for continuity (Silverman 1980; Madera 2000). The members determine policy and control resources, and they are also both providers and recipients of service. Mutual-help organizations must be distinguished from such voluntary philanthropic organizations as the American Cancer Society, where volunteers usually join in order to help others, not to solve a common problem. Yet in a hospice volunteer programme the volunteer may bring their own experience of loss to their work. In this sense such programmes can be seen as a mutual-help experience if volunteers are encouraged to use their own experience to inform their work. The Widow-to-Widow Program (Silverman 2004) in which widowed helpers reached out to the newly widowed in their community, was developed by me as a professional. However, the widowed helpers used their own experience as the basis of help and as the basis for educating me about widowhood.

They helped me understand how little I knew and how much they had to teach me from their life experience.

Accessibility to the web has changed the way people approach problems or periods of transition in their lives and how services are located to suit a particular need (Madera and White 1997; Colin 2004). It is a new way of finding each other. In an internet search of resources in the United States, two kinds of programmes appear. One is chat lines where people with similar problems can sign on and engage in an ongoing exchange with others like themselves. A good example of this is the Young Widow chat line. An online approach also makes available help for parents, for example, who have lost their only child or for grandparents whose grandchild died. The other programmes that appear are mutual help or self-help organizations such as Compassionate Friends, Mothers Against Drunk Driving, and To live Again that have local chapters where members come together on a regular basis to meet their needs and to participate in the organization's various programmes and activities. These organizations have survived over the years with new members joining as the need arises, giving new life to the organization. Organizations with a national office are more likely to survive as this office gives direction and support to local chapters. A professional organization such as the American Association of Suicidology provides information on support groups for surviving family members, helping them find a group in their own community. They have available a manual on starting self-help groups. The internet also allows people to cross national boundaries and people from all parts of the world can connect and learn from each other.

Learning is made much easier when the teacher is someone with whom you share the same experience that can provide you with a new and empowering perspective on what you can do for yourself. We must keep in mind that I am not talking about people coping by themselves, but with help from family members, their friends and their community in a caring world where people are committed to help and care for each other. Dealing with the death of someone we care about will never be easy, but with appropriate information and resources we can cope and prevail. I have suggested that a variation on a public health theme may lead to greater resilience in how people deal with their grief. I hypothesize that a different use of language could lead to a population of people being helped to cope more competently, empowering them to act on their own behalf in a manner that also supports mourners' ability to help each other.

References

Anderson R (1974) Notes of a survivor. In: *The Patient, Death and the Family*, pp. 73–82 (eds Troup SB, Green WA). New York: Scribners.

Borkman T (1976) Experiential knowledge: a concept for analysis of self help groups. *Social Science Review* **50**, 445–456.

Borkman T (1999) *Understanding Self Help/Mutual Aid: experiential learning in the commons.* Camden, NJ: Rutgers University Press.

Colin Y (2004) Technology-based groups and end of life in social work practice. In: *Living with Dying: Handbook for end of life health care practitioners*, pp. 534–547 (eds Berzoff J, Silverman PR). New York: Columbia University Press.

Etzioni A (2006) *Times* Editorial Page *New York* **10 October**, A27.

Farber S, Egnew T, Farber A (2004) What is a respectful death? In: *Living with Dying: Handbook for end of life health care practitioners*, pp. 102–127 (eds Berzoff J, Silverman PR). New York: Columbia University Press.

Foreman J (2007) When doctor's news is bad, give the crisis its due. *Boston Globe,* January 22, c1&c3.

Friedson E (1970) Dominant professions, bureaucracy, and client services. In: *Organizations and Clients*, (eds Rosengren W, Lefton M). Columbus, OH: Merrill.

Horowitz M (2007) Mediating on complicated grief disorders as a diagnosis. *Omega Journal of Death and Dying* **52**, 87–89.

Machin L (2003) Research in practice. In: *Loss, Change and Bereavement in Palliative Care.* pp. 38–52 (eds Firth P, Luff G, Oliviere D). Berkshire: Open University Press.

Madera E, White BT (1997) On-line mutual support; The experience of a self- help clearing house. *Information and Referral* **19**, 91–107.

McKnight J (1995) *The Careless Society.* New York: Basic Books.

Normand CL, Silverman PR, Nickman SL (1996) *Continuing Bonds: New Understandings of Grief*, pp. 87–111 (eds Klass D, Silverman PR, Nickman SL). Bristol, PA: Taylor & Francis.

Nickman SL, Silverman PR, Normand CL (1998) Children's construction of a deceased parent: the surviving parent's contribution. *Journal of Orthopsychiatry* **68**, 126–134.

Parkes CM (2006) Symposium on Complicated Grief. *Omega Journal of Death and Dying.* New York: Baywood Publishing Co.

Pettus A (2006) Psychiatry by prescription. *Harvard Magazine* **July–August**, 38–42, 89–92.

Prigerson HG, Maciejewski P (2006) A call for sound empirical testing and evaluation of criteria for complicated grief proposed for DSM V *Omega, Journal of Death and Dying* **52**, 9–19.

Rowling JK (1999) *The Prisoner of Azkaban.* New York: Scholastic.

Silverman PR (1980) *Mutual Help Groups: organization and development.* Beverly Hills, CA: Sage.

Silverman PR (1988) In search of new selves: accommodating to widowhood. In: *Families in Transition: Primary Programs that Work*, pp. 200–219 (eds Bond LA, Wagner B). Newbury Park, CA: Sage Publications.

Silverman PR (2000) *Never Too Young to Know: Death in children's lives.* New York: Oxford University Press.

Silverman PR (2004) *Widow-to-widow: How the bereaved help each other*, 2nd edn. New York: Rutledge.

Silverman PR, Klass D (1996) Introduction: What's the problem? In: *Continuing Bonds: New Understandings of Grief*, pp. 3–27 (eds Klass D, Silverman PR, Nickman SL). Bristol, PA: Taylor & Francis.

Silverman PR, Nickman SL (1996) Children's construction of their dead parent. In: *Continuing Bonds: New Understandings of Grief*, pp. 73–86 (eds Klass D, Silverman PR, Nickman SL). Bristol, PA: Taylor & Francis.

Silverman PR, Worden JW (1993) Children's reactions to the death of a parent. In: *Handbook of Bereavement*, pp. 300–316 (eds Stroebe M, Stroebe W, Hansson RO). Cambridge: Cambridge University Press.

Silverman PR, Nickman SL, Worden JW (1992) Detachment revisited: children's construction of their deceased parent. *American Journal of Orthopsychiatry* **62**(4), 494–503.

Stroebe M, Schut H (1999) The dual process mode of coping with bereavement. *Death Studies* **23**, 197–224.

Stroebe M, Schut H (2006) Complicated grief: a conceptual analysis of the field. *Omega Journal of Death and Dying*, pp. 53–70. New York: Baywood Publishing Co.

Walter T (2006) What is complicated grief? A social constructionist perspective. *Omega Journal of Death and Dying*, pp. 71–80. New York: Baywood Publishing Co.

White M (1988) Saying Hello Again: The Incorporation of the lost relationship in the resolution of grief. *Dulwidge Centre Newsletter*. Adelaide, Australia.

Resilient multiprofessional teams

Malcolm Payne

Introduction: resilience and teamwork

Palliative care works through multiprofessional teams to provide a holistic service to dying and bereaved people in their families and social networks. Multiprofessional teamwork tries to respond to the whole range of issues that people needing the service might face and brings to bear a wide range of expertise and knowledge. While there is evidence that this is more effective than other ways of providing the service, no one model of the membership and organization of the teams is supported by research (Gysels and Higginson 2004). Because, as a healthcare specialism, palliative care has sought to bring together different professions to respond to a wide range of issues that require engagement from many different points of view, multiprofessional teamwork has always been a particular concern within palliative care practice particularly in bringing forward psychosocial and spiritual issues (Sheldon 1997; Sykes *et al.* 2004; Speck 2006). In health and social care services generally, teamwork is a widely used way of working (Payne 2000; Borrill *et al.* 2001). How might ideas about resilience be relevant to multiprofessional teamwork in palliative care?

Multiprofessional teamwork might strengthen resilience in health and social care organizations providing palliative care and might itself be strengthened by greater resilience. There are three potential contributions:

- multiprofessional teamwork might help health and social care organizations be more resilient;
- it might help individuals in the teams or elsewhere in the organization to be more resilient, 'the protective veneer to the stress of work' as a respondent in a study of mental health teams put it (Edward 2005, p. 146);
- it might help the teams themselves be more resilient.

Fraser *et al.* (1999, p. 136) usefully define resilience as '… unpredicted and markedly successful adaptations to negative life events, trauma, stress, and other forms of risk'. This analysis points up that we only talk about resilience when people do better than expected at responding to adversity, or to the risk of adversity. We do not refer to resilience when people react in a negative way to adversity. Ideas about resilience, therefore, assume that there will necessarily be adversities in people's lives; that things will not always go well. Resilience assumes a norm of reaction that some people, whom we see as resilient, will improve upon.

The idea of resilience derives from attachment theory, which in turn comes from psychoanalytic ideas. Attachment therefore reflects the focus of psycho-analysis on the interaction of people's internal emotional responses and external experiences and on the impact of earlier on later experiences (Bower 2005). Emotions are the way our bodies, brains, and minds react when aroused by external events that have meaning for us (Howe 2005, p. 11). Attachment theory assumes that in close relationships, we 'mentalize' other people's behaviour; that is, we respond to how they behave according to our assumptions about their mental state. We base our assessment of their mental state on our previous experience, particularly with our parents and other people emotionally important to us, of how close relationships (attachments) work (Howe 2005).

Resilience and attachment theory are bodies of ideas about human development and behaviour, often used for therapeutic purposes. They have rarely been directly applied to teamwork or multiprofessional practice and the suggestion that teamwork enhances resilience or resilience enhances teamwork is often discussed in a common sense rather than theoretically informed way. However, with a proviso, this account of the main theoretical principles shows how resilience ideas might be relevant to multiprofessional teamwork, perhaps particularly in palliative care. Multiprofessional teams are situations in which people work together in continuing relationships, and in palliative care some of these relationships will involve intense emotions around the experience of death and bereavement. It is therefore possible that they will be affected by past experience of close relationships. Teamwork often involves mentalizing the reactions of other team members to events, so the attachment approach may be helpful in analysing how people behave towards each other. The major caution about applying this approach is that transferring a therapeutic psychological theory to analysis of social relations in practical teamwork in health and social care organizations is not supported by directly relevant research. In this chapter, I use ideas and analogies from work on resilience and attachment to enrich ideas about multiprofessional teamwork, rather than assuming that the research on attachment and resilience is directly applicable.

Teamwork and identity

Multiprofessional teamwork raises questions and tensions about identity, which I place at the centre of understanding resilience in multiprofessional teams.

Identity is the set of characteristics that make us like other people. Looking at people's identity involves understanding what characteristics they share with others and how that sharing takes place. Nobody, even twins who are genetically identical, is completely the same as another person; we all have social experiences that make us different from others. However, we develop our own characteristics through differentiating ourselves from and modelling ourselves on others in our social relationships. From babyhood onwards, we look at others and say 'I don't want to be like that', or 'I should like to be more like them.' Identity is thus socially constructed from our experiences of others. Our identities make us part of, that is identity attaches us to, collectivities of other people, because we may see ourselves as like them, or they may see themselves as like us. This of course means that identity may exclude us from, as well as attach us to, participation in other groups. Thus, we may be part of a family, a community within a neighbourhood, or a faith group or our attachments may exclude us from groups. For example, a Muslim is not usually considered part of a Christian faith group. However, such identities may be complex. For example, a Muslim may prefer to be cared for in a Christian hospice that recognizes the importance of faith, rather than not cared for at all, or being cared for in an avowedly humanist or atheist organization. Identities may be even more complex. For example, do we become member of our spouse's family in marriage? Do we lose that identity on divorce, when children may keep the families in touch? The answer to these questions depends, among other things, on our culture, cultural expectations and views of the families involved and personal preferences and might vary over time. Therefore, understanding peoples' identities involves complex social perceptions. Recent research on identity often focuses on social categories, such as social class, nationality, ethnicity, or gender (Alcoff and Mendieta 2004). It is clear that attachment to some social identities, for example a particular gender, faith, or nationality, may limit or help us in attachments to other identities.

We take parts of our identities from our attachments to work groups such as professions, organizations, or teams. Through involvement in such groups we develop a commitment to that collectivity of people—a feeling that our membership of that group has meaning for us and that this feeling is reciprocated in some ways by them. However, these identities may be in conflict with one another. For example, meeting the financial restrictions to keep an employing organization going may conflict with professional commitments, if we have to cut corners in our practice, or personal loyalty to team members, if some have to be made redundant for example. Also sometimes our personal, family, or community commitments may conflict with work identities; commitment to the team or professional role may get in the way of our family or social life, for example. Work-life balance is a common issue for people in employment.

In multiprofessional teamwork, two important identities, professional identity and our work group or team identity may be in tension. The aim of a multiprofessional team is to bring together people who get part of their identity from different professional groups with different intellectual and academic disciplines. The team aims to get them to work together to provide a coherent service to individual patients. Coherent service may mean changing professional practice so that it fits in with the knowledge and practice of other team members; their knowledge or approach to the situation may also be in tension. For example, a difference is sometimes drawn between a social model of disability, where disability is considered to come from social failures in accommodating the special needs of disabled people, and a medical model, which may see some disabilities as deficits in capacity to deal with a world that is assumed to be 'normal'. A doctor and a social worker might therefore take a different view of appropriate actions to respond to a person with disability.

Teamwork may bring such professional and disciplinary conflicts to the surface, so that they may be appropriately negotiated and resolved. Suppressing conflicts may store up trouble and resentment or prevent team members from being fully engaged in resolving difficult issues. However, team members can plan for how and when to raise issues, because at any particular time there may be other priorities, or because conflict resolution can be best achieved in a planned and positive way (Payne 2000, chapter 6). For that to be achieved, multiprofessional teamwork has to be organized thoughtfully: unsuccessful multiprofessional teamwork might increase rather than resolve tensions in between different aspects of our identities.

Adversities in palliative care multiprofessional teamwork

Resilience arises in the face of adversities. If we want teamwork to make us more resilient or resilience to improve teamwork, it is important to understand how our identities may be affected by adversities. To examine resilience in teams involves identifying what adversity is, the kinds of adversity that team members might face, and how these adversities might affect the team.

What is an adversity? Any situation that might be difficult to adapt to raises the risk of significant difficulties in adaptation for an individual, team, or organization; if the risk becomes reality and becomes an adversity this may cause an emotional reaction that increases the level of difficulty. In teamwork, an adversity is a situation that individuals, teams, or organizations may find it difficult to adapt to and that reduces the capacity of a team to facilitate and develop cooperation among its members in achieving collective and individual professional goals.

Adversities affecting an individual or team might come from any number of sources. First, adversities might come from an individual team member's psychological make-up, their home lives and their own interpersonal relationships. For example, Benita, a physiotherapist, was a strong trade union member and had conflicting relationships with managers as a trade union representative. However, she was well-regarded as an effective worker in the multiprofessional and physiotherapist teams. Many staff valued her for her supportive attitude towards individuals and her commitment to representing people in difficulties with the hospice. However, eventually this extended into sometimes hostile relationships with the physiotherapy manager, and a cynical and negative attitude to work in general, which upset some members of the multiprofessional team. They felt relieved when she left the hospice for another job. Later they discovered that, during this period of difficulty, she had been receiving treatment because she was unable to conceive a child and this had caused stress in her marriage. In this situation, adversities derived from personal life, possibly affecting her identity as a woman, may have affected her personal relationships in work. Her identity as a strong trade union activist may have 'leaked' from trade union activities, so that people have allowed their attitudes to the trade union role to affect other dealings with her. For example, the attitudes of the physiotherapy manager, who saw her initially as an effective professional, may have been affected by the hostile attitudes Benita engendered among her management colleagues. Also, Benita's anger, drawn from her trade union identity, began to affect her work identity. It is also possible that some of the anger felt by palliative care patients in the dying process may have connected with her own anger about difficulty in having children, her marital relationship, and her hostile relationships with managers. Perhaps the response came partly from conflicting gender identities: from dislike of working with a strong rather than pliant woman. From these examples, we can see that emotional reactions to various adversities may interact with each other and affect parts of our lives that are distant from the source of adversity.

Teams or work groups might also produce adversities. This might include the multiprofessional team and the individual's own professional group within the organization. For example, by agreement with a Primary Care Trust (PCT), the commissioner of local community services, a hospice's procedures provided for ward nurses to assess patients' suitability for funding for continuing NHS care in the community, enabling them to have care at home fully paid for. The arrangements for discharge were set out in a folder of information. A ward nurse, under pressure from a patient's relatives to help her return home quickly, helped them reinstate and improve a pre-existing package of care services. Nurses and the relatives saw this as flexible and responsive, responding to their identity as caring people. However, the consultant palliative care physician felt that it presented him with a *fait accompli* when he came to consider whether a discharge was appropriate. From his point of view, it questioned his identity as a decision-maker, and also his feeling of high status as a doctor, a senior member of the team, and his feeling of personal medical responsibility for the patients, even though he saw them less and was not seen by the patient's relatives as so personally close as the nurses. Because the procedure for getting funding was not followed through, the PCT commissioner also felt dragooned into agreeing to funding, and the social worker subsequently felt that making exceptional arrangements for future patients became more difficult as a result. So, this apparently helpful act, put several team members in a more adverse situation, and a link with an outside organization was also strained. A caring act, responding to nurses' self-identities, cut across the self-identities of the doctor, who felt he held overall responsibility, the social worker as the team member who usually took responsibility for connections with outside organizations, and the PCT commissioner's feeling of responsibility for control of the budget.

The organizations and wider society might generate adversities affecting the team and its members. This might include:

◆ The organization, for example the staff and managers in a hospice, community health service, or hospital. An independent charitable hospice may be experienced as a less-secure workplace that the National Health Service, or offering less opportunity for promotion and a variety of job experience than a hospital palliative care team. On the other hand, it may engage stronger personal commitment to its traditions and objectives.

◆ The health and social care system, including policy-makers and managers. For example, a social worker put a great deal of time helping a distant relative with learning disabilities have a good experience of the death of his aunt in the hospice. Healthcare colleagues felt he neglected the immediate need of the patient to return home. However, social work objectives include strengthening the capacity of weaker members of the family through the present experience so that they can deal with future adversity. The relative with learning disabilities was a high priority to the social worker because he would gain most future stability from a good experience with this death, and had a lot to lose, while other members of the family were not a risk for bereavement difficulties. This difference in priorities needed to be examined and understood more widely in the team. Although it was initially seen as a fairly harmless personal preference, similar decisions pursued over time without full understanding might have led to weakened relationships with the social worker. Discussing it also led to a debate about ethical priorities in long-term and shorter-term objectives, and the tension between patients' needs and family needs. This increased team members' understanding of the practical consequences of palliative care policy to care for both patients and families.

♦ Wider society, including the local community, wider ideas about what is good health and social solidarity, and socio-cultural and political ideas, such as concern about, for example, immigration or gender issues. For example, Benita's anger may also have connected with her ethnic minority identity, a shared experience with other women that they are often oppressed in social and marital relationships, in receiving healthcare, in achieving professional advancement and in employment generally.

Finally, many patients have a great deal of adversity in their lives and so may transfer that adversity into the team or its members. For example, Gary, a lorry driver experienced a rapid onset of stomach cancer after a difficult period in his life. His marriage had broken down in acrimony after his daughter had accused him of sexual abuse in her childhood, although this was unproven, and he had begun living alone in poor-quality housing alongside other isolated men. There was a good deal of drinking, and until his illness Gary had been the only man in the house with a job. When he was admitted as an inpatient, his wife and daughter refused to visit, and the reason for this refusal became known in the team. Another ill-kempt man from his house spent a lot of time at the hospice and was experienced as aggressive and sometimes under the influence of alcohol. This was very difficult for female nurses to manage, and at times it connected with their feelings about the patient as a possible abuser. The behavioural difficulties thus connected to gender identities and beliefs about how families should work: some team members felt that the women members of the family should rally round and prepare to deal with their feelings of anger and loss in bereavement, while others felt solidarity with anger about sexual abuse.

As well as the *source* of adversities, it is also important to examine the *process* by which they affect teams. Because a team consists of individuals, one person often experiences them first, and their response then affects other team members. Thus, adversities *flow* through a team, as they do through a family (Greene and Livingston 2002, p. 65). This is sometimes because work flows through a team: Øvretveit (1993) characterizes health and social care work as the progression of a service user through a pathway, in which there are gateways, where decisions are made and patients' pathways may diverge. For example, Gary's difficulties were dealt with mainly by the nursing team, referring to the ward doctor, until they were reviewed at the multiprofessional team meeting, when the social worker and consultant palliative care physician became involved: not all patients would engage the social worker.

The flow of work is often the conduit of adversity because as work passes between team members, it generates different emotional reactions and engages different identities. In Gary's case, the adversity was most strongly felt by nurses as a personal emotional experience. Doctors and the social worker, less frequently involved in day-to-day interactions on the ward, and as men, were less emotionally engaged in rejection of the lifestyle of the men and the fear of the risk of sexual abuse. Thus, gender identity and direct involvement with the patient produced particular feelings for nurses, which flowed towards the doctors and social worker who had to provide additional support and discussion with nurses. The team usefully provided support for the nurses, which would not have been available if the patient had been cared for at home. The home environment might also have been more stressful for nurses to work in than the inpatient unit, because of a mismatch between gender identities among the men sharing the house and the visiting women nurses.

Adversity may be heightened or reduced by a range of factors as adversities flow through teams in this way. One factor may be ethical issues, which often affect teams (Wilmot 1997, chapter 5). In Gary's case, various risks were present, which some team members felt strongly about: the possibility of sexual abuse, the possibility of disorder in the inpatient unit because of alcohol abuse and an associated risk of feared violence towards staff. Among the ethical factors that needed resolution in the team were the balance between the safety of staff and the provision of support to patients in need, consideration of the right of a patient to treatment, in spite of the stigma of possible involvement in a crime that had not been proved against him. There may also have been a question of gender stereotypes about the possibilities of violence from men with alcohol problems, and of discrimination on grounds of socio-economic class.

What this case draws attention to is the value of being able to use the team to reduce the difficulties that both adversity and to the risk of adversities might generate. A useful way of understanding this is to see teams as mediating the impact of adversities on team members, the team and the organization in a variety of different ways as they flow through the team. There are two elements of teamwork that might achieve this:

- ◆ establishing a team environment and practice that would engage commitment to mediating adversities;
- ◆ managing team processes so as to bring adversities to the surface and permit them to be dealt with.

Team environment

A resilient team environment is one that respects and responds to the differing identities of team members. Palliative care teams, like many teams in health and social care, are based around professional practices involving discretion and skill. Therefore, there is often an assumption that the main issue in developing multiprofessional teamwork is to deal with issues that arise between *professional* identities. However, because, as we have seen, adversities interact with each other and may come from sources outside professional practice with service users, many other identities may also be relevant in generating and responding to adversities. Professional identity thus introduces complexities to teamwork issues, and organizational identity and teamwork often raises special difficulties for professional practice. The two areas interact, and both need to be considered.

Among these issues that differing professional identities in multiprofessional teams may raise are:

♦ different perspectives and values, which may not be understood or respected;

♦ multiple lines of accountability;

♦ differing legal responsibilities;

♦ conflicting budgetary responsibilities (Martin and Henderson 2001, pp. 97–98).

Some of these issues arose in the various case situations discussed above about adversities. For example, different professionals reveal different perspectives and values in the cases, and legal and budgetary responsibility also varies, for example between the palliative care team and the commissioner in the case of difficulties about discharge. Research in health and social care teamwork has also identified such issues. For example, McGrath's (1991) research in the 1980s in multiprofessional learning disabilities teams identified, as organizational adversities, different lines of accountability and budgetary conflicts. Some staff were responsible to local authority social services departments, others reported to local health authorities and local agreement on professional decisions about patients was sometimes vitiated by disagreements among more senior staff about whose budget paid for what.

The management literature on teamwork suggests a range of factors that promote effective team working. These include achieving agreement about a clear shared purpose and clear definition of roles, creating a sense of belonging, creating an open, participative, informal atmosphere, having sound procedures and regular reviews of practice and work, having good external links supporting individuals' professional development and encouraging creativity (Payne 2002, chapter 2). This general literature is supported and focused by a range of studies in health and social care. For example, Borrill *et al.* (2001) found in a major study of a range of healthcare teams, but not including palliative care teams, that four characteristics mark successful teams:

♦ clear objectives

♦ high participation

- commitment to quality, and
- support of innovation.

Similarly, Onyett (2003), reviewing research and practice literature on mental health teams, identifies a range of interventions that provide support to staff, including:

- promoting clarity of role
- creating manageable workloads
- minimizing paperwork
- maintaining physical safety
- promoting interpersonal contact between team members
- sensitivity to gender issues
- autonomy to control work and exercise professional discretion
- promoting effective leadership
- helping people achieve a personal focus for their work
- organizing peer consultation to share expertise
- making team meetings work well.

Some resilience factors for multiprofessional teams can be connected with this literature. Shared objectives and effective leadership provide a clear context within which team members may position their professional identity and gain incorporation for their identity within the shared identity. A flexible, open and sharing atmosphere, peer consultation and effective team meetings allow team members to negotiate openly uncertainties and conflicts about their professional identity within the team. Opportunities to continue personal professional development also maintain and support professional identity within the shared team identity.

A resilient environment for multiprofessional teamwork, therefore, involves both individual and group factors. A resilient team environment aims to achieve frequent interaction among team members, sense of stability and continuity, mutual support and concern, and freedom from chronic conflict (Baumeister and Leary 1995, cited by West 2004, p. 155). The importance of sharing and working together to achieve such a climate does not negate the importance of individual professional responsibilities and development.

However, the importance of sharing aims and work raises questions. Why would people agree to cooperate and share knowledge? Government policy and the teamwork literature assumes that collaboration is a good thing, but this cannot be taken for granted. Hislop (2005) reviews a range of management studies that identify some of the factors that affect people's willingness to share knowledge. One factor is the nature of the knowledge used, particularly where much of it is tacit, personal, or embodied in the people carrying it. For example, it is possible to write down much of the medical knowledge about constipation, an important side-effect of opiate drugs, but it is not easy to convey the skills of getting patients to understand and discuss changes in bowel movements and examining faeces to identify significant factors about the patient's condition.

There are also a range of management and organizational factors such as:

- The existence of intergroup and interpersonal conflict.
- Concerns over the effect of sharing on status and recognition of expertise.
- A sense that organizational processes are fair and equitable.
- Interpersonal trust, the belief that it is likely people will honour their obligations rather than acting opportunistically. In relationships, trust is based on reciprocity or mutual benefit.
- Explicit organizational commitment.
- General organizational culture.
- Reward and recognition for collaboration.
- The visibility of knowledge, attitudes, and values about sharing in senior levels of the organization (Hislop 2005, p. 50).

Most important, adverse personal experience in the organization may conflict with a rhetoric of collaboration. We can see this in the impact of New Labour government managerialist policies in the UK, executed through its modernization agendas. For example, there were claims to establish a modernized education system with collegiate working and partnership with parents. However, this was experienced by teachers as coercion through 'managed consent', with changes imposed with a semblance of consultation. This led to bitterness and inward-looking self-interest among teachers rather than active cooperation (Ozga 2000). In the NHS, attempts to set numerical and financial targets and payment by results is experienced by some professionals as a coercive rather than respectful management regime (Waine 2000). More widely, in several industrial settings, some forms of teamwork have been used to increase the pace and pressure of work by promoting participation in decision-making. Research into these settings has shown that this participation took place within competition between teams, and limitations and targets imposed by managers. Team leader roles were used to reduce the influence of employee-led representative organizations such as trade unions and reorganizations were used to select employees carefully so that people were likely to be among the more cooperative personnel. Nevertheless, the mutual support and even limited participation through such participative structures was appealing to team members (Buchanan and Huczynski 2004, pp. 405–406). All this work tells us that participative organizations using teamwork may achieve greater productivity and effectiveness, and some aspects of participation may be improved. However, the way that this is done is important: employees will be aware of and may react against approaches to teamwork that exploit their goodwill or manipulate them, and this will lead to a decrease rather than increase in resilience.

Sharing and cooperation cannot therefore be taken for granted. Team members may in principle agree that such an approach to practice is useful, but how it is implemented in the organization, or the personal effects of implementing sharing on individuals may obstruct teamwork. One of the most important conceptions for developing resilience may be the 'community of practice' (Wenger 1998). This assumes that, rather than cooperating by adjusting or negotiating the boundaries of established professional identities, the multiprofessional team shares common knowledge, overlapping values and a shared identity as a team: this creates resilience by focusing on factors that contribute to the shared identity of the team, rather than demanding clarity of external identities, such as professional or organizational identities. Thus, while doctors may maintain clear individual professional roles and responsibilities for, for example, prescription of medication, other team members share some of that knowledge and act cooperatively. So nurses, in addition to being in some circumstances prescribers themselves, also take responsibilities for deciding when discretionary medication should be used, for breakthrough pain for example, using shared knowledge about the effects of medication, but a different professional role. Both professional groups see themselves as working for the holistic care and, in this case, pain control objectives of palliative care, and share the identity of working in a team serving patients on a ward.

By working together in this way, the members of a community of practice develop through shared learning, a way of working that is unique to them. Thus, the organization's procedures and policies are interpreted and refined in shared ways that begin to diverge from standard practices. The team, the organization, and individual team members gain resilience from greater flexibility because it is reciprocal. The response to flexibility in one part of the organization, may be flexibility in others. However, as we have seen, many adversities within the organization may reduce that flexible response, so the team processes also need to be able to deal with failures in the environment.

Team processes

A resilient team environment, therefore, may support or inhibit individual resilience through flexibility, shared learning and shared values in a community of practice: that is what a multiprofessional team is. How the team processes its work, using multiprofessional knowledge, skills and understanding affects the impact of adversities and resilience on individual members.

For example, marital difficulties between a man with prostate cancer and his wife led to a complex rehearsal of marital conflicts over more than 40 years, and a home care community nurse specialist found it hard to break into a cycle of blaming and anger, which was leading to considerable distress. However, her experience when working with the team social worker in other situations allowed her to identify some of the communication difficulties that the patient and his wife were having as something that the social worker could tackle. In a joint interview, the social worker took control of the interactions and interrupted the cycle of dysfunctional communication, requiring only one person to speak at a time, and reducing the complexity of all the issues included in each communication. This allowed some progress to be made, but the nurse, while she could see that this was required, did not have the confidence in making the psychosocial intervention in such a firm way. In this situation, the shared understanding of what was possible enabled her to call the social worker in and convince the couple that the social worker could help, but she also recognized the need for the expert skill of the social worker in relationship work. Thus, multiprofessional shared identity together with separate professional skills and identity were facilitated by the teamwork. The learning the nurse gained from the joint interview gave her greater confidence in the social worker's ability to intervene in these situations and broader understanding of the capacities of social work, which also strengthened team functioning in the future. This is how a community of practice allows separate objectives and skills while at the same time strengthening sharing and permitting flexible movement between shared work and separate work.

Resilience functions in the same way as adversities: it is not one thing that is possessed or not possessed, rather it flows through the team in response to the situations that it faces. Team members trade off various aspects of their professional understanding to mediate the adversities that affect them and others. In this case, the marital conflict was an adversity for the nurse, which by her intervention, the social worker mediated from affecting the team. Team members may assess the level of risk that adversities raise for individuals and the team by thinking about the degree of disruption to people's identities. In this case, the nurse's identity as a competent manager of the case was at risk, and the availability of a social worker in the team gave it a collective identity that could help. The intervention enhanced both the social worker's identity within the team as a specialist professional, and the team's collective identity as a group that could respond to unusual and difficult situations. Usually team members assess threats to identity fairly informally and through everyday adjustments to team functioning (Payne 2006).

Various factors facilitate the flow of resilience from one team member to another, as they mediate adversity. Opie's (2003) study of a variety of social care teams focuses on how teams process knowledge and information. Her study shows that effective teamwork aims to facilitate people in expressing to others and contributing to the joint work their own knowledge and skills. In working with patients and families, each professional group contributes their own objectives, to be added to and integrated into shared team objectives. A physiotherapist, for example, may have rehabilitation objectives, a social worker might aim to help the family plan for future care for the children, a nurse may aim to support a spouse in managing difficult symptoms, and a doctor directly manage pain control. They may share agreed objectives about the integration of these separate aims into an overall plan for supporting a family and their family member who is a palliative care patient.

Other aspects of teamwork that help to mediate adversity are the effective shared management of participation, workload, status differentials and identity conflicts around ethnicity, gender, sexuality, and nationality. All these have been discussed above as potential adversities arising from the organization and the team and from wider society.

Qualitative research in a number of healthcare settings identifies other factors that may make team processes more resilient and may apply to palliative care teams. Pollock *et al.* (2003), discussing responses to mass emergencies, argue that resilience may be fostered in preparation for events, during them as they affect the team, and afterwards. Therefore, first, prediction and building up recorded experience of the types of event that the team may have to deal with can be useful. Review of difficult situations, recording and identifying their characteristics and what strategies were successful in dealing with them may therefore be a useful approach. This codifies, for future anticipatory planning, what has been achieved in responding to the present event. Resilient teams in this setting established systems for the delegation of tasks, seeking second opinions and alternative views to the team member dealing with a situation, and planning and debating plans and actions from a variety of points of view. Bradley *et al.* (2006) examined emergency heart treatment and found that resilience was improved by an organizational culture that established clear aims for improvement and in which teams worked to identify explicitly challenges or setbacks in achieving them, which could then be overcome. Altman Dautoff (2002) identified various factors that particularly contributed to resilience in transient teams set up to achieve a short-term project, compared with other factors that did not. These were: flexibility, confidence to solve particular problems, support for shared purposes, and efficient use of organizational resources. She proposes that an effective strategy to create a more resilient organizational environment includes building individual flexibility and confidence together with the active involvement in the team of 'sponsors' of particular changes or services, so that they are aware of difficulties and can deliver organizational resources to support the objective.

Teamwork often involves a tension between the organizational objective of achieving more effective and integrated services and team members' personal objectives in having interpersonal support from their colleagues. The starting point of support is awareness and responsiveness and this is a significant element of the resilience of a team. As identity issues are crucial elements in adversity, resilience requires systems within the team to evaluate adversities and their impact on identities within the team, and on the identities of the team and organization within health and social care services. Awareness of risk to identity is a crucial element of the support that teamwork offers through its community of practice.

West (2004, pp. 158–163) identifies three different aspects of support in teamwork:

- social support, including emotional, informational, instrumental, and appraisal support;
- social climate, and
- support for individual team members' growth and development.

Emotional support means being an active, open listener when another team member has experienced strong emotions and threats to their identity. It involves stopping what you are doing, listening to the team member's story of what happened, and being prepared to accept the emotional reaction to it. Informational support means being prepared to share information about how you did something, or that will help a colleague achieve something, and not expecting credit or thanks. Instrumental support means seeing that a colleague has a pile of work, and offering to take over some of her phone calls. Appraisal support means being prepared to help a colleague talk through and look at the alternative interpretations of a difficult situation.

It helps personal resilience to recognize how these issues may interfere with a colleague's identity as a competent professional in a palliative care team. An intimidating relative or pressure of work or a struggle to understand a complex situation can damage our sense of competence and our perception that we have a contribution to make. In a team meeting, recognizing how a situation or a verbal exchange may have threatened a colleague's professional or personal identity can help us to be flexible. For example, a patient's relative rang a manager to ask a palliative care team to arrange that 'that black woman' should not visit again. This is an attack on a colleague's ethnic and possibly gender identity, and perhaps also on their professional identity, as it is being implied that a person of that ethnicity and gender cannot provide a suitable service. However, the request may reflect a genuine difficulty of poor quality work or in the relationship with a perhaps elderly patient who is unaccustomed to having people of another ethnicity in her house. The deathbed is not always the best place to change people's social attitudes: other things are more important. Nevertheless, the manager will need to consider how to respond to the relative in a way that maintains respect for all staff, and work out a way of interacting with the worker and the team. Within the team, team members demonstrating that they prepared to engage with the emotions generated by such an event, the team leader's difficulties in discussing such a complex issue, and the worker's feelings, which may raise long-standing experiences of discrimination and oppression. Trying to understand and respond to especially difficult personal experiences is an important part of resilient teamwork.

Conclusions

Achieving resilient multiprofessional teamwork in palliative care means raising awareness and understanding of how organizations, teams, and the individuals within them can respond effectively to adversities. Adversities may come from wider society, from the organization, team, and individual themselves and from the people whom the service serves. The crucial element of adversities in teamwork is their effect on personal, professional, team, and organizational identity. The emphasis of resilience and attachment theory on emotional responses based in previous relationships draws attention to the importance of dealing with team members' emotional reactions to adversities. This is so because the main purpose of multiprofessional teamwork is to facilitate more effective and co-ordinated holistic services to patients and their families. This means bringing together workers with their different personal and professional identities in a way that incorporates those identities into a team, organizational, and service identity. Resilient teamwork requires tensions between different identities to be dealt with in a planned and consistent way.

A multiprofessional team may achieve greater resilience by creating an environment that strengthens capacity to be flexible and responsive to threats to its members personal and professional identities. It is this that allows one team to be more resilient than another. The fact that adversities and resilience flow through a team, suggests that the way that teams process information, work, communication, participation, and various aspects of identity is the crucial factor. A focus on processing these aspects of teamwork allows the potential resilience generated by the team environment to strengthen team members' capacities to help each other respond effectively to adversities. In this way, a team's potential resilience may generate actual resilience through multiprofessional teamwork.

References

Alcoff LM, Mendieta E (eds) (2003) *Identities: Race, Class, Gender and Nationality.* Malden, MA: Blackwells.

Altman Dautoff DC (2002) Exploring individual and organizational resilience as factors in effective transient work teams. *Dissertation Abstracts International Section A: Humanities and Social Sciences* **62**(11-A), 3847.

Baumeister RF, Leary MR (1995) The need to belong … *Psychological Bulletin* **117**, 497–429.

Borrill CS, Carletta J, Carter CS, Dawson JF, Garrod S, Rees A, Richards A, Shapiro D, West MA (2001) *The Effectiveness of Health Care Teams in the National Health Service.* http://homepages.inf.ed.ac.uk/jeanc/DOH-final-report.pdf.

Bower M (2005) Psychoanalytic theories for social work practice. In: *Psychoanalytic Theory for Social Work Practice: Thinking Under Fire*, pp. 3–14 (ed. Bower M). London: Routledge.

Bradley EH, Curry LA, Webster TR, Mattera JA, Roumanis SA, Radford MJ, McNamara RL, Barton BA, Berg DN, Krumholz HM (2006) Achieving rapid door-to-balloon times: how top hospitals improve complex clinical systems. *Circulation* **113**, 1079–1085.

Buchanan D, Huczynski A (2004) *Organizational behaviour*, 5th edn. Harlow: Prentice-Hall.

Edward K (2005) The phenomenon of resilience in crisis care mental health clinicians *International Journal of Mental Health Nursing* **14**(2), 142–148.

Fraser MW, Richman JM, Galinsky MJ (1999) Risk, protection, and resilience: toward a conceptual framework for social work practice. *Social Work Research* **23**, 129–208.

Greene RR, Livingston NC (2002) A social construct. In: *Resiliency: An Integrated Approach to Practice, Policy, and Research*, pp. 63–93 (ed. Greene RR). Washington DC: NASW Press.

Gysels M, Higginson I (2004) *Improving Supportive and Palliative Care for Adults with Cancer: Research Evidence.* London: National Institute for Clinical Excellence.

Hislop D (2005) *Knowledge Management in Organisations: A Critical Introduction.* Oxford: Oxford University Press.

Howe D (2005) *Child Abuse and Neglect: Attachment, development and Intervention.* Basingstoke: Palgrave.

McGrath M (1991) *Multi-Disciplinary Teamwork: Community Mental Handicap Teams.* Aldershot: Avebury.

Martin V, Henderson E (2001) *Managing in Health and Social Care.* London: Routledge.

Onyett S (2003) *Teamworking in Mental Health.* Basingstoke: Palgrave Macmillan.

Opie A (2003) *Thinking Teams/Thinking Clients: Knowledge-based Teamwork.* New York: Columbia University Press.

Øvretveit J (1993) *Coordinating Community Care: Multidisciplinary Teams and Care Management.* Buckingham: Open University Press.

Ozga J (2000) Education: New Labour: new teachers. In: *New Managerialism, New Welfare?* (eds Clarke J, Gewirtz S, McLaughlin E) , pp. 222–235. London: Sage.

Payne M (2000) *Teamwork in Multiprofessional Care.* Basingstoke: Palgrave.

Payne M (2006) Teambuilding: how, why and where? In: *Teamwork in Palliative Care: Fulfilling or Frustrating?*, pp. 117–36 (ed. Speck P). Oxford: Oxford University Press.

Pollock C, Paton D, Smith LM, Violanti JM (2003) *Promoting Capabilities to Manage Posttraumatic Stress: Perspectives on Resilience.* Springfield IL: Charles C. Thomas.

Sheldon, F (1997) *Psychosocial Palliative Care: Good Practice in the Care of the Dying and Bereaved.* Cheltenham: Thornes.

Speck P (ed.) (2006) *Teamwork in Palliative Care: Fulfilling or Frustrating?* Oxford: Oxford University Press.

Sykes N, Edmonds P, Wiles J (eds) (2004) *Management of Advanced Disease* (4th edn). London: Arnold.

Waine B (2000) Managing performance through pay. In: *New Managerialism, New Welfare?*, pp. 236–249 (eds Clarke J, Gewirtz S, McLaughlin E). London: Sage.

Wenger E (1998) *Communities of Practice: Learning, Meaning, and Identity.* Cambridge: Cambrige University Press.

West MA (2004) *Effective Teamwork: Practical Lessons from Organizational Research.* Oxford: BPS Blackwell.

Wilmot S (1997) *The Ethics of Community Care.* London: Cassell.

Resilient organizations: Part 1

Peter Speck

> To live is to change, and to be perfect is to have changed often
>
> *Cardinal Newman (1845)*

There are many ways in which palliative care can be provided and, as we think about the term 'Organization', we may soon realize that the specialist palliative care provider may itself be the organization. This is often the case with a free-standing hospice unit that is independent of the NHS or of a particular national charitable body. In other cases there is usually a larger organization in the background to which the specialist palliative care team relates. This larger organization may be an NHS acute Trust, a Primary Care Trust, or a large Charitable organization with many units, of which an inpatient hospice is a constituent part. The continued existence and delivery of the service will depend to a large extent on the nature of the relationships between the service providers and the organization as a whole, as well as the interactions that take place within and outside the organization. No organization or service provider exists in isolation but is part of a wider context to which it must relate.

Many chapters in this book have offered descriptions of the term 'resilience' and I shall use it in the sense of the 'capacity of an individual person or social system to grow and develop in the face of difficult circumstances' (Vanistendael 2003). Socio-economic changes in recent years have led to major changes in how people view work and their relationship with organizations. It is no longer so common for people to leave school and enter a particular organization and stay working for that firm for the rest of their working life, knowing that there is job security and a pension at the end. Many now change jobs and may have several career changes during their working life. Coupled with the real possibility of redundancy, cutbacks, loss of pension funds, and so on, there can be much uncertainty around for those in work—even within the caring professions that were often deemed to provide 'a job for life'. Resilience, at an organizational and individual level, will therefore relate to flexibility, dynamism, and responsiveness such that innovation, development, and change can be engaged with and valued in the same way that order and stability in one's working life were valued in the past (Miller 1993).

There are many ways to describe the life, work, and structure of an organization. In considering the nature of palliative care and the various ways in which it is delivered it can be helpful to view the organization as an open system that takes input from the environment and through a series of activities, transforms or converts these into outputs that fulfil a desired objective (see chapter 2, Speck 2006). Thus patients with life-threatening illness enter the system, have their symptoms and varied needs assessed, and responded to and palliated. They will eventually leave the system, in cooperation with family and community care workers, to return home or may continue in care within the system until they die. Seeing the organization as an open, rather than a closed system, implies interaction between the organization and the surrounding environment. Few organizations have a totally unified structure and so there will usually be a number of subsystems that need to be interrelated and co-ordinated if the desired outcomes are to be satisfactorily achieved. If we translate this into palliative care provision, within an inpatient unit, we can envisage a variety of departments involved within the hospice in order to provide high-quality care to patients and families: nursing, medical staff, catering, portering, physiotherapy, psychosocial–spiritual care, cleaning, administration, finance, senior management, and others. We can also appreciate that there needs to be good relationships and cooperation with the outside world: Primary Care Teams, local Trust hospitals, purchasers of services, volunteer groups in the local community, user groups, and so on. A key objective for good palliative care is that there should be a seamless service from the time of diagnosis or referral and throughout the time the patient and family are in need of palliative care. If this is to be achieved there needs to be a sufficient level of trust and respect between the people involved to enable the patient to pass from one subsystem to another, across several boundaries, without experiencing any change in the quality of care provided. This objective is one aim within the NHS Cancer Plan (Department of Health 2000) and the NICE (2004) guidance for supportive care.

In talking about the organization in terms of systems and subsystems it is important to remember that these are human organizations and contain a complex network of dynamic relationships, which need to be held in careful balance if the desired outcome of high-quality care is to be achieved. This will depend to a large extent on the ability of those responsible for management of boundaries. It is tempting to say that this is the remit of managers and administrators alone. However, I would suggest that everyone has boundaries that they should be aware of and be managing for themselves as well as in collaboration with others. This might be the boundary between the team/department and other departments or teams within the organization; the boundary with the patient/ family; the outside world; or the more personal boundary between our own private life and our professional role at work. Central to this is the importance of each person within the organization having a clear understanding of the primary task of that organization and the way in which their work role contributes to the achievement of that task. While this clearly applies to clinical staff and those in management, it also applies to the electrician, the cook, the IT staff, the secretary, etc. As we come into work we take up our role at work in relation to the primary task of the organization or team within which we work. Much organizational stress derives from lack of clarity as to role and task as well as lack of control over the content and pace of one's working day.

If resilience relates to an ability to be flexible and responsive in the face of difficult circumstances then it also relates to the ability to remain on task, or to return to it when knocked off task by a variety of influences. Many factors may contribute to 'off-task activity' by staff and test the resilience of the individual and the organization-as-a-whole.

◆ Personal issues at home may distract and make it difficult to concentrate at work. The individual needs to take ownership of the issue and either attend to and resolve it themselves, or seek appropriate help to resolve the issue. One aspect of a resilient organization is the extent to which it provides, directly or indirectly, support and counselling facilities to individuals who are experiencing stress due to work or personal events. Such support is not necessarily designed to take ownership of everything being experienced by the staff member, but to enable them in a supportive setting to distinguish the personal from the work-related and to find appropriate help. Sometimes the bulk of the stress is work-related and the individual is experiencing what might be termed 'toxic side-effects' of the work or the work setting for which the organization should take some ownership and manage the situation to reduce the 'toxins' rather than load the full responsibility on to the individual worker. Resilience within the organization as a whole is not sustained by failure to address the dynamics that affect individuals, often at an unconscious level (see chapter 7, Speck 2006).

◆ Individuals may also be knocked off-task because of changes of personnel in terms of new team members, a new manager, a change of direction because of a team or organizational decision for which the individual did not vote. For example, many people who come to work are territorial and like to personalize their working space. A change to 'hot-desking' or an open-plan office can feel very threatening if imposed or introduced without appropriate consultation with those affected. Budget restrictions may have led to reduced staffing levels and redundancies that will affect the perceptions of those who remain in work, their morale, and any feelings (positive or negative) they may have about the loss of colleagues. The ability of the individual to adapt to the new structure or working practice will demonstrate their resilience, although the transitional period may be stormy and stressful and some may choose to leave.

♦ Many of the definitions of resilience imply the capacity of the system or individual to accommodate to change or the effect of external forces. Within palliative care the relationship between the specialist palliative care service and the external environment can have a marked effect on its ability to stay 'on task' when facing a variety of perceived threats or challenges. One example of this is the tension between being a caring organization and being a business. This can create discomfort within the organization as the various subsystems and the organization as a whole seek to sustain funding, achieve targets, manage boundaries and promote and provide their service. If a funder/purchaser switches to another provider (e.g. a new hospice unit or team), or reduces the size of their contract, the impact on the original provider may be very serious. Some changes that happen over the internal–external boundary may be predictable and strategies can be developed to enable the organization to survive and adapt in creative ways to the change. This requires the organization to be alert to 'market changes' and different expectations and demands, changes in policy by government health department or charitable bodies. This awareness may enable them to be more proactive than reactive and to actively seek to provide a modified service that will meet the new situation. Sometimes the most creative response is for the primary task to be re-defined or realigned. This realignment may also be required in response to new statements of policy, guidance, or changes in the law that impact on the service being provided. A significant test of organizational resilience is how it copes with the pace of changing external demands over which it has little or no control.

Some senior managers must, at times, feel like corks bobbing around in the ocean, unable to determine where the current will lead them and not able to steer the course for themselves. When organizations enter such periods of uncertainty it is important to maintain control over those aspects for which they do still have control, while they assess the possible effects of the new policy or demands. It is also vital that they review their primary task, either to reaffirm it or to begin to change it in the light of the new requirements. It can take courage to change the primary task at team or organizational level, and it can feel that one is reinventing oneself.

Box 11.1

For 20 years Hospice X, as an organization, saw its main task as the provision of inpatient beds with some associated services. The change in health provision locally and an increase in the availability and quality of palliative care within the local acute hospitals meant fewer referrals to the hospice, reduced occupancy and the closure of some beds. The hospice could either see this as a 'blip' and bury it's head in the sand, or re-define itself and change it's primary task to the provision of specialist palliative care out in the community and seek a closer partnership with the Primary Care Trusts within the area. The measure of their resilience would be reflected in their ability to have the courage to drastically reduce their role as an inpatient unit and enhance their community focus. Such a change would also test the resilience of the various subsystems (departments) that might need to redefine, and perhaps slim down, the service they provided. Thus the whole-time spiritual care provider may have fewer inpatients to care for, but might still have a role with the staff group and a new role to provide spiritual care to patients and families in their home setting or attending day centres, etc. He/she would need to negotiate the most appropriate way of taking up this new role in relation to community faith leaders who may either see such care as impinging on their role (which they might be providing very well, or not to the same quality as the specialist palliative care provider wished). The chaplain/ spiritual care provider may also be welcomed, especially if perceived as a collaborative colleague and resource able to relieve community faith leaders of a task that they felt unable to provide. This re-negotiation of role in relation to a changes primary task would be reflected at many levels within the organization and the extent to which this was embraced and worked with would be a measure of the resilience of both the individuals concerned and of the organization as a whole.

If an organization is to develop and retain any sense of resilience, against the backdrop of a constantly changing environment, it is essential it acknowledges that the mission, tasks, boundaries, and identity of the organization are a continuous process. The example given in Box 11.1 creates an expectation that the leadership will be 'evolutionary' in style and open to the new, rather than closed and protective of existing success. The temptation is not to engage with the dynamic created by providing a service in the context of uncertainty, which will be mirrored by the uncertainty already experienced by the patients and families. There will be a common agenda of loss, together with a mixture of hope, elation, and anxiety about the new future that is opening up. The leader is faced with the task of containing the process of change that includes a future that is uncontainable. The need for leaders who are able to work with organizational and personal unconscious processes is important for their own well-being as well as that of their colleagues, and their patients. Appropriate support structures for people at all levels of the organization is not a luxury but a necessity if the organization, and the various teams and departments are to stay on task and continue to provide a quality service both now and in the future.

Jackson (Part 2 of this chapter) develops some of these issues further from the perspective of the NHS (UK) as it seeks to implement the NHS Cancer Plan (Department of Health 2000) with its far-reaching demands and expected rapid pace of implementation, which will challenge all healthcare professionals if it is to provide the promised benefits to patients by 2010. By this date, to quote Newman (1845), we 'may have changed often' but whether the service will be 'perfect' or 'resilient' remains to be seen.

References

Department of Health (2000) The NHS Cancer Plan: a plan for investment, a plan for reform. London, DoH.

Miller E (1993) Power, authority, dependency and cultural change. In Miller E *From Dependency to Autonomy: Studies in organization and change*. London, Free Association Books.

Newman JH (1845) *Essay on Development of Christian Doctrine*, I, 1, p 40.

NICE (2004) Guidance on Cancer Services: Improving supportive and palliative care for adults with cancer. London, National Institute for Clinical Excellence.

Speck P (2006) Teamwork in Palliative Care: fulfilling or frustrating? Oxford, Oxford University Press.

Vanistendael S (2003) Humour and résilience : La sourire qui fait vivre. In: Julier CR and Amiguet O (eds). Impasse, ratages, échecs. Sources de créativité pour les pratiques systémiques et travail social. pp 75–99. IES, Geneva.

Resilient organizations: Part 2 Organizational resilience within the National Health Service and cancer care

Timothy Jackson

Following significant amounts of new investment into the United Kingdom's National Health Service (NHS) over the last 5 years, there is now increased and continued pressure from politicians to modernize, reduce overspends, balance the books, and generate a surplus. There is also an increased public expectation for a flexible NHS that is responsive in meeting their health needs as and when required. The NHS is one of the largest providers of healthcare in Europe and one of the largest employers. Current health policy is radical and the speed of change rapid. Along with the ongoing need to deliver the business of the NHS, this places seemingly impossible demands on both healthcare organizations and the individuals who work within them. Current health policy encourages competition from the private sector which is being exhorted to provide excellence and value for money in healthcare on behalf of the NHS. Existing NHS organizations must adapt in this 'New World' of healthcare delivery if they are to survive.

Resilient organizations will have horizon scanned, planned and been proactive in modernizing the way they deliver healthcare. The principles of organizational resilience need to be understood, adopted, and integrated into the organization's DNA. Organizational resilience has been described as 'an enterprise's capability to respond rapidly to unforeseen change, even chaotic disruption. It is the ability to bounce back and in fact, to bounce forward with speed, grace, determination and precision' (Bell 2002). Nowhere is the need greater for an organization to be able to achieve this, than within the current NHS in the United Kingdom.

This chapter will explore the concept of organizational resilience and apply its components to healthcare concentrating on cancer and palliative care in the United Kingdom. Organizational resilience can be considered as 'the characteristic of managing the organization's activities to anticipate and circumvent threats to its existence and primary goals. This is shown in an ability to manage severe pressures and conflicts between safety and the primary production or performance goals of the organization' (Flin 2005). It has also been described as 'the ability of organizations to respond effectively to adverse events but this is dependent on their structure, the management and operational systems they have in place and the collective resilience of these' (Brunsdon and Dalziell 2006). The ability of NHS organizations to function in the face of unexpected events is an expectation of the public, healthcare professionals, and politicians alike. Healthcare providers have to deliver services to patients with increasing expectations and often complex health needs against a background of political interference and the implementation of numerous and often conflicting health policies. For example, creating a 'patient-led NHS' is currently being implemented and is described as the most radical reorganization of the NHS since its formation in 1948. This shifts the focus onto the crucial area of commissioning where expert, imaginative commissioning is central to a patient-led NHS with changes to the organization of primary care attempting to make the NHS fit for the twenty-first century (DH 2005a). However, this needs to be implemented in conjunction with numerous other health policies and guidance, as well the need for clinicians and managers to get on with their day job delivering services to patients.

Context of health and cancer care in the twenty-first century in the United Kingdom

The NHS Plan acknowledges that 'the greatest post-war reform was the establishment of the NHS. It liberated millions of families from the fear of becoming ill and inability to meet the cost of treatment' (DH 2000b, p. 2). However, for all its strengths, the NHS has profound weaknesses. Despite having the most equitable healthcare system in the world, health inequalities have grown not diminished. 'Uniformity in provision has not guaranteed equity in healthcare outcomes and there are unacceptable variations in standards across the country' (DH 2000b, p. 2). There are significant variations in the incidence, access, standards, outcomes of treatment and care across a number of diseases, e.g. cardiovascular and diabetes. This is especially evident with cancer where 'survival rates for cancer sufferers tend to be lower than many in comparable countries' (Klein 2001, p. 223). There is inequity in the treatment and care of patients, including differences in survival rates across England.

More than one in three people in England will develop cancer at some stage in their lives and one in four will die from cancer. Every year, over 200 000 people are diagnosed with cancer and about 120 000 people die from it. Better prevention and detection of cancer, and better treatment and care, matter to everyone. As life expectancy of the general population increases in England, so does the incidence of cancer by 2% annually (DH 2000c, p. 5). To support the modernization of the NHS and cancer services in particular, a comprehensive strategy for cancer care and treatment was developed in 2000. The NHS Cancer Plan sets out the first comprehensive national cancer programme for England, and has four main aims.

The four main aims of the NHS Cancer Plan

1. To save more lives.
2. To ensure people with cancer get the right professional support and care as well as the best treatment.
3. To tackle the inequalities in health that mean unskilled workers are twice as likely to die from cancer as professionals.
4. To build for the future through investment in the cancer workforce, through strong research and through preparation for the genetics revolution, so that the NHS never falls behind in cancer care again.

   (DH 2000c, table 1.1, p. 5)

The government blames the years of underinvestment for the variable standards of treatment and inequity of services across the country. However, the NHS Cancer Plan acknowledges that money on its own is not a sufficient solution and that national and local leadership is needed to support and drive change in NHS cancer services (DH 2000c, p. 93).

Klein (2001, p. 225) supports this view, 'inadequate services may reflect either inadequate funding or poor use of existing resources and a considerable body of evidence supports the latter view, in particular a succession of reports from the National Audit Commission'.

The need for organizational resilience

In recent years it has been suggested that government has increasingly acted to disturb inherited organizational forms within healthcare, imposing waves of top down change (McNulty and Ferlie 2004). The breadth and speed of change needed for the modernization of cancer services is a significant challenge for all healthcare professionals and managers involved in cancer care. However, if services for cancer patients can be improved and modernized, there is the potential for all patients treated within the NHS to benefit. The need to deliver the NHS Cancer Plan by 2010 is a political imperative and is the responsibility of both politicians and all who work within the health service. The modernization of the NHS challenges relationships and morale and threatens clinical freedom and even the survival of some clinical teams, especially where services have evolved through the entrepreneurial clinician and are no longer compliant with best practice. Reconfiguration of services is expensive, often needing to be achieved in a cost neutral manner through the rationalization of services. These challenges are further compounded by the competitiveness and mistrust between healthcare providers; a legacy of the internal market. Modernization needs stronger leaders who can challenge, work with and inspire clinicians who have been resistant to the centralization of specialist services and who have sometimes been accused of participation in covert delays to the decision-making process (Ferlie and Addicott 2004).

The modernization of cancer services is often juxtaposed with other areas of the modernization within the health service; non-cancer 'targets' that must be achieved can place conflicting demands on supporting services such as diagnostic and pathology services. Modernization of the NHS requires clinical staff and managers to learn to work in new ways across organizational boundaries to achieve the new models of care needed. This is a significant challenge for organizations with differing cultures, priorities, philosophies, and dominance within the healthcare arena. Cancer policy in isolation is easily implementable; however, cancer care does not operate in isolation, it often clashes or conflicts with other government health policy. For example 'Patient Choice' recommends patients having the choice to decide when and where to be treated (DH 2003b). This has the potential to destabilize local healthcare commissioning especially if patients exercise choice and demand to be treated outside their local network. Organizational resilience provides a strategy to navigate these turbulent times. 'Resilience Management brings together existing risk management and business continuity planning; combining a strategy of managing identified risks with an ability to respond effectively when a crisis actually happens, irrespective of whether or not that event has been previously identified as a risk' (Brunsdon and Dalziell 2006).

Bell (2002) emphasizes five principles of organizational resilience, while underlining the agility needed to respond quickly to unforeseen and unpredictable forces: Leadership, Culture, People, Systems and Settings. The five themes interlink and are interdependent.

Leadership

Resilience begins with leaders who set the priorities, allocate the resources needed to deliver the organization's business and commit to the philosophy of organizational resilience. In a healthcare context safe patient care is essential;

however, leadership must achieve a balance between risk containment and risk taking to ensure ongoing innovation (Bell 2002). Prudent risk minimalization is essential in healthcare and especially cancer care where the ongoing introduction of new or unproven technologies is needed to reduce mortality and morbidity. These two apparently conflicting objectives for leadership create tensions that need to be managed. NHS organizations need a model that clearly identifies roles and responsibilities for staff along with clearly defined levels of authority to manage risk in order to promote decentralized decision making, individual and organizational growth. Manthey and Miller (2003) identify 'responsibility as ownership; a two way process, both allocated and accepted. Authority is the right to act in areas where one is given and accepts responsibility.' Strong leaders need to articulate clearly their expectations of the workforce and organizational strategy in relation to risk taking.

Organizations must prepare or recruit professionals with a track record in leadership or who have the potential to develop into these demanding roles. Succession planning for future leaders must not be forgotten. Leadership development is important at all levels. Situational leadership is defined by Buchanan and Huczynski (1997, p. 619) as 'an approach to determining the most effective style of influencing by supporting and building on the expertise of those being led. It considers the direction and support the leader needs to give, and the readiness and maturity of those being led to perform a particular task.' The approach helps the leader and follower to map their own development in a mature adult-to-adult behaviour and is especially useful with new leaders who need to develop their leadership portfolio. Mullins (2002) believes that transformational leadership is dependent on engendering higher levels of motivation and commitment from followers by giving them new tasks in which they are sufficiently supported to succeed. The emphasis is on generating a vision for the organization and the leader's ability to appeal to higher ideals and values, thereby creating a feeling of justice, loyalty, and trust in followers. The agenda is too big to deliver alone, therefore recognizing and supporting other leaders to emerge is essential. Leaders need to have an understanding of group development to enable them to support the group to mature and become effective, as outlined by Tuckman (1965).

To support risk-taking, organizations need to adopt leadership interventions that allow them to move from autocratic to decentralized systems. The model presents a developmental approach enabling decentralization by supporting self-directed risk taking teams that work in line with the business of the organization. However, this approach needs commitment at all levels within the organization, takes time and requires recognition that at times of crisis there may be a need to move back along the continuum.

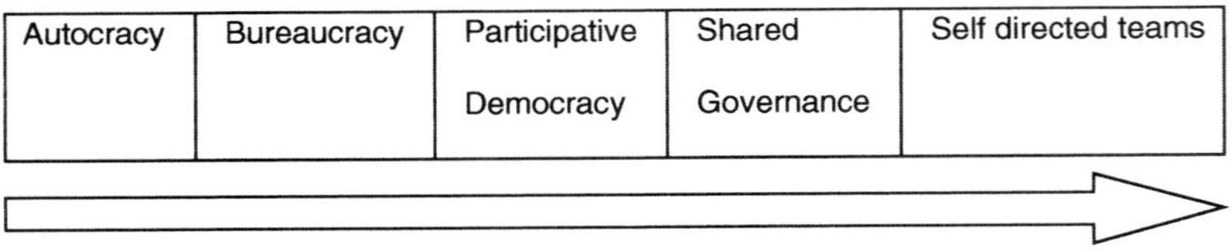

Autocracy	Bureaucracy	Participative Democracy	Shared Governance	Self directed teams

Figure 11.1 Organisational Development Continuum (Manthey & Miller 2003:10). Reprinted with permission. *Leading an Empowered Organization: Participant Manual.* Copyright 2007, Creative Health Care Management, Inc. Minneapolis: MN. USA.

Keane (2006) suggests that there are a number of strategies leaders can employ to build both individual and organizational resilience: accept change as a reality, be a positive role model for openness, honesty, and authenticity in all communications and meetings, and encourage open and honest dialogues about success and failures.

The NHS recognizes the need for diverse leaders. Byram (2000) argues that leadership is defined by skill sets not job titles. In some instances leadership may reflect the personal qualities of the post-holder rather than position-based power. Other leadership qualities, such as emotional intelligence, honesty, and a sense of humour are highlighted as essential for leaders (Manthey and Miller 2003, p. 34). Mullins (2002) believes that an effective leader requires sufficient influence to bring about longer-term change in people's attitudes and to make change acceptable.

The education and training of current and future leaders is essential to the development of organizational resilience. The new NHS Knowledge and Skills Framework (DH 2004), when combined with The NHS Leadership Qualities Framework (DH 2002), has the potential to facilitate the competency framework needed for developing current and future leaders. There are 15 qualities within the Framework covering a range of personal, cognitive and social qualities arranged in three clusters- Personal Qualities, Setting Direction and Delivering the Service.

A number of leadership courses have been developed and implemented across the NHS. These include the National Cancer Nursing Leadership programme hosted by the Royal Marsden Hospital, which supported the development of cancer nurse leaders. The 3-day 'Leading an Empowered Organization' (LEO) programme developed by Manthey and Miller in 2000 was successfully rolled out across the NHS by Leeds University. The purpose and outcome of the programme was to improve the skills of front-line leaders with a range of practical leadership tools. In 2002 Woolnough and Faugier reported that over 32 000 clinical staff had completed the LEO programme. However, there is the need for continued development of leaders and succession

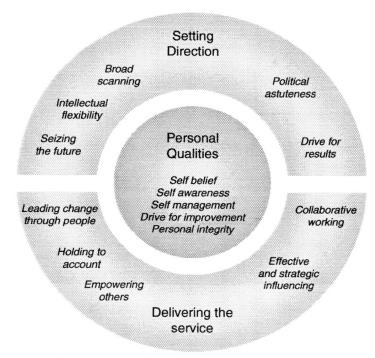

Figure 11.2 NHS leadership qualities framework, Department of Health, 2002.

planning for future leaders. Formal courses are often costly; organizations therefore need to be creative and utilize local leaders and experts to develop opportunities for shadowing, mentoring, and coaching from within their own networks. Current leadership programmes have been accessed by nurses, allied health professionals, and managers; it is essential that medical leads are also encouraged to undertake these programmes.

Culture

Keane (2006) believes that 'in the NHS and its constituent parts there is a tremendously powerful culture. Although there are similarities in achieving sustainable change in public and private organizations, public sector organizations have a unique challenge. They are inherently complex, have entrenched traditions and hierarchical structures and have a culture and power dynamic not conducive to change!' Handy (1993) supports the view that barriers to organizational resilience include ingrained cultural and structural diversity. London teaching hospitals have been described as having well established and dominant medical hierarchies (Klein 2001). Walter (2001) suggests that the loyalty of clinicians to their profession, to their independent clinical judgement and to themselves makes them immune to the normal organizational hierarchy. This is true in areas such as cancer care where national guidance describing best clinical practice has been developed by clinicians for managing site-specific cancers; but when clinicians have been tasked to implement the guidance they have resisted for some of the reasons mentioned above.

The second component of organizational resilience is the creation of an enterprise culture build on principles of organizational empowerment, purpose, trust, and accountability. This must evolve systematically into networks of employees (action learning sets) who self-organize into communities of practice for learning and mentoring, and who are empowered to participate, lead, and organize virtual teams (Manthey and Miller 2003). Bell (2002) explains, 'It is those networks of empowered and connected employees that form the bedrock of the resilient organization. The resilient organizational culture has a strong sense of enterprise purpose that cascades down and across the enterprise. It is that strong sense of purpose that glues the resilient organization together and aligns individual, workgroup and enterprise goals as a continuum'. A resilient culture is built on a strong sense of trust between employees, management, suppliers, and partners. Finally, Bell (2002) suggests 'the resilient organization inculcates a strong culture of accountability up and down the organization. People assume responsibility without question. People commit to action and do what has to be done—regardless of rank, title, or job description. A resilient organization is a passionate organization, and it is this culture of passion that drives, achieves and rewards personal and team accountability.'

This approach can be used to introduce change at all levels within the organization, however, small. Over time numerous small changes have impact. Within the NHS there is clinical guidance that supports the direction of change. A number of nationally agreed protocols of care have been developed by the National Institute for Health and Clinical Excellence (NICE) known as Improving Outcomes Guidance, which outline evidence-based practice and technologies for differing diseases. Although national experts have often developed the guidance, it still requires good, strong clinical leadership and good performance management to ensure implementation and compliance. Bridges (2001) comments 'In managing change and transition ..., it is important to recognise and value what has gone on before and value the past, resilient organizations recognise this'.

McNulty and Ferlie (2004, p. 63) believe that because physicians remain dominant among professional hierarchies, they enjoy a higher degree of organizational power and autonomy over their work than other health professionals and managers. This can further hinder the formation of new organizational structures such as cancer networks that require a multiprofessional, non-hierarchical team approach and a softening of the dominant person culture. Macbeth (2002) believes that the power base of such clinicians has made it difficult and expensive to achieve quite modest local changes in the processes of clinical care. One reason he offers is the opposition of many clinicians to the systematization of clinical care (an essential part of all quality improvement methods), because of a perceived threat to their autonomy. The challenge for organizations is how to overcome the professional cultures that prevent change and waste resources. Resilient organizations possess shared beliefs, attitudes, values, and norms of behaviour, developed through working together and recognised collectively as 'the way that things get done around here' (Davies *et al.* 2000). This approach needs strong leadership and management by clinical champions and peer pressure to comply. One model is the site-specific tumour working groups whose terms of reference are the implementation of the guidance. These groups consist of stakeholders, clinicians, managers, commissioners, service users and nurses who all share the responsibility for the implementation of the guidance. Where there is maverick behaviour this is managed within the group. Leaders must be proactive in managing this process to avoid the emergence of unhealthy cultures or behaviours that are not compatible with the organization's philosophy. Resilient organizations have a strategic plan, which outlines the direction of travel and time-scales. Therefore, leaders must set individual employee and team objectives with defined timeframes to ensure achievement of corporate aims and objectives. Personal development must be linked to these corporate objectives and not at the whim of the individual; however, individuals' talents should also be developed to support their future career aspirations, even if they are not needed in their current role.

Organizational values

The NHS is increasingly using a 'no blame' approach to adverse incidents and is attempting to create a new national system for learning from adverse events (DH 2001). Punishment is seen as negative; it makes organizations, patients, and staff vulnerable, and induces blame and denial. The 'no blame' approach allows leaders to 'recognise good performance but confronts poor performance' (Grote 1995). This approach, known as 'Positive Discipline', teaches adult to adult behaviour where there is a co-owned expectation from the employer and employee to take responsibility to improve their behaviour or performance. Empowering staff to learn from their mistakes requires calculated risks whereas a culture of blame reduces risk taking for fear of punishment

(Manthey and Miller 2003). However, rather than talk in terms of success and failures, a more positive articulation for leaders to use is; 'What went well?' 'What could be improved on or done differently?' Positive discipline involves teaching rules, boundaries or limits for both behaviour and performance. It promotes and increases risk taking, growth, learning, and self-esteem, and fosters the adult to adult relationships essential for empowered and resilient organizations (Manthey and Miller 2003). Garratt cited in Mullins (2002) states that 'A learning organization needs to promote the philosophy of self-directed learning and also learn from other organizations.' Nowhere is this more important than within the NHS, where mistakes and failures to learn from mistakes, cost lives. In cancer care, fatalities occurred following the inappropriate intrathecal administration of the chemotherapy drug 'Vincristine'. The government recognized that the NHS should learn from its mistakes and developed guidance (An Organization with a Memory, Building a Safer NHS for Patients, DH 2000a). Within the author's own unit, there was an anonymized approach to incident reporting. The incidents were analysed on a monthly basis. This highlighted a pattern in the number of drug incidents or near misses that occurred between the hours of 1600 and 2100 hours on a Saturday and Sunday, when there was a reduced number of competent nurses skilled in intravenous therapy administration. The analysis provided the basis of a successful business case for increasing the skill mix of nurses at weekends. If a blame culture had existed there would have been the potential for under-reporting and consequently a reactive rather than a proactive approach.

People

The bedrock of organizational resilience is the enterprise of its workforce. People who are properly selected, motivated, equipped, and led will overcome almost any obstacle or disruption. During this challenging time within the NHS, it is important to harness people's incredible ability to lead and respond during trying circumstances. This requires a systematic strategy for people selection and people support (Bell 2002). Within the NHS staff often go the extra mile in terms of their belief in what they do and in times of crisis. This is well recognized by politicians and the public, 'NHS staff are the biggest asset the health service has ... they do a brilliant job' (DH 2000b). NHS policy recognizes that 'modern health services require modern employment services and staff work best for patients when they can strike a healthy life work balance, are valued and supported and have access to personal and professional development opportunities' (DH 2000d).

There has been significant new investment within health, cancer, and palliative care services. However, new investment is not simply replacing existing old technology, but rather increasing capacity. Examples include the development of nurse prescribing and case management by community matrons for patients with long-term conditions. The workforce needs to evolve and develop new skills; traditional healthcare professionals need to recognize the need for new and differing roles. The workforce is a major challenge, with ongoing recruitment and retention problems facing the NHS at all levels. New models for delivering care need to be explored, supported by the development of new roles such as the assistant practitioner role, which aims to support registered healthcare professionals. The assistant practitioner is someone who works under the guidance of a registered nurse or allied healthcare professional, delivering elements of care, but not responsible for prescribing or evaluating the care.

However, these new roles can be seen as a threat to professional identity; further challenging traditional professional values, ways of working and boundaries. Read *et al.* (2001) recommend that role clarity is vital for all new roles, including role boundaries. However, as Miner (1971) has observed, role ambiguity may result from an idiosyncratic perception of role; either the role prescriptions are unclear, or misunderstood, or deliberately distorted. Klein (2001) discusses the fact that the close definition of 'role' and delineation of duties, have never featured in the medical profession's service to the NHS. Only an enthusiastic workforce can create a resilient organization. The NHS Plan and NHS Cancer Plan acknowledge the need to build for the future through investment (DH 2000c). The new 'Knowledge and Skills Framework' (KSF) supports the development and acquisition of competencies for all staff working within healthcare. A new pay and remuneration system for all NHS staff, 'Agenda for Change', has been introduced to reward all staff who embrace new skills and roles in recognition for their input and value to the modernization of the NHS and patient care. New roles are being created such as Assistant Practitioners in radiotherapy or endoscopy and Multidisciplinary Team Co-ordinators, who provide administrative support to the healthcare team so that the scarcity and the skills of healthcare professionals and doctors can be used more fully in patient care. The KSF supports competency development of all NHS staff including non-clinical staff such as porters and ancillary staff, who have patient contact but little in the way of training. The KSF supports them acquiring skills in communication with patients in order to improve patient experience but also so that this invaluable group of staff feel invested in, developed, and rewarded for their contribution to patient care. Within cancer care, experienced healthcare assistants are being trained to take on additional technical roles that were previously the responsibility of the registered nurse. The new roles include phlebotomy, peripheral venous cannulation, and taking down infusions. 'The evaluation from Hinchingbrooke Hospital, Cambridge where this new role was piloted, has demonstrated reduced waiting times and improved patient experience.' (Taylor 2004).

While career advancement and remuneration are important motivators for staff recruitment and retention, it is also vital to recognize and support staff with the emotional burden of caring for patients and carers. It has long been acknowledged that working within healthcare, and especially cancer and palliative care, is stressful and that staff need to feel and be supported. Staff working within cancer and palliative care often form intense relationships with their patients and carers, which may expose staff to the risks of burnout from a repeated sense of loss, and eventual futility, in their role' (Kelly *et al.* 2000). A number of support strategies can be employed. Clinical supervision is a means of supporting nursing staff, developing practice and enabling the maintenance and improvement standards of care. Clinical supervision is a practice-focussed professional relationship, involving a practitioner reflecting on practice guided by a skilled supervisor (Nursing and Midwifery Council (NMC) 2002). Wilkin *et al.* (1997) believe that clinical supervision supports nurses and helps them survive the tremendous pressures of a demanding profession and encourages a high standard of care to patients. The potential benefits and impact of clinical supervision on the nursing profession and beyond are far reaching; 'the establishment of clinical supervision is an important part of clinical governance and in the interests of improving standards of patient care' (NMC 2002).

The benefits of clinical supervision (NMC 2002) are thought to include:

+ safer practice
+ reduced untoward incidents and complaints
+ better targeting of educational and professional development
+ better assessment of patient/client opinion
+ reduced stress among staff
+ improved levels of sickness or absenteeism
+ improved confidence and professional development
+ greater awareness of accountability
+ better input into management appraisal systems
+ better managed risk and better awareness of evidence-based practice.

However, clinical supervision has been introduced and integrated into practice in a very *ad hoc* manner across the country. Were clinical supervision to be systematically used and evaluated by leaders and managers, its success could be measured through data on recruitment and retention. Butterworth *et al.* (1996)

suggest it may be possible to audit clinical supervision through existing mechanisms, such as rates of sickness and absence, recruitment and retention of staff. This has yet to be achieved.

Action learning is another methodology for problem solving and resolution but currently there has been little evaluation of this in relation to nursing. Other support strategies for lead cancer nurses include preceptorship. The Nursing and Midwifery Council (NMC) recommend that all staff in a new role, whether newly registered or a more experienced practitioner, should receive a period of preceptorship; 'many people find transitional or new roles a daunting prospect' (NMC 2002, p. 4). While clinical supervision has been predominantly used with nurses, it can be adapted and used for all staff working within the NHS. Other support strategies managers need to utilize include allowing staff the choice to work part time, full time, or flexible annualized hours. Job shares, career breaks, carer's leave, paternity leave, and flexible phased retirement can also be offered and are all examples of good human resource practices, which enable staff to achieve a work life balance. Some organizations are now offering full-time staff the choice to work 4 days a week rather than the traditional 5 days, to reduce travel time and high levels of absence. This was previously an option developed for nurses and is now being extended to other healthcare professionals, non-clinical staff and managers. Other examples of good practice exist across the country. One such initiative by the Christie Hospital in Manchester is 'Improving stressful working lives', where the Trust has introduced free of charge complementary therapies, counselling, and clinical supervision for its entire staff (Mackereth et al. 2005).

Increasingly patients and carers (users) are playing a pivotal role in the modernization of health and cancer services by working in partnership with healthcare professionals. Users of the service can ensure that we move away from a 'service that does things to and for its patients, to one which is patient led, where the service works with patients' (DH 2005). However, healthcare professionals and users need clear guidance and training for this to become a reality rather than merely another source of stress. Macmillan Cancer Support has developed a training programme known as CancerVOICES, which is being implemented across the country (Bradburn 2003).

Systems

Organizational resilience builds on the infrastructure and philosophy of clinical governance and includes many interlinked quality initiatives. Within the governance agenda there is the need to modernize and strengthen self-regulation and build on the principles of performance. Nurses, midwives, and health visitors have been strengthening and improving professional self-regulation since 1992. 'However, this is still a relatively new concept for doctors and allied health professionals' (Smith 1998). This approach protects the public from unsafe practitioners. It is also important that when a practitioner breaches professional standards, the regulatory body, where possible, will work with the individual to meet the standard. Where there has been a breach due to ill health, temporary suspension from practice until a period of rehabilitation is undertaken is often imposed. This allows practitioners the opportunity to return to practice rather than past practice where removal from the professional register made return to practice impossible.

Within the NHS there is much guidance developed by clinical experts to support managers and clinicians to implement, or commissioners to purchase, services that are considered best practice. The development of service standards to ensure equity and access to evidence-based service specifications across the NHS is referred to as National Service Frameworks (NSFs). These include, for example, Care of Older People, Long Term Conditions and the Cancer Plan. This is complemented by further guidance developed by the NICE. 'NICE will procure clear guidance for clinicians and commissioners of healthcare about which treatment works best for patients. It is envisaged that NICE should standardise care and equity of care so that regardless of postal code, patients will have the confidence that they are receiving a national standard of care' (DH 1998). Within cancer care there is 'Improving Outcomes' guidance for all site-specific cancers, which is further supported by new treatments and technologies such as cytotoxic chemotherapy and biological therapies approved by the NICE. The purpose of the guidance is to ensure equity and access for patients and to avoid a postcode lottery of care and treatment for patients. The guidance outlines to clinicians, managers, and commissioners what should be provided for their patients. Peer review within cancer facilitates the review of cancer services in an open, supportive manner, helping identify and acknowledge good practice and develop prompt action plans, to manage non-compliance and patient risk. NHS organizations are now beginning to accept that to maintain organizational resilience through good clinical governance, they must be compliant with national guidance, so that they can be monitored and benchmarked against their peers. In this way patients can be confident that they are getting the best treatments regardless of their postcode.

Settings

The final component of organizational resilience is the physical deployment of the workforce and combines a number of factors that support resilience. In terms of service delivery healthcare professionals should where possible develop services nearer to patients to improve access; however, this must not compromise safety. The principle must be that of 'safe and effective services as locally as possible, not local services as safely as possible' NICE (2005). The work should include: identifying and building good practice, assessing and minimizing the risk of untoward events, investigating problems as these arise and ensuring lessons are learnt and supporting health professionals in delivering quality care (DH 1998). In developing new ways of deploying staff, resilient organizations must undertake a comprehensive assessment to ensure workplace security and safety.

Another example of a change in care delivery and how staff work is the Marie Curie 'Cancer Care Delivering Choice' programme (www.delivering-choiceprogramme.org.uk) This programme aims to meet the challenge of improving community based end of life care and consequently to help more people to achieve their wish to die at home. This is achieved through working in partnership in communities and local statutory and voluntary organizations to improve planning, co-ordination, and delivery of key services. The end of life care programme is aimed at young people and adults with life-threatening illnesses not just those affected by cancer. It offers innovative, responsive solutions such as running a rapid response team of nurses. This team co-ordinates access for all patients needing palliative care across all the services—healthcare, social care and home care, together with managing the vital task of handling the discharge of patients from hospital to home.

Conclusions

The NHS is challenged by the need to achieve financial balance; resilient organizations cannot exist without consideration of finances. A resilient organization is one that anticipates potential risks in terms of income and expenditure. As the NHS adopts market principles and competes with a variety of independent healthcare providers, it must (Bell 2002):

- be without boundaries
- be impassioned by a strong sense of leadership
- build a culture of purpose, empowerment, trust and accountability
- select, motivate, and support people who have the requisite skills to flourish in ambiguous and uncertain environments
- exploit systems to connect and inform the organization
- move to highly distributed settings that diffuse and disperse enterprise assets and operations.

All resilient healthcare organizations will have 1–3-year strategic directions of travel; these must be shared with all employees at all levels in the organization.

Leaders and managers then need to articulate what is expected from employees, build individual employee's personal objectives and performance manage all employees, so that each employee understands what is expected from them, and can deliver their unique contribution to ensure the business of the organization is successfully executed. If the healthcare organization is people centred, and supports excellence in patient care, and values the contribution of its staff and contributes to their development, it will have the ability to move forward and survive challenging times. Based on its reputation of how it supports both patients and staff, the resilient organization will attract and retain the best staff. The concept of organizational resilience is essential for healthcare organizations; if they are able to pre-empt, respond, and take control during turbulent times and recognize change as inevitable, they will survive and meet patient need.

References

Bartlett A, Ghoshal S (1990) Matrix management: not a structure, a frame of mind. *Harvard Business Review* July–August.

Bell MA (2002) *The Five Principles of Organisational Resilience*. Gartner Research. http://www.gartner.com/DisplayDocument?doc_cd=103658 accessed on 18/09/2006.

Bradburn J (2003) Developments in User Organisations. In: *Patient Participation in Palliative Care. A Voice for the Voiceless*, pp. 23–38 (eds Monroe B, Oliviere D). Oxford: Oxford University Press.

Bridges W (2001) *Managing Transition: Making the Most of Change*. London: Nicholas Brealey.

Brunsdon D, Dalziell E (2006) *Making Organisations Resilient: Understanding the Reality of the Challenge*. Accessed on 18/09/2006 www.resorgs.org.nz/Resilient_Infrastructure-Brunsdon%20Dalziell.pdf.

Butterworth T, Bishop V, Carson J (1996) First steps towards evaluating clinical supervision in nursing and health visiting. Theory, policy and practice development. A review. *Journal of Clinical Nursing* 5(2).

Byram D (2000) Leadership: a skill not a role. *Clinical issues American Association of Critical Care Nurses.* 11(3).

Davies T, Nutley SM, Mannion R (2000) Organisational culture and quality of health care. Special Article. *Quality in Health Care* 9, 111–119.

Department of Health (1998) *A First Class Service, Quality—The New NHS*. London: Department of Health.

Department of Health (1999) *Improving Working Lives Standard*. Department of Health. London: Department of Health.

Department of Health (2000a) *Building a Safer NHS for Patients: Implementing an organisation with a memory*. London: Department of Health.

Department of Health (2000b) *The NHS Plan; a plan for investment, a plan for reform*. London: Department of Health.

Department of Health (2000c) *The NHS Cancer Plan, a plan for investment, a plan for reform*. London: Department of Health.

Department of Health (2000d) *Improving Working Lives for Those People who Work in the NHS*. London: Department of Health.

Department of Health (2002) *NHS Leadership Qualities Framework*, p. 5 www.nhsleadershipqualities.nhs.uk. London: Department of Health. Accessed on 20/09/2006.

Department of Health (2005) *Creating a Patient Lead NHS: Delivering the NHS Improvement Plan*, p. 3. London: Department of Health.

Department of Health (2006a) *Safety First, a report for Patients, Clinicians and Health care Managers*. London: Department of Health.

Department of Health (2006b) *Our Health, Our Care, Our Say*. London: Department of Health.

Ferlie E, Addicott R (2004) *Determinants of Performance in Cancer Networks. A Process Evaluation*. Cardiff University. p14. www.ewan.ferlie@rhul.ac.uk and r.addicott@imperial.ac.uk. Accessed on 14/06/2005.

Flin R (2005) *Erosion of Managerial Resilience. The Vasa Effect*. Aberdeen: Industrial Psychology Research Centre, University of Aberdeen.

Grote D (1999) *Discipline without Punishment*. New York: American Management Association.

Handy C (1993) *Understanding Organisations*, pp. 97, 178. London: Penguin Business Management.

Jackson T (2006) Staff support and retention. In: *Nursing in Haematological Oncology*, 2nd edn, p. 554 (ed. Grundy M). London: Baillière Tindall–Elsevier.

Keane K (2006) Resilience and organisational change. Resilience in organisations. *Journal of Holistic Healthcare* **3**, 1.

Kelly D, Ross S, Gray B, Smith P (2000) Death, dying and emotional labour; problematic dimensions of the role the bone marrow transplant nursing role. *Journal of Advanced Nursing* **32**(4), 952–960.

Klein R (2001) *The New Politics of the NHS*, 4th edn, pp. 223–239. Pearson and Prentice Hall.

Lugon M, Secker Walker J (1999) *Clinical Governance. Making it Happen*, p. 5. London: The Royal Society of Medicine Press Limited.

Macbeth FR (2002) *How Effective is the Cancer Collaborative?* bmj.com at http://www.bmk.bmjjournals.com/cgi/eletters/3247330/164#19234. Accessed on 15/06/2005.

Mackereth P, White K, Cawthorn A, Lynch B (2005) Improving working lives: complementary therapies, counselling and clinical supervision for staff. *European Journal of Oncology Nursing* **9**, 147–154.

Manthey M, Miller D (2003) *Leading an Empowered Organisation, Responsibility, Authority and Accountability Equals Decentralisation*, pp. 6–7. Leeds: University of Leeds School of Health Care Studies.

Marie Curie Delivering Choice Programme. www.DeliveringChoiceProgramme.org.uk. Accessed on 28/12/2006.

McNulty T, Ferlie E (2004) *Re-engineering Health Care. The complexities of organisational transformation*, p. 63. Oxford: Oxford University Press.

Miner JB (1971) *Management Theory*. Basingstoke: Macmillan.

Mullins LJ (2002a) Qualities and competencies for the 21st Century Board of Directors. Appendix 2. In: *Management and Organisational Behaviour*, pp. 882–885, 6th edn (ed. Garratt B). London: Prentice Hall.

Mullins LJ (2002b) *Management and Organisational Behaviour*, 6th edn. London: Prentice Hall.

National Institute for Health and Clinical Excellence (2005) *Improving Outcomes in Children and Young People with Cancer*, p. 9. London: Department of Health.

Nursing and Midwifery Council (2002) *Supporting nurses and midwives through life long learning. Protecting the public through professional standards*, p. 7. www.nmc-uk.org. Accessed on 18/12/2004.

Read S, Cameran A, Collins K, Doyles L, Dowling S, Furlong S *et al* (2001) *Exploring New Roles in Practice*. Sheffield: Universities of Sheffield and Bristol and The King's Fund.

Stewart R (1989) *Leading in the NHS: A Practical Guide*. Basingstoke: Macmillan.

Smith R (1998) Regulation of doctors and the Bristol Inquiry. *British Medical Journal* **317**, 1539–1540.

Taylor L (2004) *Hinchingbrooke Health Check Annual Report 2004. Cancer Care gets International Recognition*, p. 2. www.hinchingbrooke.nhs.uk. Accessed on 12/02/07.

Tuckman BW (1965) Development sequence in small groups. *Psychological Bulletin* **63**, 384–399.

Walter M (2001) Organisation and management. In: *Health Studies. An Introduction* (eds Naidoo J, Wills J). Basingstoke: Palgrave.

Wilkin P, Bowers L, Monk J (1997) Clinical supervision, managing the resistance. *Nursing Times* **93**(8), 48–49.

Woolnough H, Fragier J (2002) An evaluative study assessing the impact of the leading and empowered organisation programme. *Nursing Times Research* **7**(6), 412–417.

Resilient communities

Allan Kellehear and Barbara Young

The relationship between palliative care and the communities they serve is crucial to the successful support of both. Palliative care services need communities to be actively involved in dying, death, loss, and care issues so that support for patients and their families is maximized beyond the simple provision of services. Effective and supportive care during and after dying, death, and loss depend heavily on effective and timely medical and nursing services but also on support from members of the broader community.

An individual's capacity to withstand the stresses of serious illness, loss or the demands of caring for someone seriously ill, depends on the support they receive from friends, family, workmates, employers, club members, parishioners, and many others who have regular contact with patients and their families. Communities, in their turn, need their local palliative care services for technical and professional support during times when they require specialized care and support. Palliative care services are often one of only a handful of community service leaders that are able to supply important information, supports or education to their surrounding community about end-of-life matters that people may encounter every day. Death, dying, and loss, like the matter of good health and its maintenance, is everyone's responsibility—not simply the sole responsibility of healthcare professionals and the services that employ them. For example, we need oncology services, but we also need people to give up smoking. We need accident and emergency departments in our hospitals, but we also need people to wear their seat belts while driving, to moderate their daily alcohol consumption, or to develop better eating and exercise habits in the whole community. Good services and good community development and education promote good health and safety.

This chapter focuses on how community resilience is enhanced by a health promoting palliative care approach that makes community development initiatives a crucial part of its offerings. Our aim is to provide a brief theoretical and practical introduction to health promoting palliative care by showing how this approach makes an important contribution to community development and resilience. We will first discuss the relationship between community and resilience and link this to popular initiatives in community development. We will then show how community development goals are intrinsically linked to a health promoting palliative care approach. The final part of the chapter will illustrate this link between resilience, community development and health promoting palliative care by describing a health promoting palliative care programme developed by an Australian palliative care service.

The relationship between resilience and community

The terms 'resilience' and 'community' have a lot in common. For one thing there is significant and continuing debate about what these words mean. Community was a term much favoured by sociologists at the turn of the twentieth century. Ferdinand Tonnies, Emile Durkheim, Max Weber, and even Karl Marx were all social critics and theorists who believed that 'community' was endangered by the accelerating and destructive forces of industrialization in Europe in the late nineteenth and early twentieth centuries. For the writers of these times, community was an intimate, face-to-face network of workers and families living and dying together in one physical locale—a small village, hamlet, or local area. In those places, and amid that web of social relations, people would find daily support for one another, share a common core of values and attitudes, and relate to each other around a common economy despite their different status or social class. This romantic idea of community as place, and as a style of social relations, received considerable criticism during the 1960s and 1970s (Mayo 1994, 2000) but is now undergoing something of a revival, or perhaps we should say a rehabilitation among social commentators (Wellman and Wortley 1990; Crow and Allan 1994).

Communities are now rarely described in singular terms of place or of broad commonalities of occupation, economy, or values. We have moved our definitions toward the idea of social networks, co-operation and partnerships despite differences, shared services and resources for different needs and at different times. The recent revolution in communications in telephone and computer means that 'communities' can be spread across vast distances, can in fact be global, but still perform the intimate functions of support and resource-sharing formerly associated with more socially closed and physically closer interpersonal relations. However, although a diversity of personal needs are addressed in several locations, sometimes over vast distances, the regular satisfaction of many other personal needs remains local, from seeking veterinary advice for pets, attending local schools or churches, or simply being a member of the local library or neighbourhood watch programme.

Resilience, recently described as an 'academic fad' idea, is a concept whose definition is also highly contentious (Tremblay 2005). Initially, resilience was described as successful coping (Werner 2005), or positive adaptation (Riley and Masten 2005), or good performance (Agaibi and Wilson 2005) in the face of adversity, disadvantage or impediments. However, these introductory remarks about resilience also quickly disperse and become vague in their meaning when they become inclusive of other ideas about maintaining identity (Bonanno *et al.* 2002), or recovering well or easily from adversity, or a recovery from trauma that returns individuals or communities to 'normal' (Tremblay 2005; Riley and Masten 2005).

Clearly, the idea of resilience is the development, protection and thriving of *positive* character in the face of threats to overwhelm, even to destroy, these positive traits. Yet, rather ironically, to develop, protect, or help these positive features of an individual personality or community also assumes that these features are there in the first place, however modestly. These features may be present in the form of supports, role models, or crucial bonding with a special caretaker, or in some community sources such as a school or church group. Despite what often appears to be a catastrophic social background; family abuse, discord or break-up, poverty, or parental dysfunction; positive influences manage to strengthen and then dominate an individual response and subsequent personal lifestyle. Even in communities torn by violence, dysfunctional neighbourhoods, poor welfare and health supports, some communities are able to show positive lifestyles and outcomes based on alternative social behaviours and cultural world views. To some extent then, the problem of defining resilience can be a rather circular problem of definition for the field of resilience research.

All researchers in the field of resilience argue that the personal qualities of resilience, however defined and understood, are contextual. This is the case whether we are speaking about the crucial developmental relationship of infant and the primary caregiver; or the importance of the wider social relations of that core relationship (family); or the even wider relationship to that family itself (community, school, or workplace). The psychology of resilience, whatever its definitional problems, is a *social psychology*. Resilience is a social quality, of individuals or communities, forged in the face or in the wake of adversity by the unwavering co-presence of positive social influences that strengthen and promote, not only survival but an ability to thrive despite trauma and insults to the host.

Maton (2005) and DeV Peters (2005) argue that for communities to be resilient they must demonstrate changes, structures, and processes of positive support that work alongside negative social influences. This not only maximizes the social conditions under which individuals might access crucial positive resources for personal development, support, and life direction but also acts against the detrimental social forces themselves. Of course, resilience would be far less a community issue if adverse circumstances were not there in the first place; if poverty, community violence, or lack of human services were fully addressed by the governments and private interests responsible to those communities. However, in the absence of such ideal political circumstances and social harmony, most of the programme development and experiment in community resilience has been drawn from ideas of community development.

Central to these ideas of community development to promote resilience has been the need for community building efforts to be holistic, in other words, to take a whole community approach; to be inclusive of all parties within a community; for any community building efforts to be community-led; and for the relationships between the different players to be of a collaborative, participatory and partnership character (DeV Peters 2005; Maton 2005, pp. 122–126).

In Australian palliative care circles these assumptions have circulated as health promoting palliative care ideals (Kellehear 1999). Health promoting palliative care assumes that care of people with life-threatening illness, those living with loss and those caring for one or both of these former people can benefit from health promotion ideas that focus on prevention, harm reduction, and community partnerships. Health-promoting palliative care services recognize the limits to direct service provision. Most Australian services now acknowledge that most of the time spent by most patients and their families when dying or living with loss and care is done so outside the influence of professionals or services. To promote positive and supportive experiences for people while they live with serious illness, loss or care, therefore, requires a community development approach as the majority of time is spent in the usual routines and networks of work, school, clubs, or churches and temples. With this recognition has come state (State of Victoria 2004) and national (Palliative Care Australia 2003, 2005) policy guidelines that encourage health promotion and community development in all palliative care services in Australia.

Resilience, community and health promoting palliative care

Health promotion, including health promoting palliative care, recognizes that all community initiatives must be participatory. Health services must work in partnership with community sectors and groups. Advocates of health promotion recognize the social character of health and illness, in other words, that experiences of health and illness can frequently be traced to social sources.

For example, illnesses such as cancer might be linked to social habits of smoking, ultraviolet exposure or high fat diets. Quality of health services is linked to problems of access, equity, and welfare in different populations. Experiences of health relate not just to access to services but also access to quality housing, effective sewerage systems, adequate income and education levels, or local policies that protect the health and safety of people at work or school, or while travelling by car, using drugs and alcohol, or engaging in sex.

Health promotion initiatives in all these areas emphasize education, information, and policy development, and direct and design these initiatives for the well and the ill. Health promotion, or to put it another way, the task of promoting good health and well-being, is everyone's responsibility. Health promotion is not simply promoting good health service provision but also promoting healthy and safe lifestyles in every sector of society (Kellehear 1999, p. 12).

The goals of a health promoting palliative care are to facilitate education and information for health, dying, death, and loss; to facilitate social supports both personal and community; to encourage interpersonal reorientation that adds value to people's ability to cope and develop alongside their experiences of dying, death, and loss; to encourage palliative care services to reorient towards health promotion rather than simply confine themselves to clinical service offerings; and to combat death-denying health policies and attitudes in the general community, media, and community health colleagues and services (Kellehear 1999, p. 20).

Some of the ways to address these goals lie in providing health and death education programmes to the community and in increasing the number and type of supports that any palliative care service might offer their patient/family clients. Other ways to address these goals relate to creating professional and intersectoral partnerships with services outside palliative care such as accident and emergency, community health, or disaster management. However, a key methodology for increasing resilience toward experiences of dying, death, or loss is to engage in the participatory exercise of community development (Kellehear 2005).

Community development is 'any set of initiatives designed to develop the social resources of the community in order to enhance its quality of life' (Kellehear 2005, p. 118). Such initiatives may be introduced in health, welfare, recreational, educational, or workplace settings but they are always developed in partnership with members of those settings and the needs, wants or desires for those improvements derived or identified by people from there. The idea is to increase or enhance the community's ability to cope with, or recover from, the traumas, harms, or personal difficulties associated with dying, death, or loss. Community development programmes are designed to maximize the community conditions; people, information, awareness levels, or key networks; under which resilience may thrive, develop, or protect individuals that encounter death and loss. 'All community development initiatives have as their main aim the desire to deepen the quality and extent to which a community may look after its own members.' (Kellehear 2005, p. 118).

There are many ways to engage in community development. Some services choose to employ a community development worker for the purposes of leading the service's offerings in this regard. That community development worker may be from an education, social work, or nursing background. At other times, a service may create a 'community panel' of members drawn from a cross-section of interested parties; local schools, chamber of commerce, the mayor's office or trade union. This committee then engages further networks, or may hold a public forum to discuss the community's perceived needs around dying, death, and loss. From such meetings come further volunteers, as well as possible programme suggestions and sources of funding. Yet other services simply add this function to their 'community services' reorienting outpatient/day care services to work more closely with schools or workplaces or to cultivate new relationships with clubs such as Rotary, Apex, or Lions. Other palliative care services have forged new relationships with their volunteers employing them as community partners in their joint attempts to develop outreach towards non-'traditional' carers; the trade unions, golf clubs, radio stations, or art galleries; organizations that might play innovative but leading roles in education, support, or raising public awareness.

In Australia, palliative care services have adopted all three of these 'models' of community development in one form or another and there seems no shortage of creative ideas to forge community partnerships with whatever time and personnel shortages or restrictions each service experiences as their own particular constraints. A range of health promoting and community development examples can be found within the pages 'Social Networks'—the national newsletter of the public health and palliative care network in Australia (www.latrobe.edu.au—palliative care unit).

We provide the following example of a rural-based palliative care service in the Australian state of Victoria. Although Victoria is the second smallest state in Australia, covering only 1/34th of its land area, it nevertheless remains, by world standards, a very large geographical area in its own right, slightly smaller (220 620 km^2) than the total land area of the United Kingdom (244 103 km^2) (Macquarie Library 1984). Hume Palliative Care (formerly known as 'Hume Regional Palliative Care' (HRPC) from the Hume region in North-East Victoria) has been a leading health promoting palliative care service for some years now and is widely recognized for its innovative community development programmes.

Community development programmes of Hume Palliative Care

An opportunity to explore health promoting palliative care arose when HRPC (a partnership of a Northeast Health Wangaratta and Ovens and King Community Health Service) was one of the successful projects (*Building Rural Community Capacity through Volunteering*), funded for 2 years under the Commonwealth (Australian) Department of Health and Ageing (DoHA) 'Caring Communities' Programme (CCP). HRPC covers a large rural region in Northeast Victoria of 40 000 km². Much of this area is rurally isolated. HRPC managed and co-ordinated a programme that subcontracted five agencies to facilitate the equitable delivery of community-based palliative care across the whole HRPC region. This was achieved through a partnership of existing local services (doctors, district nurses, hospital, community health, and home care staff) and specialist palliative care services. The five specialist services consisted of specialist palliative care nurses, a loss and grief co-ordinator and a region-wide network of 17 local palliative care volunteer services. These services were supported by the regional consultancy team (manager, visiting medical physician, clinical nurse consultant, loss and grief consultant, volunteer support and community development worker, and an education officer).

This community capacity building project set out to demonstrate that a well resourced and supported palliative care volunteer service can assist in raising awareness that death, dying, loss, and care is a shared concern for all communities and not just health professionals alone. It involved establishing a health promoting palliative care delivery model utilizing the volunteer services. However, as the process unfolded, it was found that groups beyond the palliative care volunteer services could also be encouraged to contribute to building community resilience in this area. The question then arose: what could be changed within the existing HRPC structure so that community members had a better way to respond to the issues that surround death, dying, loss, or care? The resources of a community-based palliative care team can be limited by the constraints of funding, position descriptions, and availability of professionals who can provide a holistic range of services. These limitations are often heightened in rural areas along with greater travel distances to access services.

This project looked at whether health professionals and palliative care volunteers working in the palliative care sector and the community health arena might work together to assist, mentor, and encourage other community members to develop activities utilising a public health approach to support the work of the palliative care service and its community. This subgroup or team could act as a resource to enable the wider community to become an integral part of health promoting palliative care service delivery. This team would be the vehicle that could drive the momentum towards achieving these goals as defined by Kellehear (1999, p. 20):

- provide education and information for health, dying and death
- provide social supports—both personal and community
- encourage interpersonal reorientation
- encourage reorientation of palliative care services
- combat death-denying health policies and attitudes.

The formation of this cross-agency team or partnership relied on interested people to 'volunteer' their time and energies. The team was supported by their auspice agencies allowing attendance at meetings and time availability regarding telephone mentorship. Outreach into the community was vital to the success of this health promotion resource team's work, as community development is based upon identified need at the local level.

Research also informs us that 'the use of volunteers in various palliative care service models is both traditional and innovative ... the resources needed to support volunteers are substantial ... and volunteers are crucial elements in any public health approach that involves community partnerships.' (Palliative Care Australia 2003, p. 30). The social support strategies within a health promoting palliative care programme for those people living with a life-limiting illness and their families and carers, 'must emerge from the everyday worlds of families, workplace and church.' (Kellehear 1999, p. 105). A recent study found that 'the utilization of volunteers to facilitate partnerships with community groups who have shared values may provide community health with new opportunities to generate community health and wellbeing' (O'Donnell 2002, abstract).

Creating the interest and the passion

Education and training around health promoting palliative care was crucial to the development of health promoting palliative care in the region. It was, and is continuing to be, provided by the La Trobe University Palliative Care Unit.

Initially, a presentation on the public health approach to palliative care was given as part of the HRPC annual palliative care volunteer regional day. One volunteer wrote a report of her learning from the day that included 'it is time we brought back to the people and the community themselves the responsibilities of caring, education and health ... death is ordinary and common-place and so we need to talk about it, and educate all people everywhere.' Another participant commented that: 'I see the need for community involvement.' One co-ordinator of volunteers who was unable to attend the day shared: 'my volunteers came back so enthusiastic to go ahead with a palliative care information day we had thought about … I'm trying to catch their mood'. The scene had been set with the volunteers.

The next step was to create interest among regional health professionals to attend an education and training workshop around health promoting palliative care. A colourful and informative flyer was sent out to palliative care service providers and community health centres across the region. After follow-up phone calls, e-mails, and some site visits, 19 people registered to attend the day. It was at this workshop that the Big 7 Checklist (Kellehear 2005, p. 156) was presented as a way of developing a good idea into a health promoting palliative care activity. A truly health promoting initiative needed to meet one of the first three criteria documented below and include all of numbers 4–7:

1. prevention of social difficulties around death, dying, loss or care;

2. harm minimization of current difficulties around death, dying, loss or care; or

3. early intervention strategies along the journey of death, dying, loss or care experiences.

4. changes to community settings or environments for the better in terms of our present or future responses to death, dying, loss or care;

5. partnerships proposed, partnered and sustained by community members;

6. sustainable impact beyond the intervention; and

7. evaluation of how successful or useful the intervention was.

A key comment from the workshop expressed the mood of the day: '[the workshop] made me look outside the square … ideas and framework for planning future palliative care/health promotion … more understanding of community development and a community supporting itself'.

Establishing a regional team to champion health promoting palliative care

Those who attended the workshop were then invited to become a part of a Health Promotion Resource Team to support, mentor, and encourage health promoting palliative care activity planning across the region for the life of the project. The ongoing sustainability of the team would become part of the evaluation process. A group of 10 people joined this team, eight from the palliative care ranks and two from community health.

This team developed a 'terms of reference' document and met quarterly under the support and co-ordination of the project worker. For this to work a pool of funds was required for health promotion activities. Guidelines for accessing these funds were developed in partnership with La Trobe University and were utilized by the Health Promotion Resource Team in determining their distribution. The criteria to access funding were based on the Big 7 Checklist. This checklist became a way to guide discussion with applicants in the development of activities and also facilitated education around the public health approach. The application form was written with minimum reporting requirements so as not to be too daunting, to allow flexibility to fund smaller projects or larger-scale initiatives and freedom for the applicant to develop initiatives according to locally perceived need. The funding sought ranged from less than a hundred dollars for small projects to over two thousand dollars for larger ones. The guidelines were distributed widely to community groups, health centres, and neighbourhood houses in January 2004 and repeated in July 2004. The resource team members identified that they needed further education on how to assist others to discuss the activity against the Big 7 checklist. A short workshop, facilitated by the La Trobe University Palliative Care Unit, was held during the June 2004 meeting of this group.

Local communities responding to the challenge

The culmination of this project was seeing the broader general communities embrace health promotion around the areas of death, dying loss, or care. The health promotion concept was filtering through all of the five specialist palliative care service subregions that operate across the Hume Region. These services were providing networking and partnering opportunities with other health and community organizations that would otherwise not have occurred. This resulted in improved networking between specialist palliative care service providers, palliative care volunteer services and with many local community groups. These links may otherwise have not been identified. The HPRT assisted with or mentored 25 funded mini projects. Of the 12 first round projects, 10 were proposed by palliative care service providers and/or members of the HPRT and two by other community groups. Of the 13 second round projects this trend was reversed with five proposed by palliative care service providers and/or members of the HPRT and eight by other community groups. The following are examples of this diverse array of innovative activities:

- One larger rural town explored how young people can communicate creatively about the reality of loss and grief in their lives. The partnerships involved in developing a performance event included local youth service workers, a school nurse, community health workers, a church minister, the local palliative care loss and grief co-ordinator and volunteer service, a music therapist, and other community members with creative talents.

The event has been linked with other youth funding schemes that increases its potential as a sustainable project. This large project was often overwhelming for the person leading the arrangements who found that cross-agency partnerships can be fraught with risks. However, the 8-month journey culminated in an art exhibition and dramatic performance, increased learning about loss and grief issues by the community service providers and provided great links for future community/agency partnerships.

◆ In another small rural community, an older adult day activity programme explored how to assist their clients reflect on personal and family resources that have been used throughout their life span. This was done through photos, stories, memory boxes, and the commencement of an illustrated journal, including each participant's life story as shared. They involved the local primary school, the adult learning centre, and the community health centre as partners in the project making it sustainable and accessible to others within their community.

◆ An adult education centre in a small town ran two courses for carers in their community. The aim was to strengthen their knowledge of available community support, to inform about loss and grief, to provide resources and skills and access to a sustainable self help network.

◆ Six 'World Café' style discussions (see www.theworldcafe.com) were held targeting a range of population groups in local communities through partnerships between the local palliative care teams and community groups. The first café applicant invited general community members and attracted 25 people to an evening with supper provided to discuss a series of five open questions around grief, loss, and life-threatening illness. Another targeted palliative care volunteers and the open question was around death through the eyes of a child. A third café applicant targeted men and partnered with a community health centre to host an evening at a local winery to raise awareness around death, dying, loss, and grief with 25 attendees. A fourth café applicant attracted 20 and 22 general community members respectively to attend a café in two small town locations. The fifth café applicant drew on the wisdom learnt through these and successfully conducted two cafés at a local restaurant and targeted accidental listeners in the community (businesses, taxi drivers, reception staff, hairdressers, etc.) and people who work with children (schools, sporting clubs, youth groups, guide and scout leaders, etc.). Each café was followed with the offer of basic grief support education 2 weeks hence with overwhelming success. Of the 75 who attended these two cafés, approximately two-thirds went on to attend the skills session.

◆ Other groups have involved local craft and woodwork groups to create memory boxes for children of clients on the palliative care programme. This allows the child, along with their parent who has the life-threatening illness, to fill these boxes with personal memorabilia to support enduring relationships beyond the death of the parent.

◆ One palliative care volunteer service commenced discussion with their local government council to establish a reflective space at the city cemetery to shelter families and carers visiting people who have died on the palliative care programme and who are buried there. A partnership between them and the local cemetery trust, the local hospital and the palliative care service saw a rotunda and garden area built.

◆ The project supported a church pastoral care group, in partnership with the local palliative care volunteer service, to run a 'Celebrating Life' education session that included discussion on funeral celebrations, bereavement support, legal aspects, and other practicalities and choices to do with death and dying. This type of death education increases the capacity of community members to better support their own when called upon in the future.

◆ Palliative care services have organized palliative care information stands and sessions during local events such as festivals and horse races. Another partnered with the Alzheimer's Association to run a session conducted by a music therapist.

◆ A palliative care volunteer service sought community support from business houses to run a 'Care for the Carer Day' for the volunteers during palliative care week to acknowledge their work. Business houses and services were approached to provide items that would nurture these local people; support provided included massage, gifts, food and a venue.

◆ A group of interested palliative care workers and volunteers are now building on the development of a regional biographer or memoir service for clients on their programme. This service allows the client an opportunity to reflect on what their personal legacy to others has been. The biographer transcribes the oral biography into written form.

The outcomes and future of the Health Promotion Resource Team

The HPRT team identified ways to resource the specialist palliative care services' and palliative care volunteer services' ability to become more health-promoting in their palliative care practice.

- Health Promoting Palliative Care Resource Kits are now under development and will be made available to the subregional specialist palliative care services, the 17 palliative care volunteer services and the members of the health promotion resource team.

- Materials and boards for a static display were provided to the five subregional specialist palliative care services for use at events where their service can be given a more public face.

- Death education occurred through the establishment of journal or reading groups. They discussed topics that dealt with death, dying, loss, and care within the palliative care and healthcare settings. A set of 10 copies of 'Seven Dying Australians' (Kellehear and Ritchie 2003) containing the seven very personal stories of seven people living in end of life circumstances were purchased for loan as a lead in to encourage the formation of such groups. During the project one health service took up the offer. Hopefully more will take this on in the future.

- The Centre for Grief (now known as the Australian Centre for Grief and Bereavement), based in Victoria's capital city, Melbourne, was contracted to provide grief education and best practice resources to local professionals from a wide range of disciplines. Twenty-four people (including a general practitioner, social workers, nurses, funeral directors, clergy, loss and grief co-ordinators, and personal care attendants) attended a 1-day course on how to conduct a public seminar around adult grief support. This ensured 'basic' grief education was available at the local level across the large rural region. It also increased the pool of skilled educators who could assist in normalizing loss and grief.

- This Commonwealth (Australian) Department of Health and Ageing 'Caring Communities Program' project sought to develop an innovative capacity-building model of health promoting palliative care in a rural setting. Through the development of a Health Promotion Resource Team, the community has been invited to participate in building resilience around death, dying loss, and care. The activities listed in this chapter illustrate ways that the community can share the care as an integral part of a local palliative care team. The project findings recommended the continuation of the HPRT team. However, it must be remembered that the membership of this team is reliant on the capacity of the membership to include public health responsibilities within their usual paid or volunteer role. The availability of the small grant seed funding was also essential to the establishment of partnerships within local communities.

The findings from the impact research report (Rumbold and Gear 2004, p. 3) sum up the results well. '... the HPRT has been most effective in its task of promoting and supporting community development activities that have increased understanding and knowledge of dying, loss, and grief in general, and palliative care in particular across the region. Many of these activities have also developed skills that contribute substantially to their local community's capacity to care for those in their midst living with loss and grief, or life-threatening illness.' This project should encourage others to have a go at this very rewarding health promoting approach. Community and palliative care services can work alongside each other and together strengthen their local community's ability to assist those living with a life-limiting illness.

Conclusions

Every health service in industrial national settings attempts to develop and enhance their communities' resilience against disease, trauma, and disability. This is a fundamental axiom of all public health. That public health approach has always been characterized by a two-pronged approach. The first priority has been to address crises, to deal with illness, accident, or impairment through medical, surgical, or pharmacological repair and support. Increasingly, over the last 150 years, our concerns with repair have been gradually balanced by a parallel concern with prevention, first, of specific disease-borne problems related to infectious diseases, polluted water and food. But later these concerns with prevention, harm reduction and early intervention turned to non-infectious diseases such as cancer and heart disease, and later still, to the problems of psychiatric and physical disability, domestic violence, sexual abuse, drug and alcohol use, and a host of other sources of social disruption and poor health. The spread of these ideas of prevention, harm reduction and early intervention through innovative healthcare initiatives such as health education, intersectoral partnerships, and community development has been slow to reach the health services in end-of-life care. Nevertheless, the last decade in Australia, Britain, and the USA has witnessed major progress in these developments as each of these countries attempt to enhance their own communities' resilience to the morbidity and mortality associated with death, dying, and loss.

We have long recognized that the experiences of death and loss can continue to create yet other death and loss in a community. Deep sorrow and grief can disable for a time, a long time, and for some people it can even take away the will to live. People who live with life-threatening illness are subject to social and emotional difficulties such as depression or social rejection and stigma whether they are living with HIV or cancer. Health promoting palliative care programmes recognize the social character of these difficulties, recognize their impact on the quality and even longevity of patients and their families, and attempt to strengthen a community's resilience against these through community development initiatives such as the one described here. A broad public health approach to death and loss is crucial to the resilience of every community in their ongoing attempts to make sense of mortality, and in helping each other to enhance the quality of their lives in its shadow.

References

Agaibi CE, Wilson JP (2005) Trauma, PTSD and resilience: a review of the literature. *Trauma, Violence and Abuse* **6**(3), 195–216.

Bonanno GA, Papa A, O'Neill K (2002) Loss and human resilience. *Applied and Preventive Psychology* **10**, 193–206.

Crow G, Allan G (1994) *Community Life: An introduction to local social relations.* Hertfordshire: Harvester-Wheatsheaf.

DeV Peters R (2005) A community-based approach to promoting resilience in young children, their families and their neighbourhoods. In: *Resilience in Children, Families and Communities*, pp. 157–176 (eds DeV Peters R, Leadbeater B, McMahon RJ). New York: Kluwer Academic.

Kellehear A (1999) *Health Promoting Palliative Care.* Melbourne: Oxford University Press.

Kellehear A (2005) *Compassionate Cities: Public health and end-of-life care.* London: Routledge.

Kellehear A, Ritchie D (eds) (2003) *Seven Dying Australians.* Bendigo, Victoria: St Lukes Innovative Resources.

Macquarie Library (1984) *The Macquarie Illustrated World Atlas.* Sydney: Macquarie Library and Division of National Mapping.

Maton KI (2005) The social transformation of environments and the promotion of resilience in children. In: *Resilience in Children, Families and Communities*, pp. 119–135 (eds DeV Peters R, Leadbeater B, McMahon RJ). New York: Kluwer Academic.

Mayo M (1994) *Communities and Caring: The mixed economy of welfare.* London: Macmillan.

Mayo M (2000) *Cultures, Communities, Identities: Cultural strategies for participation and empowerment.* Basingstoke: Palgrave.

O'Donnell G (2002) *Enabling the Community: The Role of Volunteers In a Rural Health Setting.* Unpublished Master of Public Health Thesis: University of New South Wales, Sydney.

Palliative Care Australia (2003) *Palliative Care Service Provision in Australia: A planning guide.* 2nd edn. Canberra: Palliative Care Australia. www.pallcare.org.au/.

Palliative Care Australia (2005) *A Guide to Palliative Care Service Development: A population based approach.* Canberra: Palliative Care Australia. www.pallcare.org.au/.

Riley JR, Masten AS (2005) Resilience in context. In: *Resilience in Children, Families and Communities*, pp. 13–25 (eds DeV Peters R, Leadbeater B, McMahon RJ). New York: Kluwer Academic.

Rumbold B, Gear R (2004) *Evaluation of Health Promotion Resource Team: Hume Regional Palliative Care Caring Communities Project 'Building Rural Community Capacity Through Volunteering'*. Melbourne: La Trobe University Palliative Care Unit.

State of Victoria (2004) *Strengthening palliative care: A policy for health and community care providers 2004–09*. Melbourne: Continuing Care Unit, Programs Branch, Metropolitan Health and Aged Care Services Division, Department of Human Services. www.dhs.vic.gov.au/ahs/concare.htm.

Tremblay RE (2005) Disruptive behaviours: Should we foster or prevent resilience? In: *Resilience in Children, Families and Communities*, pp. 27–45 (eds DeV Peters R, Leadbeater B, McMahon RJ). New York: Kluwer Academic.

Wellman B, Wortley S (1990) Different strokes from different folks: community ties and social support. *American Journal of Sociology* **96**(3), 558–588.

Werner EE (2005) Resilience research: past, present, and future. In: *Resilience in Children, Families and Communities*, pp. 3–11 (eds DeV Peters R, Leadbeater B, McMahon RJ). New York: Kluwer Academic.

13

Resilience in trauma and disaster

Stephen Regel

Introduction

The past decade has seen an increasing focus and consensus on the importance of providing psychosocial support following disasters and complex emergencies. Many health and social care professionals with expertise in palliative care are being increasingly called upon to use their experience of working with loss to assist in post-disaster interventions. Many non-governmental organizations (NGOs) have been actively involved in the delivery of Psychosocial Support Programmes (PSPs; sometimes also referred to as Psychological Support Programmes) in varied contexts and settings, whether it is following natural disasters, as in the case of the recent Tsunami or in the wake of armed conflict. The term 'psychosocial' has become the preferred term when describing interventions designed to positively impact on the mental health needs of those individuals and communities affected by complex emergencies and will therefore be used throughout this chapter. In addition, the field of psychosocial interventions is relatively young and inevitably there have been calls to determine the evidence base for such interventions. There have also been critiques of the notion of PSP, as there is a view that many communities affected by complex emergencies are resilient and thus have an innate capacity to heal themselves without external intervention. Inevitably, there have also been critiques of the appropriateness and what has often been perceived as the 'medicalized' nature of such interventions.

In the context of this chapter, the psychosocial well-being of individuals and communities can be defined with reference to three core domains: human capacity, social ecology, cultures and values. These domains form the conceptual framework for mapping the human, social, and cultural resources available to people responding to the challenges of complex emergencies such as natural or man-made disasters and armed conflict (Psychosocial Working Group 2003). Nevertheless, there is an increasing recognition that individuals, families, and communities affected by adversity can also be vulnerable. Therefore, the key question is how to deliver effective psychosocial support and thus promote resilience and coping following exposure to extreme traumatic events.

There are numerous definitions of the concept of resilience that have relevance dependent on the context in which they are used. The definition of the International Resilience Project as '... universal capacity which allows the person, group or community to prevent, minimise or overcome the damaging effects of adversity' (Newman and Blackburn 2002) has utility for the concept of resilience in or following disasters and other complex emergencies. Resilience is sometimes attained over the long term at the expense of resilience in the short term. The extreme tenacity of the poor in developing countries in taking the long-term view to preserve their future livelihood is often observed in areas severely affected by famine, drought, or other hazards. An example of this would be the case of a woman in Sudan's Darfur region, who during a recent famine preserved her millet seed for planting by mixing it with sand, to prevent her hungry children from eating it. During the same famine, people were also reported to be leaving food aid centres to return home in time for planting. Resilience can be regarded as a common characteristic of all human beings, yet what may be regarded as deprivation and hardship in one context or country, may simply pass for a way of life in another. For example, disruption of electrical power in a Western context creates serious disruptions to everyday life and work. However, in many parts of the developing world, the mere search for raw materials to prepare food and provide other necessities is a daily chore to be faced with stoic acceptance.

These examples point toward a common theme. That is the importance of understanding the innate ability of individuals, communities, and societies, not only to cope with, but also to adapt to adversity and to focus psychosocial interventions at building on these strengths. While it may be a common perception that emergency appeals and media representations of disasters concentrate on identifying the vulnerable and their needs, there is little attention paid to what communities have achieved for themselves. There has been an inevitable shift from vulnerability to capacity, particularly in the area of PSPs and how they attempt to address mental health needs. There have indeed been detractors and critiques of PSP and these will be addressed later in the chapter, but these have since been superseded by innovative and challenging approaches to PSP in areas affected by complex emergencies. In 1991 the International Federation of Red Cross and Red Crescent Societies (IFRC) launched the Psychological Support Programme (PSP) as a cross-cutting programme under the Health and Care Division. To assist the IFRC with the implementation of the programme, the Danish Red Cross and IFRC established the Reference Centre for Psychological Support as a centre of excellence in 1993. From November 2004 the centre changed its name to the Reference Centre (RC) for Psychosocial Support, which has the following guiding principles (IFRC Reference Centre for Psychosocial Support 2006):

- assisting local initiatives, which will lead to a durable and meaningful change in the psychological well being of people affected by disasters and stressful life events;

- collaborating with Red Cross/Red Crescent National Societies to build sustainable psychosocial support programmes that are based on genuine local ownership, avoiding the creation of aid-dependent parallel structures;

- working on the basis of locally identified needs, rather than on the reflexes of the aid community;

- paying special attention to women and children who are often the most vulnerable groups in a post-conflict situation, as well as to families with missing members;

- any discussion on the relationship between humanitarian aid providers and recipients should be based on the concept of respect for the prevailing culture and its mental health or psychosocial healing practices.

It is also inevitable that the notions of resilience and the impact of traumatic events have become inextricably linked, but as yet this has not been addressed by the literature in any specific way. In the development field, the idea of sustainable livelihoods (SL) approach has become an important framework for the NGOs, donors, agencies, and government bodies (Chambers and Conway 1992). The SL approach is primarily concerned with the potential competence, capacities, and strengths, rather than weaknesses and needs of communities. This model also takes the view that even the worst off have some potential, so the focus of interventions must be on removing constraints to the realization of this potential. The SL approach recognizes a range of strengths and assets, which it calls 'capitals', essential for sustaining a livelihood. These include;

- **natural** capital: water, land, rivers, forests, and minerals;

- **financial** capital: savings, income, remittances, pensions, credit, and state transfers;

- **human** capital: knowledge, skills, health, and physical ability;

- **social** capital: networks, relations, affiliations, reciprocity, trust, and mutual exchange;

- **physical** capital: infrastructure, shelter, tools, transport, water and sanitation, and energy.

The complex relationship between assets, capacities, resources, and strengths together provide people with what has been called 'layers of resilience' to deal with adversity, including disasters protecting individuals and communities from various adversities, each kind of capital has something vital to offer, although different combinations of capital will be called upon to cope with and recover from different kinds of adversity (Glavovic 2002). As yet, the role of mental health and mental resilience has yet to enter the equation. Though it may be implicit in the human and social capital referred to above, it has never been really articulated. Ill health and/or lack of education are recognized as core dimensions of poverty as well as of vulnerability to disaster. Let us also look at the notion of 'social capital'. In the sustainable livelihood context, it is taken to mean the forms of mutual social assistance upon which people draw. These include networks such as clan or caste; memberships of more formalized groups such as women's associations; or affiliations of religion or ethnicity. These social networks can provide an informal safety net during difficult times and often play a crucial part in helping affected individuals and communities access urgently needed resources after a disaster. If we accept this, then mental ill health or suffering must also play a part in this vulnerability. One of the most important characteristics of resilient communities is the extent to which they work together toward common aims and goals, a function of social cohesion. These themes will be explored in more depth below in the context and framework of providing psychosocial support following complex emergencies.

Mental health, resilience, and trauma

The role of mental health in the context or promotion of resilience has also become somewhat contentious. Let us first deal with resilience in the face of trauma within a western European context. At the time of writing, the impact of the recent London bombings of 7 July 2005 have been the focus of much attention, both in terms of the emergency response and the psychological impact on the survivors. While it is yet too early for the research emanating from a 'Screen and Treat' programme of psychological care conducted by a major London National Health Service (NHS) hospital to be published, there have been some interesting public and professional responses to the provision of psychological or psychosocial support. The service described as an NHS Trauma Response, was conducted through a large NHS mental health service and offered free and confidential advice, help and treatment to anyone experiencing emotional problems as a result of the London bombings. The Screening Team was staffed by mental health professionals with the aim to screen as many people as possible who may be emotionally affected by the bombings in order to offer them advice, support, and psychological treatment where necessary. It was estimated that approximately 4000 people were exposed to the events of that day. However, it has been reported that only about 516 survivors came forward to avail themselves of the service. Estimates from previous research for those who go on to develop a diagnosis of post-traumatic stress disorder (PTSD) following a major disaster are in the region of 25–28%, with many experiencing chronic levels of anxiety that remain high for 2 years or more (Raphael 1986). If this were the case then approximately 1000 people would be at risk for developing longer-term psychological sequelae. There have been no epidemiological studies to assess PTSD in the community, but a survey, designed to study the distribution, correlates and consequences of psychiatric disorders in the United States (The National Co-morbidity Survey), estimated lifetime prevalence of PTSD at 7.8%. Survival analysis showed that more than one-third of people with an index episode of PTSD fail to recover even after many years (Kessler *et al.* 1995).

This leaves the obvious question: what of the other hundreds (potential PTSD sufferers) exposed to the incident? And what of other survivors who may be undergoing a psychological crisis as a result of their exposure to the event? One of the possible reasons given for the lack of uptake of the service is that there was a deliberate strategy not to be proactive in support, arguing that symptoms and problems should only be picked up and treated when people had started to display distress. As one eminent mental health professional was quoted as saying,

> What we've lost in the PTSD discourse is what they knew in the Second World War, par excellence ... Which is that people's reactions to trauma, adversity, war and terror are determined by the group psychology and not individual psychology. Now we're beginning to remind ourselves that normal people are pretty resilient. They have their own resources; they can maximise their social support

> The Guardian Weekend (17 June 2006)

However, mental health statistics tend to suggest another side to the face of resilience. A recent report on mental health in the UK, indicated that 16.5% of people aged 16–75 suffer from some form of mental illness, with depression and anxiety, making up the largest proportion of sufferers (Centre for Economic Performance 2006). What this suggests is that while many people will be resilient and cope well with adversity, there may be many who do not have the human or social capital to draw upon. For example, it is well known that significant risk factors for the development of PTSD are a lack of social support and previous psychological problems (Brewin *et al.* 2000; Perkonigg *et al.* 2000). Studies of disaster victims in Britain have also highlighted the importance of social support for trauma victims (Joseph *et al.* 1992). It is generally believed and understood that societies in western European countries have changed and that there is greater sense of isolation, alienation, and withdrawal, among some communities. Social structures and support networks are no longer as robust, with a greater emphasis on the individual. Therefore, assumed resilience may not always be a given. This leads to the challenge that faces many aid organizations and agencies following disaster, of how to facilitate and promote resilience following trauma.

The concept of PTSD is contentious and it is not the intention within this chapter to engage in an extended discourse on the presence or absence of the condition, but is nevertheless important to address some of the issues raised in the context of resilience in disaster. PTSD is a relatively new diagnostic category, but persistent pathological reactions to traumatic experiences have been recognized for a considerable period of time (Trimble 1985). The American Psychiatric Association included PTSD as a diagnostic category in the third edition of the Diagnostic and Statistical Manual (DSM-III) in 1980 (APA 1980). The growing body of empirical work on PTSD has led to the refinement of the conceptualization of the disorder. The developments in thinking about and understanding the impact of trauma have, in turn led to two revisions, the most recent being the fourth edition of the DSM (APA 1994) and its inclusion in the 10th edition of the International Classification of Diseases (WHO 1992). PTSD as a condition is characterised by three clusters of symptoms: (1) re-experiencing the event; (2) avoidance of triggers and reminders; and (3) symptoms of increased arousal (see Appendix). The contentious nature of the diagnosis and its use has divided the academic world into what Brewin (2003) describes as 'Saviours and Sceptics'. This is an enlightening treatise of the condition and the views of its 'Saviours and Sceptics', are well articulated in a balanced view of the current debate on the relevance of PTSD, in both western European contexts and other cultures.

It has also been argued that PTSD is a socially constructed concept of Western origin (Young 1995; Summerfield 2001). Young (1995) locates the origins of the trauma discourse in the late nineteenth century, when the word trauma, previously understood in terms of physical injury, was extended to include the psychological sequelae of exposure to extremely stressful events. He further suggests that the concept of PTSD has been constructed and shaped over time and has not always existed, but was waiting to be discovered by psychiatry: 'The disorder is not timeless, nor does it possess an intrinsic unity. Rather it is glued together by the practices, technologies and narratives with which it is studied, treated and represented and by the various interests, institutions and moral arguments that mobilised and these efforts and resources' (p. 5).

However, Young also goes on to say (though never quoted) within the space of a sentence of two:

> On the contrary, the reality of PTSD is confirmed empirically by its place in people's lives, by their experiences and convictions. My job as an ethnographer is not to deny its reality, but to explain how it and its traumatic memory have been *made* real, to describe the mechanisms through which these phenomena penetrate people's life worlds, acquire facticity and shape the self knowledge of patients, clinicians and researchers. (p. 5)

Summerfield (2001) argues that the diagnosis of PTSD 'lacks specificity … DSM IV criteria are subjective and that the diagnosis of PTSD can be made in the absence of objective dysfunction' (p. 97). In addition, he makes the assertion that there is 'more social utility attached to expressions of victimhood than to "survivorhood"' (p. 96). Shephard (2000) discusses the 'culture of trauma' in the context of psychiatry and war, and charts the rise of post disaster interventions in the wake of high profile disasters that occurred in the UK. Shephard cites the Bradford football ground fire in the UK as a turning point in the way healthcare professionals and the public regarded disasters because of the very public witnessing of the event on television. This meant that millions of viewers were able to witness the horror first hand and thus identify more easily with victims and their families. The destruction of the World Trade Centre on 11 September 2001 could not have demonstrated this more graphically. There was significant empathy for the victims, survivors, and their families and widespread recognition and acceptance that some form of psychological support be provided for the survivors, families of the bereaved, emergency services workers, the rescue workers and others involved in the rescue, and recovery operations.

The discussion and debate about PTSD inevitably influence the nature and provision of post-disaster psychosocial interventions and have led to a divided opinion as to the provision of such support. It is pertinent then to consider this in a cross-cultural framework and how this influences and impacts on mental resilience in complex emergencies.

The concept of psychological trauma and cultural differences across cultures

Across cultures, people differ in what they believe and understand about life and death, what they feel, what elicits those feelings, the perceived implications of those feelings, their expression and appropriateness of certain feelings and strategies for dealing with feelings that cannot be directly expressed (Rosenblatt 1993). A cross-cultural perspective demonstrates the variety, for example, in people's responses to death and dying and the process of mourning. Rather than being process orientated, mourning is seen as an adaptive response to specific task demands arising from loss that must be dealt with regardless of individual, culture, or historical era (Hagman 1995). Stroebe (1992) challenges the belief in the importance of 'grief work' for adjustment to bereavement. She examined claims made in theoretical formulations and principles of grief counselling and therapy concerning the necessity of working through loss. Grief reactions are also patterned by the culture, formed by one's society's belief systems, and expectations, values and norms for relationships and bonds. This will influence both expression and duration of grief reactions across different cultural settings. In essence, sensitivity to the culturally appropriate needs for ritual in responding to grief and providing for privacy and personal needs are paramount.

Research on post-traumatic reactions in non-Western groups has mostly been conducted in western Europe and the United States to meet the needs of refugees from developing countries (Klebe *et al.* 1995). Differences in the prevalence of PTSD across ethnic and cultural groups have been reported (Marsella *et al.* 1996). However, there are several conceptual issues related to cross-cultural trauma research. One of the reasons for discrepancies in cross-cultural studies is that Western diagnostic criteria are not always applicable in non-Western cultures. For example, a recent study on Tibetan refugees in India, demonstrated that in this population the destruction of religious symbols was a major stressor. If culturally defined stressors are not heeded, the amount of stress experienced would be evaluated lower than it actually was. The same group of workers also noted that some symptoms common to trauma survivors such as guilt were displayed far less than would be expected, explained by the fact that the word *guilt* does not even have a Tibetan equivalent. A further illustration can be seen in the above study within a religious context. Buddhism implies that 'hopelessness lies in the nature of the world'. Therefore, a good Buddhist would present with generalized feelings of hopelessness similar to depression. The acknowledgement of the all pervasive presence of suffering in the world is almost 'endorsed' by Buddhism. A 'non-disorder' frame of reference for 'depressive' symptoms is therefore present within Buddhist cultures (Terheggen *et al.* 2001). A recent study that attempted to assess PTSD in a radically non-Western culture, that of Kalahari Bushmen found that the results compared closely with PTSD assessments in other non-Western societies (McCall and Resick 2003).

In addition, the absence of culturally sensitive instruments and rating scales make accurate assessment difficult. The development of instruments with acceptable psychometric properties faces numerous methodological challenges.

First, the massive trauma experienced by refugees and torture victims raises ethical and clinical questions about the potential negative impact upon them of a checklist or questionnaire. Secondly, the diverse ethno-cultural and political backgrounds require assessment instruments sensitive to a wide range of traumatic events and experiences (Mollica 1989). For example, the traumatic experiences of Chilean political prisoners are dramatically different to those of Indo-Chinese refugees. Finally, while specific symptoms have been clearly linked to the trauma of torture, the DSM-IV criteria for PTSD has not been established as a valid disease construct in non-Western cultures. Cross-national comparisons by the World Health Organization (WHO) suggest that, despite core features of major depression, each culture has its own specific symptoms. PTSD criteria may reveal a similar pattern across cultures; however, a central universal core of PTSD remains to be established. There are issues concerning the definition and nature of traumatic stressors in different cultures. These are often different depending on the cultural settings (Kleber *et al.* 1995). Therefore, a standardized checklist could under- or overestimate the prevalence of traumatic stressors if the list was not sensitive to the cultural values of the population studied (Manson 1997).

Nevertheless, there have been a number of studies conducted with disaster survivors (Canino *et al.* 1990; de la Fuente 1990; Zhang and Zhang 1991; Escobar 1992; Guarnaccia *et al.* 1993; Joh 1997), refugees and asylum seekers (Lavik *et al.* 1996; Silove *et al.* 1997; Terheggen *et al.* 2001) survivors of torture (Morris and Silove 1992; Ramsay *et al.* 1993; Allodi 1994; Carlson and Rosser-Hagan 1994) earthquakes, and political violence (Goenjian *et al.* 2000), which used the most culturally appropriate assessment methods available. It would appear that the most common symptoms displayed across the cultures sampled in the above studies, were those associated with the diagnoses of depression, anxiety disorders and PTSD. They manifest themselves in different ways within cultures, but the symptoms tend to fit the general diagnostic criteria for the disorders mentioned above. In recent years there have also been studies that have attempted to address the issue of assessment and the use of culturally sensitive measures with some degree of success (Mollica *et al.* 1987, 1992).

Recently, critics of the concept of PTSD as applied to non-Western settings have also argued that data are lacking that suggest mental health morbidity is higher in populations exposed to conflict and other complex emergencies, citing Northern Ireland as one such example (Almedon and Summerfield 2004). The authors further suggest that over the last 30 years of civil conflict there has been little evidence of significant impact on referral rates to mental health services. However, a recent published epidemiological survey to assess the effects of the civil unrest (the Troubles as they have come to be known) on the general population concluded that exposure to the Troubles has resulted in a significant and independent detrimental effect on the mental health of the population in Northern Ireland (O'Reilly and Stevenson 2003). Secondly, it has only been since the start of the Peace Process that many of those affected have been able to discuss the emotional and psychological impact of the Troubles and begin to seek help, as the conflict engendered a culture of silence (Healey 2004). These factors were further supported in a recent review of mental health and learning disability in the Province, which supported the view that psychological trauma, had not been sufficiently addressed as a specific health issue (Northern Ireland Office 2004).

In the most comprehensive work about ethnocultural aspects of PTSD to date, Marsella *et al.* (1996) write in their concluding chapter: 'It should be noted, in this regard, that trauma seems well understood by people from non-Western cultural backgrounds, as noted throughout this book, even in the face of variations in concepts of health and healing' (Marsella *et al.* 1996, p. 533). There is reason to believe that there is a universal biological response to trauma (see Marsella *et al.* 1996) where at least the re-experiencing and arousal symptoms have a biological basis. The significance of these studies indicate that reactions to traumatic events do have a degree of universality, but the implications for early intervention are primarily based on a clear understanding of culturally specific reactions to trauma and the sophistication in the applicability of psychosocial interventions as outlined below.

Psychosocial interventions and enhancing resilience in complex emergencies

If there is a recognition and acknowledgement that in complex emergencies such as major disasters, especially those involving severe injuries, bereavement, and loss, there will indeed be mental health consequences for many survivors. This would be specially so where the social infrastructure has been compromised, whatever mental health systems existed prior to the emergency that may be insufficient to meet the multifaceted needs of communities affected. Mollica *et al.* (2004), only a few days before the Asian tsunami of 2004, urged countries throughout the world to prepare themselves to deal with '*Mental health in complex emergencies*'. It is noteworthy that the authors were not calling for armies of counsellors to be drafted in or for Western models of therapy to be utilized, but acknowledging the impact that disasters can have on the three core domains as mentioned above. Nevertheless, there remains a body of criticism of PSP, which argues that interventions cause more harm than good and do not promote the natural mental resilience of individuals and communities affected (Almedom and Summerfield 2004). The criticism often hinges on the debate as articulated above as to whether those affected by disasters and other traumatic events suffer from what we know as PTSD and other psychological sequelae, e.g. depression and anxiety and how that should be addressed.

Despite the sceptics, the concept of PSP has become firmly established in the canon of humanitarian organizations' interventions following complex emergencies. There is an expectation that individuals and communities following catastrophe are resilient, but, there is also an understanding borne out by a considerable body of evidence (as outlined above) that there are mental health consequences for some survivors. The loss of life and forced migration suffered by many communities following the Asian tsunami focused national and international agencies on the need to provide appropriate psychosocial care from the very beginning. The early arguments and criticisms surrounding PSP and early interventions paled into insignificance when faced by the urgent need to reduce distress and prevent the development of longer-term mental health problems. In the wake of the death, destruction, multiple bereavements and losses, including homes and livelihoods, doing nothing was not an option. Lessons had also been learned following the mental health response after the earthquake that devastated the city of Bam in Southern Iran, destroying 85% of the city. An estimated 26 000 people were killed and a further 30 000 injured. This response was delivered early and was the product of much planning and preparation for just such a disaster. Knowing that the region was vulnerable to earthquakes, the Department of Mental Health in the Ministry of Health in Iran in collaboration with the Iranian Red Crescent started conducting a series of workshops for relief workers in the basic skills of psychosocial support. Further training was also facilitated by UNICEF and the Centre for Crisis Psychology in Norway (Yule 2006).

This example is of course one of among many illustrating that PSPs do not focus on PTSD and are not restricted to a conventional Eurocentric view of suffering and distress. All PSPs are designed in collaboration with local agencies and communities, especially those conducted through the International Red Cross and Red Crescent Societies' Reference Centre for Psychosocial Support. A key element is, and always has been, the facilitation and enhancement of local resources and communities, together with capacity building. Requests for PSPs come from a wide variety of Red Cross and Red Crescent National Societies and a recent example has been the author's experience of working with the Somali Red Crescent in developing a culturally sensitive framework for the development and delivery of psychosocial training for volunteers. In many developing countries the local Red Cross/Red Crescent provides basic health and social care, something in the West that is taken for granted.

The request for a PSP came from the Somali Red Crescent and was developed using the framework of a 'programme development' workshop. The materials used were adapted and developed by the workshop participants, all members of the Somali Red Crescent health teams and this will be utilized and delivered as part of a community based first aid programme.

Some have argued that the transfer of Western concepts and techniques, for example to war-affected societies, risks perpetuating the colonial status of non-Western mind-sets as every culture has its own frameworks for mental health and norms for help-seeking at times of crisis (Summerfield 1999). This argument is based on making distinctions between Western 'eurocentric' cultures and cultures in non-industrialized countries and while it may appear a straightforward distinction, it is far from being the case. Many societies have chosen to adapt mental health concepts developed by Western psychology and prefer corresponding intervention methods, often in combination with traditional healing (Straker 1994). Similarly, in many rural areas in European countries traditional healing techniques for physical and mental complaints have remained popular.

Concerns continue to be expressed about psychosocial responses to disasters and the lack of an evidence base for such interventions. Inevitably, these remain focused on the apparent lack of awareness by practitioners of local cultural practices, needs, and religious rituals for facilitating the process of recovery from loss or multiple losses. However, these reports continue to remain anecdotal (Ganesan 2006). Elsewhere, similar reports are based on isolated instances, often by some of the smaller NGOs, for example, following the Kosovo conflict (Pupavac 2001). There is evidence that there are some instances whereby an integrated model of intervention using the framework described above has had significant utility. As referred to earlier, following the earthquake in Bam, of 2003, the Children and War Recovery Manual (Smith *et al.* 1998) was adapted with local collaboration and used by the psychosocial teams, based on previous experiences and training. This formed the basis for trauma counselling interventions based on cognitive behavioural exercises and included brief group exercises over four sessions with about 960 children and 742 adults. About 1500 local mental health professionals and teachers were trained to provide brief interventions. The evaluations and post intervention questionnaires and clinician reports indicated that 85% (some 55 000) of the survivors benefited from the sessions (Yule 2006). Many interventions utilise psycho-educational strategies, such as information about the psychological impact of traumatic events and related supportive advice. Support and guidance are likely to cover reassurance about immediate distress, information about the likely course of symptoms, strategies for effective coping, signposting for further help and self-help activities based on facilitating individual and community resilience.

Other recent developments in the field have been the development of Narrative Exposure Therapy (NET) (Schauer *et al.* 2005). NET has been developed as an integration of cognitive-behavioural therapy (CBT) and Testimony Therapy (TT) (Cienfuegos and Monelli 1983). TT is a short-term psychological treatment method that was especially developed for survivors of torture and other severe human rights violations. TT aims at the construction of a detailed and coherent report of the survivor's biography including an explicit description of the traumatic events. The written testimony created by the survivor in co-operation with a therapist is used for documentary and political purposes in support of the survivor. The procedures of CBT and TT share many common features. As in CBT, prolonged exposure to the traumatic material is realized through reporting about it. This promotes the habituation of emotional and physiological reactions to reminders of the traumatic events and so reduces symptoms. But the focus of TT is not on habituation, but on the reconstruction of the shattered autobiographical memories of the traumatic experiences. NET is therefore a combination of these two approaches and has been used successfully in many cross-cultural settings, again by working closely with and training local professionals, especially teachers (Schauer *et al.* 2005). It has been also developed for children and again used in the wake of recent disasters (Schauer 2004) and in refugee camps (Neuner *et al.* 2002). Therefore, there is evidence to indicate that there is room for diverse approaches to facilitate and support resilience following disaster and that these approaches, now being shown to be effective and with a sound evidence base need to be accommodated within the context of psychosocial approaches.

Many of the criticisms of PSP and other interventions following complex emergencies have also been based on isolated cases of inappropriate mental health responses, fundamental misunderstandings of the principles of PSP, together with little active involvement or knowledge of a significant body of field activity conducted over the past 10 years. It has offered little in the way of positive or constructive contributions to our understanding or what works in the field of psychosocial support. Furthermore there has been a significant void in the academic discourse about what happens in practice. The current evidence is that these criticisms are not only outdated, but also redundant in the light of numerous developments by international humanitarian agencies and centres such as the IFRC Reference Centre for Psychosocial Support. Currently there are initiatives based on the experiences by agencies following emergencies from armed conflicts to natural disasters. These are being created by a growing set of lessons, tools and principles that can guide effective mental health and psychosocial support in emergency settings. The aim is to systemize the field by development of coherent practice-based guidance. This work is currently being done by the Inter-Agency Standing Committee (IASC) Task force on Mental Health and Psychosocial Support in Emergency settings (IASC 2006). The IASC is a unique inter-agency forum for co-ordination, policy development, and decision-making involving the key UN and non-UN humanitarian partners. The IASC was established in June 1992 in response to a United Nations General Assembly Resolution on the strengthening of humanitarian assistance. The General Assembly Resolution affirmed its role as the primary mechanism for inter-agency co-ordination of humanitarian assistance. Under the leadership of the IASC, the United Nations develops humanitarian policies, agrees on a clear division of responsibility for the various aspects of humanitarian assistance, identifies and addresses gaps in response, and advocates for effective application of humanitarian principles. Together with the Executive Committee for Humanitarian Affairs (ECHA), the IASC forms the key strategic co-ordination mechanism among major humanitarian agencies.

Psychosocial support following disasters: a case study

On 8 October 2005, a powerful earthquake measuring 7.6 on the Richter scale hit Northern Pakistan and Northern India; the tremors were felt across the region from Kabul in Afghanistan to Delhi. In less than a minute, whole towns and villages were reduced to rubble and landslides had washed away roads and villages on mountain sides. The death toll was more than 80 000, with over 70 000 people injured and 2.6 million people made homeless, with 145 000 being internally displaced in official and ad hoc refugee camps. The European Commission Humanitarian Office (ECHO) funded a Psychosocial Programme following the disaster, as the government of Pakistan and all relevant stakeholders involved in the relief operation recognized the urgency of addressing not only the physical and material needs of those affected but also the emotional and psychosocial needs of the population. The funding allowed the Danish Red Cross (DRC) and the Pakistan Red Crescent Society (PRCS), supported by the IFRC to initiate a Psychosocial Programme in four refugee camps in the North-west frontier and in Islamabad in November 2005. The initial assessment, carried out immediately after the earthquake, found the disaster had also caused enormous psychological distress because of significant loss of life, shelter, and livelihood, not to mention multiple losses in many cases.

The immediate priority following the earthquake was to provide food, shelter, and medical aid to all those affected. The majority of the population in the area affected by the earthquake lived in remote and scattered villages with a limited and basic infrastructure in terms of communication, transport, and other services. The small and isolated communities affected, sustained a living through the land, often eking out a basic and simple existence. The literacy rate in the most affected areas was low, with women leading secluded lives, often rarely interacting with the outside world other than their extended family. In addition, some of the affected areas had been isolated as a result of the long-lasting conflict between India and Pakistan in Kashmir. The harsh winter conditions hampered immediate reconstruction, prevented the population from regaining their livelihoods and other day-to-day activities. A large part of the affected population also had to spend the winter months in temporary camps away from their place of origin.

The psychosocial team's assessment indicated that many were experiencing what would be considered normal responses to a disaster of such proportion. Many felt disbelief at what had happened, finding it difficult to absorb the enormity of the situation and assess the damage and loss for themselves, their families and communities. Initially the emphasis was on practical issues such as recovering the remains of loved ones, arranging burial ceremonies and other cultural rituals. In this remote area of Pakistan religion plays an important part in the traditional lifestyle of these isolated communities.

At assessment, the psychosocial team were able to establish many of the challenges presented when organizing a PSP to facilitate culturally appropriate coping strategies. It was decided at an early stage that it was of great importance to involve individuals, families, and communities within the camp in the decisions regarding psychosocial initiatives so that they could express what they regarded as helpful in the facilitation of a healing process and to enhance their natural resilience. The team were also very aware of the significance of religion and the role of women in a very traditional and rural setting of Pakistan.

The programme began in November 2005 and was implemented within the biggest refugee camps, utilizing 16 PRCS field workers, a programme manager and a field team co-ordinator. All these individuals were recruited and trained using context specific psychosocial models and working in collaboration with local NGOs who agreed to provide training, professional supervision, and support to field workers during the project period. Within 3 months, four teams had generated awareness about the psychological reactions to trauma, established a variety of social activities and organised volunteers in four of the large camps. The volunteers were initially supported until they felt able to work independently before other similar activities were established in surrounding villages and communities. Activities were all based on participatory assessments and knowledge gained from focused interviews and multiple meetings with the target communities. The most common activity was psycho-educational sessions for different groups, e.g. children of different ages, women, and men. Social activities were also initiated, aimed at creating a safe and culturally appropriate environment, where different groups could meet, share problems, concerns, and be actively involved in the recovery and rehabilitation process.

The PRCS had not previously been involved in psychosocial activities and subsequently did not have any staff who were trained in this area, or who could be transferred to the new programme. In the event, all field workers were new employees having been newly introduced to the PRCS and the Red Crescent movement, receiving intensive training in required knowledge and skills. The psychosocial team found that experience and lessons learned from other PSPs meant it was important to create specific modules designed for each of the project areas. For example, women in the affected areas, not being used to attending groups where they shared feelings and feedback, were in groups facilitated by women. Widows and orphans were often absorbed into extended families and not seen as particularly vulnerable. However, the new dynamic created by social, emotional, and economic situations in a new family can be extremely problematic and result in violence and abuse. Therefore, this was a significant challenge and was addressed by using field workers and volunteers drawn from the local communities. At the time of writing the projects continue and there are plans to further develop expertise for staff, to strengthen the PRCS and engage in capacity building, ultimately incorporating psychosocial support and activities within the PRCS heath department.

At the time of writing, initiatives are under way to develop indicators to audit progress and change within PSPs. Indicators within a psychosocial paradigm are important because they (1) provide information on the process of implementing PSP; (2) give the organization and beneficiaries an indication of the effects of the programme; and (3) the amount of transparency and accountability to both local and international stakeholders. The purpose of PSPs is not to medicalize or pathologize what is often normal suffering in the context of catastrophe but to facilitate and enhance resilience and recovery. It has often been observed that up to 70% of a given population may display emotional reactions that could be addressed through PSPs. The concept and importance of thorough analysis and assessment of local conditions during the early phase of disaster is now well recognized. It is also well recognized that emotional responses and behaviours observed differ across cultures and societies and that individuals respond very differently on the basis of these socio-cultural needs. Given that PSPs are focused on bringing about qualitative changes in the lives of individuals and communities, the development of meaningful indicators is a significant challenge. Therefore, working closely with affected communities and engaging them in being proactive in defining possible solutions based on their own needs is clearly a constructive development.

Resilience in disasters: future directions in research and practice

There is ample evidence that individuals and communities are resilient in the face of disasters and other complex emergencies (Nikapota 2006). There is also an emerging literature on the observations that stressful and traumatic events can provoke positive psychological changes, an aspect also contained in the major religions Buddhism, Christianity, Hinduism, Islam, and Judaism. Growth has been reported following a wide range of stressful and traumatic events. The positive changes observed after these events have been variously described as post-traumatic growth (Calhoun and Tedeschi 1999). This has been developed further by Joseph and Linley (2005) who propose a positive psychological theory of growth through adversity, positing an intrinsic motivation towards growth, showing how this leads to the states of intrusion and avoidance that are characteristic of cognitive and emotional processing, following exposure to traumatic events. Their theory illustrates how human valuing processes, i.e. that human beings are active and growth oriented, will automatically lead to the actualization of positive changes in psychological well-being, through positive accommodation of trauma-related information, i.e. all incoming stimuli related to the traumatic experience, such as thoughts, sensory impressions, attribution, and meaning. This is facilitated if the social environment is able to support this positive accommodation process.

These developments in our conceptualization of how human beings deal with extreme trauma further build on our understanding of resilience in relation to surviving a trauma. Flach (1990) discussed the concept of resilience in relation to surviving a trauma by defining it as: 'Psychobiological resilience is the efficient blending of psychological, biological and environmental elements that permits human beings ... to transit episodes of chaos necessarily associated with significant periods of stress and change successfully' (Flach 1990, p. 40). Resilience is not therefore viewed exclusively in terms of internal characteristics but in terms of an interactive process.

Thus the notion of resilience in disaster, while often implicit in our understanding of how individuals recover following exposure to catastrophic trauma and loss, needs a greater, far more explicit exposition of the factors that account for individual and cultural differences. There is an understanding and acceptance that there is universality to human responses to trauma and loss. We know that different cultures respond in very different ways to traumatic events for multifaceted reasons. However as human beings, while our reactions to distressing, stressful, and traumatic events may differ, so do the interventions that facilitate the process of recovery and growth. The work of key players in the field such as the IFRC Reference Centre for Psychosocial Support and other major NGOs is constantly developing to take account of new understandings of resilience and growth following trauma. This investment is welcome and promising in order to aid our understanding of what influences coping to aid integration of the meaning of a traumatic experience, both on an individual basis and in a cross-cultural context. The debates and criticisms of psychosocial and mental health interventions following complex emergencies are no longer valid. The need for an integrative theory of cultural responses to trauma, positive growth, and resilience in adversity, which further enhances the quality of such interventions, is paramount and deserves to be the focus of key actors in the humanitarian agencies.

References

Almedom AM, Summerfield D (2004) Mental well-being in settings of 'Complex Emergency': An overview. *Journal of Biosocial Sciences* **36**, 381–388.

Allodi FA (1994) Post-traumatic stress disorder in hostages and victim of torture. *Psychiatric Clinics of North America* **17**(2), 279–288.

APA (1980) *Diagnostic and Statistical Manual for Mental Disorders*, 3rd edn. Washington DC: American Psychiatric Association.

APA (1994) *Diagnostic and Statistical Manual for Mental Disorders*, 4th edn. Washington DC: American Psychiatric Association.

Brewin CR (2003) *Post Traumatic Stress Disorder: Malady or Myth*. New Haven: Yale University Press.

Brewin CR, Andrews B, Valentine JD (2000) Meta-analysis of risk factors for posttraumatic stress disorder in trauma-exposed adults. *Journal of Consulting and Clinical Psychology* **68**(5), 748–766.

Calhoun LG, Tedeschi RG (1999) *Facilitating Post Traumatic Growth: A Clinician's Guide*. London: Lawrence Erlbaum Associates.

Canino GJ, Bravo M, Rubio-Stipec M (1990) The impact of disaster on mental health: Prospective and retrospective analyses. *International Journal of Mental Health* **19**, 51–69.

Carlson EB, Rosser-Hagan R (1994) Cross-cultural response to trauma: a study of traumatic experiences and posttraumatic symptoms in Cambodian refugees. *Journal of Traumatic Stress* **7**, 43–58.

Centre for Economic Performance–Mental Health Policy Group (2006) The Depression Report: A New Deal for Depression and Anxiety Disorders. Centre for Economic Performance, The London School of Economics and Political Science, http://cep.lse.ac.uk/research/mentalhealth.

Chambers R, Conway GR (1992) *Sustainable rural livelihoods: Practical concepts for the 21st Century*. IDS Discussion Paper No. 296, Institute for Development Studies, University of Sussex.

Cienfuegos J, Monelli C (1983) The testimony of political repression as a therapeutic instrument. *American Journal of Orthopsychiatry* **53**, 43–51.

Escobar JI, Canino G, Rubio-Stipec M, Bravo M (1992) Somatic symptoms after a natural disaster: a prospective study. *American Journal of Psychiatry* **149**(7), 965–967.

Flach F (1990) The resilience hypothesis and post traumatic stress disorder. In: *Post Traumatic Stress Disorder: Aetiology, Phenomenology and Treatment* (eds Wolfe ME, Mosnaim AD). Washington DC: American Psychiatric Press.

de la Fuente R (1990) The mental health consequences of the 1985 earthquake in Mexico. *International Journal of Mental Health* **19**, 21–29.

Ganesan M (2006) Psychosocial response to disasters—some concerns. *International Review of Psychiatry* **18**(3), 241–247.

Goenjian AK, Steinberg AM, Najarian LM (2000) Prospective study of posttraumatic stress, anxiety, and depressive reactions after earthquake and political violence. *American Journal of Psychiatry* **157**(6), 911–916.

Glavovic BC, Scheyvens R, Overton J (2002) Waves of adversity. layers of resilience: exploring the sustainable livelihoods approach. In: *Proceedings of 3rd Biennial Conference of the International Development Studies Network of Aotearoa, New Zealand, Massey University.*

Guarnaccia PJ, Canino G, Rubio-Stepic M (1993) The prevalence of ataques de nervios in the Puerto Rico Disaster Study: the role of culture in psychiatric epidemiology. *Journal of Nervous and Mental Disease* **181**, 157–165.

Hagman G (1995) Mourning: a review and reconsideration. *International Journal of Psychoanalysis* **76**, 909–925.

Healey A (2004) A different description of trauma: a wider systemic perspective—a personal insight. *Child Care in Practice* **10**(2), 167–184.

IASC Task Force on Mental Health and Psychosocial Support in Emergency Settings (2006) http://www.humanitarianinfo.org/iasc/content/documents/.

Joh H (1997) Disaster stress of the 1995 Kobe earthquake. *Japan Psychologia* **40**, 192–200.

Joseph S, Linley A (2005) Positive adjustment to threatening events: an organismic valuing theory of growth through adversity. *Review of General Psychology* **9**(3), 262–280.

Joseph S, Williams R, Yule W, Andrews B (1992) Crisis support and psychiatric symptomatology in adult survivors of the Jupiter Cruise ship disaster. *British Journal of Clinical Psychology* **31**, 63–73.

Kessler RC, Sonnega A, Bromet E, Huges M, Nelson CB (1995) Posttraumatic stress disorder in the national co-morbidity survey. *Archives of General Psychiatry* **52**, 1048–1060.

Kleber RJ, Figley CR, Gersons BPR (1995) (eds) *Beyond Trauma: Societal and cultural dimensions.* New York: Plenum.

Lavik NJ, Hauff E, Skrondal A (1996) Mental disorder among refugees and the impact of persecution and exile: some findings from an out-patient population. *British Journal of Psychiatry* **169**, 726–732.

Manson SM (1997) Cross-cultural and multiethnic assessment of trauma. In: *Assessing Psychological Trauma and PTSD*, pp. 239–266 (eds Wilson JP, Keane TM). New York: Guilford.

Marsella AJ, Friedman MJ, Gerrity ET, Scurfield RM (1996) (eds) *Ethnocultural Aspects of PTSD: An Overview of Issues Research and Clinical Applications.* Washington DC: American Psychiatric Press.

McCall GJ, Resick PA (2003) A pilot study of PTSD symptoms among Kalahari Bushmen. *Journal of Traumatic Stress* **16**(5), 445–450.

Mollica RF (1989) What is a case? In: *Refugee Resettlement and Wellbeing* (ed. Abbott A). Auckland, NZ: Mental Health Foundation of New Zealand.

Mollica RF, Wyshak G, de Marneffe D (1987) Indochinese Versions of the Hopkins Symptom Checklist-25: a screening instrument for the psychiatric care for refugees. *American Journal of Psychiatry* **144**(4), 497–500.

Mollica RF, Caspi-Yavin MAR, Bollini P (1992) Validating a cross-cultural instrument for measuring torture, trauma, and posttraumatic stress disorder in Indochinese refugees. *Journal of Nervous & Mental Disease* **180**(2), 111–116.

Mollica RR, Lopez Cardoza B, Osofsky HJ, Raphael B, Ager A, Salama P (2004) Mental health in complex emergencies. *Lancet* **364**, 2058–2067.

Morris P, Silove D (1992) Cultural influences in psychotherapy with refugee survivors of torture and trauma. *Hospital & Community Psychiatry* **43**(8), 820–825.

Newman T, Blackburn S (2002) *Transitions in the Lives of Children and Young People: Resilience Factors*. Summary (Interchange 78). Edinburgh: Scottish Executive Education Department.

Neuner F, Schauer M, Roth W, Elbert T (2002) A narrative exposure treatment as intervention in a refugee camp: a case report. *Behavioural & Cognitive Psychotherapy* **30**, 205–209.

Nikapota A (2006) After the tsunami: a story from Sri Lanka. *International Review of Psychiatry* **18**(3), 275–279.

Northern Ireland Office (2004) *A Review of Mental Health and Learning Disability Services in Northern Ireland*. Northern Ireland Office.

O'Reilly D, Stevenson M (2003) Mental health in Northern Ireland: Have 'the troubles' made it worse? *Journal of Epidemiology and Community Health* **57**(7), 488.

Perkonigg A, Kessler RC, Storz S (2000) Traumatic events and post-traumatic stress disorder in the community: prevalence, risk factors and co-morbidity. *Acta Psychiatrica Scandinavica* **101**, 46–59.

Psychosocial Working Group (2003) Psychosocial Intervention in Complex Emergencies: A Conceptual Framework http://www.forcedmigration.org/psychosocial/PWGinfo.htm.

Pupavac V (2001) Therapeutic governance: psycho-social intervention and trauma risk management. *Disasters* **4**(4), 358–372.

Raphael B (1986) *When Disaster Strikes—A Handbook for the Caring Professions*. London: Hutchinson.

Ramsay R, Gorst-Unsworth C, Turner S (1993) Psychiatric morbidity in survivors of organised state violence including torture. *British Journal of Psychiatry* **162**, 55–59 of Psychiatry Vol. **152**(4), 555–563.

Reference Centre for Psychosocial Support (2006) Guiding Principles.(http://psp.drk.dk/sw26837.asp).

Rosenblatt (1993) Cross cultural variation in the experience, expression and understanding of grief. In: *Ethnic Variations in Dying, Death and Grief: Diversality in Universality*, pp. 13–19 (eds Irish DP, Lundquist KF). Washington DC: Taylor and Francis.

Schauer E, Neuner F, Elber T, Ertl V, Onyut L, Odenwald M, Schauer M (2004) Narrative exposure therapy in children—a case study. *Intervention* **2**, 18–32.

Schauer M, Neuner F, Elber T (2005) *Narrative Exposure Therapy: A Short-Term Intervention for Traumatic Stress Disorders after War, Terror, or Torture*, Vol. 1, pp. 1–68. MA: Hogrefe and Huber.

Shephard B (2000) *A War of Nerves*. London: Cape.

Silove D, Sinnerbrink I, Field A (1997) Anxiety, depression and PTSD in asylum-seekers: associations with pre-migration trauma and post-migration stressors. *British Journal of Psychiatry* **170**, 351–357.

Smith P, Dyregrov A, Yule W, Perrin S, Gupta L, Gjestad R (1999) *A Manual for Teaching Survival Techniques to Child Survivors of Wars and Major Disasters*. Bergen, Norway: Foundation for Children and War (see www.childrenandwar.org).

Straker G (1994) Integrating African and Western healing practices in South Africa. *American Journal of Psychotherapy* **48**, 455–467.

Stroebe MS (1992) Coping with bereavement: a review of the grief work hypothesis. *Omega: Journal of Death and Dying* **26**, 19–42.

Summerfield D (1999) A critique of seven assumptions behind psychological trauma programmes in war affected areas. *Social Science and Medicine* **48**, 1449–1462.

Summerfield D (2001) The invention of post traumatic stress disorder and the social usefulness of a psychiatric category. *British Medical Journal* **322**, 95–98.

Terheggen MA, Stroebe MS, Kleber RJ (2001) Western conceptualisations and eastern experience: a cross-cultural study of traumatic stress reactions among Tibetan refugees in India. *Journal of Traumatic Stress* **14**(2), 391–404.

Trimble MR (1985) Post traumatic stress disorder: history of a concept. In: *Trauma and Its Wake: The Study and Treatment of Post Traumatic Stress Disorder* (ed. Figley CR). New York: Brunner Mazel.

World Health Organization (1992) *The International Classification of Diseases*, 10th edn. Geneva: WHO.

Young A (1995) *The Harmony of Illusions: Inventing Post-Traumatic Stress Disorder*. Princeton, NJ: Princeton University Press.

Yule W (2006) Theory, training and timing: psychosocial interventions in complex emergencies. *International Review of Psychiatry* **18**(3), 259–264.

Zhang H, Zhang Y (1991) Psychological consequences of earthquake disaster survivors. *International Journal of Psychology Special Issue: The Psychological Dimensions of Global Change* **26**, 613–621.

Appendix: Post-traumatic stress disorder (PTSD) diagnostic criteria

Both of the following criteria need to be met in order for this diagnosis to be made:

I. The person has experienced, witnessed, or was confronted with an event/ events that involved actual or threatened death or serious injury, or a threat to the physical integrity of themselves or others.

II. The person's response involved intense fear, helplessness, or horror.

The following symptom clusters must also be present, for more than 1 month, with disturbance causing significant distress/impairment in social, occupational, or other important areas of functioning:

Re-experiencing symptoms(1 or more needed)	Avoidance and dissociative symptoms (3 or more needed)	Increased arousal symptoms (2 or more needed)
Recurring, upsetting intrusive memories of the event (e.g., images, thoughts)	Avoidance of thoughts and feelings, or conversations reminiscent of the trauma	Difficulty falling/staying asleep
Recurrent distressing dreams of the event	Avoidance of activities, people, or situations, that is reminiscent of the trauma	Increase in irritability/anger
Behaving/ feeling as if the traumatic event were recurring (e.g. flashbacks)	Inability to recall an important aspect of the trauma	Difficulty concentrating
Intense psychological distress on exposure to internal or external reminders of the trauma	Diminished interest in usual activities	Hypervigilance
Intense physiological arousal to internal or external reminders of the trauma	Feeling detached or estranged from others Restricted range of affect Sense of foreshortened future.	Exaggerated startle response

Resilience in resource-poor settings

Amanda Bingley and Elizabeth McDermott

Providing palliative care in resource-poor settings demands a considerable measure of resilience in healthcare professionals and volunteers involved in responding to the often formidable needs of vulnerable local communities. In this chapter we explore the ways providers of palliative care engage in the 'dynamic process' of resilience as defined by Egeland *et al.* (1993) and Luthar *et al.* (2000) using the 'protective attributes' of positive adaptation, functioning, and flexibility in the face of significant adversity. Such challenges can include the negative impact of globalization, political and military conflicts, or environmental hazards that leave vulnerable communities in the developing world struggling with social and economic inequalities. Using examples from our research undertaken as part of the global development programme with the International Observatory on End of Life Care (IOELC), Lancaster University (Clark *et al.* 2003), we examine the strategies and limits of individual and community responses in attempting to deliver palliative care when challenged by poor levels of education, long-term conflict, and chronically under-resourced healthcare systems.

Much of the key writing on the concept of resilience arises from research into developmental processes of children and adolescents who appear to survive and overcome severely adverse and deprived family or community situations (Rutter 1985, 1993; Garmezy 1991; Cichetti *et al.* 1993; Bluglass 2003). However, discussing palliative care provision in terms of resilience we draw on literatures in community psychology (Sonn and Fisher 1998), which explore how communities find the capacity to maintain resourcefulness, identity and function in situations of chronic socio-economic disadvantage, cultural oppression (Elsass 1992; Hernandez 2002), political and military conflict (Kimhi and Shamai 2004), and environmental disaster (Wisner 2003). In the writings on resilience at the end of life and in old age we see descriptions of individual resilience dependent on a complex interrelation between individuals and their community (Byock 1997; Walter-Ginzburg *et al.* 2005). Key factors, many of which can translate across into palliative care provision in resource-poor settings, include an individual's capacity to maintain or regain self-esteem, having a realistic outlook of abilities and needs, a strong sense of spiritual meaning in life and the need for self-fulfilment, and positive relations with others (Ramsey and Blieszner 1999; Nakashima and Canda 2005). In the context of palliative care provision in resource-poor settings, it is also possible to observe what we term 'professional resilience'. By this we mean that healthcare professionals demonstrate resilience through the ways they use their professional judgements and skills, including a capacity and vision to make use of, and create, educational and care provision opportunities with determination and patience, despite adverse opinions and opposition from other colleagues.

Resource-poor settings in context

The term 'resource-poor settings' refers to a wide range of situations from chronic underfunding of healthcare services in otherwise relatively stable developing countries to settings where there is extreme and continuing hardship involving a whole region or areas within countries. There may, as we note above, be a number of reasons for such inadequate resources and poverty. For example, complex and negative effects of globalization on vulnerable populations in developing countries can result in a decline in the capacity of communities to be socially and economically sustaining and supportive (Baumann 2000). In this context there are adverse effects for professionals attempting to support palliative care needs. Lee and Zwi (2003) make the point that the ability of individuals, societies and countries to adapt to the process of globalization is unequal, with those less able to adapt engaging in behaviours under conditions of poor access to healthcare, that have made them, for example, more susceptible to HIV infection.

We observe that in settings with fewer resources, particularly where social networks are threatened, palliative care need increases but is less likely to be met. Wright and Clark (2006) note in their study of service provision in 47 African countries that 21 countries in the continent have no reported hospice or palliative care provision. In such regions where social welfare and healthcare systems are in an extreme, fragile state palliative care providers, if they exist at all, have to be exceptionally resilient, able to champion and campaign for training and services. They may derive such resilience in part from their ability to utilize human and social capital, including seeking their own education, working sensitively with different cultural needs, capable of providing some basic palliative care training for healthcare colleagues and developing social networks from which to draw volunteers. In part this resilience is dependent on the individual's capacity to be flexible, adaptive, perceptive, and realistic. Stjernswärd and Clark (2003) suggest that: 'finding ways to empower families and communities ... is an urgent priority and in this socio-economic and cultural solutions will be as important as medical ones if meaningful palliative care is to be achieved.' (p. 1202). From this perspective, healthcare professionals and volunteers are more likely to develop resilient systems of provision when they are able to engage with local knowledge and local cultural values and needs (Altman 2003).

Other more extreme examples of resource-poor settings include those struggling with military and political conflict and continuing hardship. These communities are often on the edge of potential collapse with subsequent failure to provide a modicum of adequate healthcare. Where a community is forced to employ multiple strategies to maintain their very existence palliative care needs may be quickly subsumed in the pressing need for basic survival. Hence an individual's dying process may not be considered a priority when the whole community is under threat. In this situation the focus is more likely to be on distribution of food and water, the urgency of feeding infants to prevent malnutrition and avert a threat to the survival of the next generation. Such are the situations faced by many healthcare professionals and volunteers in many regions of Africa and South America, parts of India, and certain regions of the Middle East.

In the following two sections of the chapter we reflect on the nature of individual, community, and professional resilience in three different resource-poor settings in India, the Occupied Palestinian Territory, and Turkey, where each region presents different obstacles and challenges. We explore the relationship between these different forms of resilience and the key factors that benefit the development of palliative care services. In this context we examine the interaction between resilient individuals, professional resilience, and how this builds and works with community resilience. Our observations in the following sections are drawn from research undertaken for the IOELC global development programme, which aims to map the development of hospice and palliative care services in regions around the world, focusing in particular on resource-poor and transition economies. A key aspect of the programme is the production of in-depth 'country reports' using a common template to map palliative care development, history, and current services. The reports are published freely on the IOELC website (www.eolc-observatory.net) providing a resource for current and future policy, education and training, and service development. Reports are compiled using a multi-methodological approach of quantitative and qualitative analysis, including statistical information, ethnographic interviews and narrative accounts, referenced peer-reviewed and grey literature. Interviews are conducted wherever possible in each country with key healthcare professionals and others involved in service provision.

The research for the country report on India was undertaken between 2004 and 2006; research for reports on the Occupied Palestinian Territory and Turkey was conducted during 2005.

Resilience and palliative care in India

India is a challenging country for those involved in developing palliative care. In 2000, the World Bank Development report notes that India contains one-sixth of the world's population, of which 89% live on less than US$2 a day and 53% on less than US$1 a day (International Bank for Reconstruction and Development/World Bank 2000). The impact of globalization has generated substantial gains in economic investment and yield but India faces serious problems such as widespread poverty, enormous pressures of overpopulation, environmental degradation, and religious and ethnic conflict (The World Factbook http://www.cia.gov/cia/publications/factbook/geos/in.html).

In terms of palliative care needs an estimated 1 million new cases of cancer are diagnosed each year in India, with over 70–80% of patients presenting at stage III and IV and in need of supportive and palliative care (Kumar and Rajagopal 1996; Seamark *et al.* 2000). Palliative care provision in the country has grown over the last 20 years but progress has been slow and uneven. Our research identified hospice and palliative care services in only 16 of the total 35 Indian states and union territories (IOELC Country Report: India http://www.eolc-observatory.net/global_analysis/india.htm). Overall, coverage is poor and usually concentrated in large cities; opioid availability is limited and there is no national palliative care policy. Resilience at an individual and community level has proved to be crucial in order to successfully develop palliative and supportive care services at the end of life in communities around India. One element of this resilience appears to stem from the capacity of healthcare professionals and volunteers to adapt Western models of hospice and palliative care into the different cultural contexts of India. In his discussion about the challenges of providing palliative care in India, Dr M.R. Rajagopal, a founder of the Neighbourhood Network of Palliative Care (NNPC), Kerala, makes clear why this adaptation is critical to the successful delivery of services:

> Our suffering people need a system of palliative care delivery that is suited to our social and cultural milieu. It has to be inexpensive: we cannot possibly have enough expensive inpatient facilities for a million people. We can learn from the hospice system of the West, without duplicating it in its entirety. We have a strong point in our favour and that is the family structure in India. People generally prefer to live and die at home. If we have a system of delivery of palliative care based on treatment at home, with the relatives being empowered in the care of the patient, it has a definite chance of succeeding.
>
> Rajagopal (2001, p. 66)

Two examples of services which have shown exceptional resilience and positive adaptation in the face of immense difficulties are 'CanSupport', located in New Delhi, northern India, and the NNPC, in Kerala, south-west India. CanSupport is a palliative care home care service, set up through the efforts of a single woman, Harmala Gupta, as she recovered from cancer. This is an example of a resilient individual working to build community resilience. The NNPC has been highly successful at developing a community participatory model of palliative care. The NNPC story demonstrates how existing community strengths and resilience have been utilized and developed by individual volunteers and healthcare professionals.

CanSupport, Delhi

CanSupport, founded by Harmala Gupta in 1997, was the first palliative care home care support service in Delhi, northern India (CanSupport 2004). The organization provides free home-based palliative care, day care, and counselling services, including bereavement support for patients and their families. There are four home care teams of specialist trained doctors, nurses, and counsellors working from different centres in Delhi. Each team visits the homes of about 80–85 patients with advanced cancer every week (Hind 2004). Family members are trained in simple nursing tasks so they can keep the patient comfortable until the next home visit. The entire service is funded through donations and grants. Harmala Gupta speaks of the challenges for CanSupport:

> … any area you touch there is a problem, which is why we have, as you suggest, gone beyond the traditional palliative care support and provided dry rations, dried food rations to people, sometimes help with transportation, we provide them with all kinds of medical aids. Really I think we also perform a much needed social function, because families tell us that even their relatives have stopped visiting them. We realise there is so much ignorance around cancer; a number of people believe it is contagious and they stop visiting.
>
> Gupta (2004, pp. 32–38)

CanSupport was set up as a result of Harmala Gupta's own personal illness journey requiring her considerable determination and resilience. In 1986, she was diagnosed with non-Hodgkin's lymphoma while studying for a PhD in Canada. The experience of dedicated cancer patient support services in Canada was in stark contrast to the stigma Harmala encountered when she returned to India. This spurred her to instigate a cancer patient support service, which eventually led to collaboration with a hospital pain and palliative care clinic and the CanSupport homecare programme. Harmala's inner resources are central to her resilience as a cancer survivor and as a palliative care pioneer. In the extract below, her personal resolve is evident as she describes her motivations and early struggles:

> I felt very strongly that it was important for me as a survivor to identify myself and to go out and let people know that you could still continue to live after cancer, and I approached the Indian Cancer Society in Delhi and was alarmed to realise that as a survivor I could not become a member … I mean it was just crazy … Well I joined the society nevertheless and I tried to persuade them that there was value in investing in patient support services, because there were people who recovered.
>
> Gupta (2004, pp. 32–38)

Harmala Gupta has shown great tenacity in overcoming the difficult circumstances of her illness, which can be attributed in part to her ability to positively adapt to adversity. However, as Luthar *et al.* (2000) argue exposure to adversity is mediated by cultural and socio-economic factors as well as individual psychology. In the following extract we see the kind of difficult socio-cultural dynamics Harmala faced, given the paternalism of healthcare professionals she encountered during her treatment and the cultural perception of cancer as a stigma:

> … there is a very patriarchal relationship between the doctor and the patient where the patient isn't really supposed to ask questions. They just obey orders, they are told what they are supposed to do. So given the situation a lot of people found themselves quite disempowered and had a sense of helplessness and hopelessness, and it was important to break through that and I really had to struggle with the doctors and tell them that there was value in having someone who had been through this experience to talk to people who were going through it …
>
> Gupta (2004, pp. 32–38)

Harmala Gupta has the advantage of being highly educated and of speaking fluent English. To some extent she feels able to 'struggle' with the medical profession because she enjoys a high social position, similar to medical professionals within Indian society. She has access to significant economic, social, and cultural resources in addition to her inner strength. She goes on to describe the gender-specific aspects of adversity that she discovered in the course of her experience as a woman faced with a cancer diagnosis, which demanded another level of resilience and determination:

> I realised that people are not told their diagnosis. Especially for a woman, there is this belief somehow that women can't take bad news. And the doctors being predominantly male tend to ask the woman to leave and discuss the diagnosis with the husband or the male member if any male member has come. Of course there is a lot of suspicion because if you are asked to leave the room you realise immediately that it must be something quite serious. But when you ask questions you are immediately brushed aside and told no, no, no, there is nothing to worry about, everything's under control.
>
> Gupta (2004, pp. 32–48)

The resilience required by Harmala Gupta to overcome and make good use of these challenges in order to set up a functioning palliative care home care service may be due to a number of factors. As an individual Harmala Gupta demonstrates certain important 'protective attributes' identified as indicators of individual resilience, such as flexibility, self-awareness, a strong sense of social awareness and support (Nakashima and Canda 2005). She has also drawn upon her high social status, educational advantages and inner resources. She has the capacity to inspire other committed individuals to join together to build new palliative care services. CanSupport services in turn help to develop community resilience. In the following account of palliative care service development in Kerala we describe an example of a community response to adversity that draws on existing community dynamics to build community resilience.

Neighbourhood Network in Palliative Care (NNPC), Kerala

In the state of Kerala, south-west India, there are impressive innovations in palliative care that have been achieved against a background of extremely limited resources (Rajagopal and Palat 2002). The development of palliative care services in this state appears to be shaped by community resilience; defined by Sonn and Fisher (1998) as a community's capacity and resourcefulness to cope positively with adversity and therefore generate effective ways of coping with the challenges of living and, in this case, dying.

The NNPC is a network of 63 palliative care clinics across Kerala, providing care free of charge to patients in need. The NNPC is a joint venture with four other non-government organizations (NGOs) attempting to develop a sustainable 'community led' service capable of offering comprehensive long-term care and palliative care to those in need (Kumar 2004). Volunteers from the local community are trained to identify the problems of people in their area who are chronically ill or dying and to intervene effectively, with active support from a network of trained professionals. NNPC aims to empower local communities to look after chronically ill and dying patients within their community (NNPC 2005).

At the beginning of the 1990s, there was only one pain clinic in Kerala at the Regional Cancer Centre in Trivandrum in south Kerala (Bollini et al. 2004). Palliative care services were initially set up in 1993 by a small group of doctors and social activists. The idea was swiftly taken up by local communities, the project going beyond what the originators had anticipated. NNPC programmes appear to have been exceptionally successful wherever they have been launched in Kerala. The programme was first 'ground tested' in Malappurum, a poor district in Kerala with a population of 4 million. Within 2 years a rate of 70% coverage in provision of long-term care and palliative care was achieved. There is an NNPC clinic at roughly every 10 km, which means patients should not have to travel more than 5 km to their nearest clinic (NNPC 2005).

The success and growth of palliative care provision appears to be, in part, due to the capacity of local communities to adapt positively to difficult circumstances. There is also a cultural tradition in Kerala of community involvement. In January 2005, NNPC physician Dr Suresh Kumar reflects, in an interview, on 10 years of developments in palliative care in Kerala:

> I think that the definite trend, as far as northern Kerala is concerned, is palliative care moving out from the institution into the community, and this has been happening much faster than even some of us who are part of it expected. And from '93 when the first palliative care clinic was started in Calicut, it was a very much institution-based, doctor/patient model. We had a few volunteers but they were doing odd nursing jobs after training, and the whole team was centred around the doctor and there was some support from the community, financial, like some of the donations. Now we have reached the stage where most of the care is delivered in the community and the doctor in many palliative care units in northern Kerala is somebody who looks after or takes care of the physical problems, and most of the other issues like social support, the spiritual issues, other emotional problems are taken care of by the volunteers. Most of the units now are run by the local groups and they employ the doctor, that's against the earlier clinics initiated by doctors and the volunteers and other people acting under him.

> IOELC interview (14 January 2005)

Community resilience can be thought about in terms of communities being capable of providing members with opportunities to be meaningfully engaged in activities and social relations. In other words, to feel a sense of belonging and identification that meets the psychological needs and material requirements of involved individuals (Sonn and Fisher 1998). In Kerala, this process can be seen in the ways different local communities have developed effective coping strategies to deal with the challenges of living and supporting those who are dying. Mr T.S. Babu, a NNPC volunteer, explains the role of volunteers in the organization:

> They can console the family to boost their morale, this thing is more important because the patients which we go and see are very, very poor; the rate of survival is a problem. More than the medicine they need the moral support and the financial help; that is what they need—so I collect money also from others.

> IOELC interview (19 January 2005)

As Dr M. Numpeli, programme executive of NNPC notes, the extent of this collectivization of palliative care can be illustrated through the voluntary nature of the service delivery and funding (IOELC interview: 12 January 2005). Dr Suresh Kumar gives examples of two highly successful fundraising ventures in Malappuram, through small community donations such as 'Palliative Care in Campus' where students contribute one rupee every month or in another example the bus drivers entering Nilambur bus station each day contribute two rupees per bus (Presentation at Lancaster University, UK: 26 September 2005).

The success of NNPC relies upon existing community resilience, partially sustained by the state's investment in education and healthcare for local people. This investment provides the social context and resources that facilitate a community cohesion or social consciousness (Sanders and Chopra 2003). The way in which an effective palliative care service has been developed in Kerala is an example of resourceful, far-thinking individuals building on existing community resources in order to provide low-cost end of life care to large numbers of people.

Resilience and palliative care in two settings in the Middle East region

Providing support at the end of life in settings, for example, where healthcare services are affected by political and military conflict or chronic poverty requires a particular flexibility and willingness in health workers to seek diverse strategies to effectively use local and community resources. In the following two examples we describe the resilience observed in healthcare professionals and volunteers providing care provision in very different situations: the West Bank and Gaza in the Occupied Palestinian Territory, and Turkey. Healthcare professionals in both regions, and for a range of different reasons, report problems in finding adequate resources with which they can provide effective palliative care services. Consequently, where services are provided, in however basic a form, we observe individuals and communities demonstrate certain resilient characteristics of resourcefulness, a positive sense of self and community values and identity, and the capacity to grasp opportunities and to make good use of social resources. These characteristics are well documented in other similar contexts (Sonn and Fisher 1998; Hernandez 2002; Wisner 2003). As we observed above, however, a key resilience characteristic in palliative care provision is the ability to 'champion the cause'.

Occupied Palestinian Territory

In the West Bank and Gaza ongoing and increasingly serious conflict has resulted in a crisis for all healthcare services (WHO 2006a,b). Healthcare professionals are unable to provide palliative care beyond the most basic pain relief and symptom management. Their efforts are further hampered by lack of available medication (IOELC Palestinian Authority country report http://www.eolc-observatory.net/global_analysis/palestinianauthority.htm). This situation forces providers of healthcare to test their resilience to the limits and draw on a range of survival tactics, or risk facing the collapse of any effective health service.

From our work in the region mapping palliative care services we identified one key service, the Patient's Friends Society-Jerusalem (PFS). Situated in East Jerusalem PFS acts to 'champion' and actively promote a range of services such as breast cancer and osteoporosis screening and support services for patients with cancer, including where possible, patients at the end of life. Carol El Jabari, director of PFS, works with local women who have, or have survived, breast cancer. The women are almost all from the West Bank. Carol is a firm advocate of self-help and education, working with women in the West Bank to run self-help support groups and a telephone helpline. She also organizes study days for physicians and nurses. As Carol notes the first requirement for the success of self help groups is commitment: 'it was important to identify women that were as keen or as committed as me to make it a reality.' The second crucial element is flexibility:

> For those women that can't get to us from the West Bank, we go to Ramallah, Jericho, Hebron and Bethlehem. My coordinator contacts women, or women contact us, and we try to gather a few to make a group session. We have a fixed meeting scheduled every month but often have other meetings as well depending on people's need. While not structured the meetings are conducted based on the women's interests … Access is a major barrier for women from areas outside Jerusalem and dependant on the 'authorities' issuing, and honouring, a permit. If we want to go to the West Bank we never know if there will be restrictions or delays, and women don't always have the financial resources to get to meetings. So there are many difficulties. Despite the misery of living under occupation, we have a group of women living with cancer and other co-morbidities that are committed to the 'group' and want to help others. That this has continued and grown is really great! It shows the women are committed, and they're so keen and it's changed their lives for some of them.

IOELC interview (10 March 2005)

In terms of palliative care, though, PFS can only help in indirect ways. Because there are no government resources to deliver formal palliative care services in the West Bank or Gaza families are called upon to care for their relatives. PFS volunteers will offer psychosocial support and help to get prescriptions, access medication, and make home visits where possible. How well these patients manage is uncertain. They are dependent on the resilience of family members having to deal with the cancer, which is still regarded as a stigma. One important factor lies in the strength of family networks, with family members willingly supporting their sick relatives despite difficulties accessing medical care, and often with their own health problems. Carol El Jabari outlines the situation:

> Those that are terminal or a late stage of the disease are just on the margins and get pretty minimal care. This has been my experience. The families are not prepared; they don't have enough medical or financial support. It's really up to them to look after

their very ill or dying relatives. They don't have the skills or the knowledge. They do their best but there's no psychosocial support for them. Doctors and nurses are not specialized in palliative care so the quality of care varies. At present there are little if any resources and no mechanisms in place for change. Healthcare is under the Palestinian Authority and they're stretched just to look after diabetics and hypertensives. Cancer isn't high on the list.

IOELC interview (10 March 2005).

Her experience is echoed by other healthcare professionals in the region, such as Dr Fouad Sabatin, a haematologist at the Augusta Victoria Hospital in East Jerusalem (IOELC interview: 2 May 2005).

Cancer appears, historically, in the West Bank and Gaza, to be a low priority in public health, with the more pressing needs of child and maternal health, problems of endemic infectious illness, sanitation, and nutrition taking precedence (Giacaman 1988). Over half of all deaths are due to cardiovascular disease, but cancer is one of the other major causes of deaths. With few resources for treatment, however, of either condition, palliative care need is high. As part of a strategy used over several decades by international NGOs and aid agencies to provide general healthcare across the West Bank and Gaza, hundreds of small local clinics are found throughout the West Bank and parts of Gaza. Although fraught with supply problems the clinics do offer some mechanism for provision of medication and equipment. Unfortunately, without specific palliative care training, clinic staff are unable to offer skilled support and patients have to attempt difficult journeys to get help as Dr Fouad Sabatin, oncologist at the Augusta Victoria Hospital, East Jerusalem explains:

People living in Ramallah [West Bank] are unlucky when it comes to having a diagnosis of cancer because there is no centre in Ramallah with the facility to treat these patients; and typically, these patients need to be referred to Beit Jala hospital or to Nablus, and all of them are far away, and there are several checkpoints in between. So getting to the hospital is really difficult, and usually it takes several days for these patients to be sent in the right direction ... And if you're asking about how these patients will do and their management, if they have a pain crisis or something like that, it's really very tough because, as I said, there is no place in Ramallah that's really able to treat these patients. They end up being treated by general practitioners at government hospitals until they can be referred to another place. It's a sad situation.

IOELC interview (2 May 2005).

The situation in Gaza presents an even greater challenge of human need; a densely populated area of 1.3 million people struggle to survive in a serious conflict with dwindling basic resources in a land area of less than 360 km². Oncologists there report that although there are three hospitals with oncology units, their efforts to support patients at the end of life are hampered by erratic supplies of opioid medication. Oncologists demonstrate professional resilience in their flexibility within continually changing situations, for instance having to adjust prescribing according to available medication supplies.

An important development in improving palliative care skills in the region has been increased opportunities for education and training. As noted above PFS offers short study days in cancer and women's health, promoting self-help and support. The organization is committed to supporting research and training, and funds volunteers and professionals to attend international conferences. Since 2004, the Middle East Cancer Consortium (MECC)[1] has run two palliative care seminars open to oncologists, physicians, nurses, social workers, and academics in the region. Well-attended by healthcare professionals, the seminars have proved highly supportive, encouraging dissemination of skills and acting to develop resilience in those involved in providing palliative and supportive care. In these various ways PFS and MECC directly and indirectly help to build and nurture individual (volunteers and professional) resilience through education and training, and external support. This approach, it is hoped, will thereby benefit and in the longer term, build community resilience.

Turkey

Healthcare in Turkey is a complex system of provision by government, military, and university facilities. This large country (land area 750 580 km^2) has a population of about 73 million, and significant numbers live in resource-poor rural areas. The major centres of healthcare tend to be most advanced in the two largest cities Ankara and Istanbul. Palliative care is not well-developed in Turkey. Healthcare professionals and academics have a complex and difficult task ahead to educate and change professional and public attitudes. The nature of the challenge is less obvious in Turkey than in the previous examples of India and the Occupied Palestinian Territory; there are no unifying factors that demand survival tactics in the sense that communities are not engaged in active conflict or facing extreme poverty. However, the government as the largest health provider is proving slow to respond to palliative care needs. Consequently, the people are reliant on the health professionals to take the lead in providing support. There are no palliative care NGOs and virtually no known charitable organizations that are involved in care of the dying. The onus is on physicians, oncologists and specialist nurses, and social workers to

---

[1] MECC was established in 1996 with the aim of setting up population-based cancer registries for member countries in order to monitor cancer incidence, mortality and epidemiology, promote preventative health policy, and encourage research and educational links. MECC members are Cyprus, Egypt, Israel, Jordan, Palestinian Authority, and Turkey. Since 2004 MECC has run two seminars on palliative care (Silbermann 2001).

find ways to provide palliative care within the context of general care and support at the end of life.

The most effective strategies appear to arise from professional resilience, in that healthcare professionals demonstrate their capacity and vision in order to grasp educational and clinical opportunities. Professionals wanting to develop services encounter a major problem of a lack of data. Professor Yasemin Oguz, a medical ethicist who has a particular interest in palliative care, reported in 2003 that:

> As the director of the needs assessment project for palliative care in Turkey I may say that our main problem is the lack of national data on the subject. Without essential data it is not possible to convince the Turkish Ministry of Health and National Health Insurance Organizations about the importance of the subject. Palliative care and end of life issues are a kind of no man's land in Turkey. Although many healthcare professionals encounter the problems and are aware of the need, they do not see the subject as their business. There are financial and legal restrictions. Our initial objective is to establish a continuous communication between interested professionals and patient advocacy groups.

> IOELC questionnaire survey (2003)

Another major problem faced by Turkish physicians is lack of resources, as the government fails to provide adequate funding for specific end of life care. The other key issue is widespread fear of opioid prescribing. Against this background we observe positive changes emerging with oncologists in seven university hospital oncology units now actively developing palliative care skills. There are a few oncologists and physicians specializing in pain relief who are also 'champions' of palliative care. Almost all these physicians have gained skills by going overseas to complete specialist training. Much of their resilience in practice is apparent through a combination of their professional and individual resilience, shown by a determination to gain skills and then to return to the country to train others and create local resources.

Pain specialist Professor Serdar Erdine aims to improve pain and symptom management (in the absence of active services in palliative care). As he says: 'pain is underestimated' in Turkey. He relates how the Ministry of Health (MoH) restricted his prescribing of opioids but when he told his patients that he was prevented from prescribing, they protested to the MoH, who gave permission for the drugs to be prescribed. Thus, with encouragement from committed healthcare professionals and public education, people can put pressure on government to improve services. Professor Erdine has focused on developing skills in pain relief and has been instrumental in the development of 'algology' or the study of specialist pain relief. With 25 years of experience and extensive knowledge of pain relief, he explains that through TV and articles in journals and newspapers he and other colleagues are trying to alleviate people's cancer fears by raising public awareness of the effectiveness of opioids in relieving cancer pain. He is also organizing a campaign to educate physicians about the safety and efficacy of using opioids (IOELC interview: 11 July 2005).

Professor Erdine gives an example of his individual ability to grasp positive opportunities as they arise. Following the severe Turkish earthquake in August 1999, thousands of opioids were sent as medical aid by other countries. Turkish doctors, however, did not make use of this medication because of widespread opioid phobia and lack of awareness. As Professor Erdine observed, 'An estimated 100,000 people were suffering but physicians did not feel confident to give opioid pain relief'. After the emergency was over the authorities offered Professor Erdine some of these morphine stocks, which he accepted. He is still using the medication in his pain clinics. As he notes: 'Turkey is one of the biggest manufacturers of opioids in the world but uses less than some countries like the US.' (Presentation at Open Society Institute palliative care seminar, Budapest: 5–7 September 2005).

In another example of education supporting and building professional resilience Dr Deniz Yamaç, oncologist at Gazi University Hospital in Ankara, explains how she was introduced to the concepts of palliative care while completing training in oncology at Arkansas Cancer Institute, USA. Since 2000, she has been inspired to develop training in her oncology unit and has run short sessions and day workshops designed for other medical faculty members and resident physicians. There is a separate programme for medical students. She is especially interested in improving communication skills and sees this as an integral part of good palliative care training and practice. She also makes an important point about skills development helping to prevent 'burnout'. Healthcare professionals in palliative care can be particularly susceptible to burnout, a state that can seriously undermine even the most apparently resilient individual and reduce the effectiveness of organizations and communities. This is an example of 'professional resilience' supporting and building individual resilience:

> I can see my way how to act, how to talk but I don't think that all Turkish doctors, especially concerned in cancer, do know this. So this is the thing we are trying to do: the workshop was about this … You should tell it, they [the patient] *must* know, it's their life. I believe in that, so I try to tell it, not to break their heart maybe, without breaking their heart, but they must know their future, I think. So you *must* tell it but the way and the condition and the time is important. So I think I can manage it and I want to learn more or I want to teach people about that. It's something to prevent your burnout I think also.

> IOELC interview (6 July 2005)

In 2005, Dr Yamaç set up workshops for nurses in the oncology unit and is also involved in a project—funded by private health insurance—to train nurses in home care for cancer patients. Part of her plan is also to encourage the development of an inpatient unit. Physicians and other health professionals involved in the Turkish Oncology Group (TOG) are also committed to the development of palliative care skills, despite the ongoing problem of a slow uptake of ideas that presents less chance for effective change or support. TOG demonstrates a commitment towards building professional resilience by creating educational opportunities. The group has, to date, organized two conferences bringing interested Turkish healthcare professionals together with several key, international specialist palliative care professionals. As oncologist Dr Seref Komurçu explains, the hope is to encourage more professionals to take an interest in developing palliative care around the country (IOELC interview: 18 April 2005).

Conclusions

When reflecting on the phenomenon of resilience as a 'dynamic process' in the development and maintenance of palliative care services in resource-poor settings we are struck by the pattern of specific characteristics or requirements observed in individuals, in people's professional practice, and in communities, that help to overcome, at times, formidable obstacles and challenges. Successful palliative care development requires the building of resilience at all levels, within the individual, professionally, and from within communities. Different situations and cultural contexts, however, demand strategies that may draw variously on the attributes of one individual, professional skill, or on existing community resources.

Of the three sources of resilience we would argue that the key is individual resilience, although there are resilience factors common to all three sources (see Figure 14.1).

Without some 'one' or some 'small group' inspired by one or two highly motivated individuals there can be no grasping at opportunities, no strategic moves to involve the community or educate and motive colleagues, however active the professional and community spirit. Key 'protective attributes' include a certain element of charisma, meaning a person who is sociable, altruistic, has vision and intelligence, the courage to confront authority and be diplomatic, shrewd and far-thinking (Clark *et al.* 2005). The capacity to 'champion' seems to be mediated by gender to some extent—as yet underresearched—as a significant number of women are found in palliative care acting as 'champions', challenging oppressive regimes, poorly resourced healthcare, and adverse social or environmental conditions. Champions, whether men or women achieve change by clearly identifying end of life needs, encouraging social networking, and developing strategies to campaign at community and government level for new services or improvements to existing services. They successfully seek out other committed individuals and

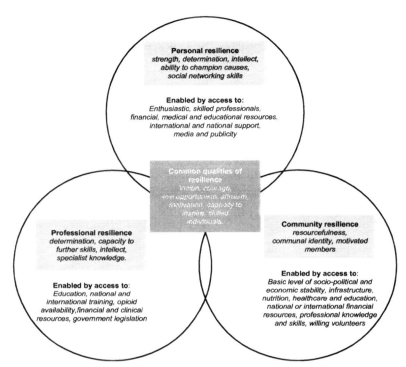

Figure 14.1 Interrelationship of personal, professional and community resilience in resource-poor settings.

have the ability to create palliative care support that utilizes local and community networks or existing healthcare services. The power of inspirational persuasion is a crucial factor in the development of successful organizations.

A second key pattern is that the individual has been 'nourished' from some outside source, by some inspiring educational experience or encounter. For example, many professionals and volunteers report that they were originally inspired by attending a lecture by Dame Cicely Saunders or by coming across her writings. This is often described as a life-changing experience and if coinciding with training or opportunities to work in a hospice has been the starting point for several 'champions' of palliative care, supporting and developing their inner resilience and resolve. The process of overseas training in building professional resilience has also proved to be a point of inspiration. However, we also observe examples, such as in the worse affected war zones in the Occupied Palestinian Territory, where educational opportunities alone will not necessarily build resilience or translate it into developing local services on return to the home country, despite great personal courage in the face of daily active conflict with many obstacles and difficulties to overcome.

Thus we come to the third and pivotal element of building resilience and the effects of resilient individuals: the relationship between the individual with personal and professional resilience and their community. In India, for example, palliative care would not have developed without the persistence and determination of dedicated non-professional individuals and healthcare professionals throughout the country. In the cases of CanSupport and the NNPC, this resilience is evident through the work of individuals in relation to their communities and social systems. For example, Harmala Gupta's work in developing CanSupport, a homecare service, is an astonishing display of individual resilience, where she is able to draw upon her inner resources and her social and economic advantage of a reasonable privileged position within India's social hierarchy. However, her story clearly shows that for her individual resilience to translate into action beyond her own daily life, she had to have vision, altruism, flexibility, and sociability. She also had the opportunity to travel away from her home situation, experience a very difficult encounter with a life-threatening illness that provided great insights, which she was able to grasp and use by returning to her home country and 'championing' the cause.

In much the same way we observe Carol El Jabari, in her work with PFS, Jerusalem, bringing a combination of professional competence, vision, sociability, altruism, and flexibility into a very challenging situation, with a community whose members are frequently overwhelmed by despair. She saw ways she could utilize social resources within the community by working with existing family and social networks to encourage women with breast cancer to join the self-help group, which builds individual and community resilience by supporting women and training them to support others. Adapting to overcome adverse political situations that limit free access through the region, the group is set up to run as flexibly and self-sufficiently as possible. The PFS phone helpline is an important link for those women in Gaza who are unable to access any other psycho-social support.

The proliferation over a 10-year period of a community-led palliative care service in Kerala provides a different lens through which to consider resilience in palliative care development. In these circumstances, resourceful professionals have been able to work with existing social cohesion and awareness, encouraged by state welfare provision. Another aspect of NNPC's success is the professionals who have explored ways to effectively adapt Western concepts of hospice and palliative care to fit resource-poor settings. The role of resilience in a global context is complex, and specific to different countries, states, communities and individuals; influenced by ethnic, socio-cultural, and economic differences.

The success stories presented in this chapter demonstrate that nurturing individual, professional and community resilience, in all its complexity, is a crucial element in the development of palliative care provision in resource-poor settings.

References

Altman D (2003) Understanding HIV/AIDS as a global security issue. In: *Health Impacts of Globalization: towards global governance*, pp. 33–46 (ed. Lee K). Hampshire: Palgrave Macmillan.

Baumann Z (2000) *Community. Seeking safety in an insecure world*. Cambridge: Polity.

Bluglass K (2003) *Hidden from the Holocaust. Stories of resilient children who survived and thrived*. London: Praeger.

Bollini P, Venkateswaran C, Kumar S (2004) Palliative care in Kerala, India: a model for resource-poor settings. *Onkologie* 27, 138–142.

Byock I (1997) *Dying Well*. New York: Riverhead Books.

CanSupport (2004) *Newsletter*, September. New Delhi, India.

Cichetti D, Rogosch FA, Lynch M, Holt K. (1993) Resilience in maltreated children: processes leading to adaptive outcomes. *Development and Psychopathology* 5, 629–647.

Clark D, Wright M, Bath P, Gatrell AC (2003) The International Observatory on End of Life Care: a new research and development initiative in end of life care. *Progress in Palliative Care* 11, 137–138.

Clark D, Small N, Wright M, Winslow M, Hughes N (2005) *A Bit of Heaven for the Few? An oral history of the modern hospice movement in the United Kingdom*. Lancaster: Observatory Publications.

Egeland B, Carlson E, Sroufe LA (1993) Resilience as process. *Development and Psychopathology* 5, 517–528.

Elsass P (1992) *Strategies for survival: the psychology of cultural resilience in ethnic minorities*. New York: New York University Press.

Garmezy N (1991) Resilience in children's adaptation to negative life events and stressed environments. *Pediatrics* 20, 459–466.

Giacaman R (1988) *Life and Health in Three Palestinian Villages*. London: Ithaca Press.

Gupta H (2004) A journey from cancer to CanSupport. *Indian Journal of Palliative Care* 10, 32–38.

Hernandez P (2002) Resilience in families and communities: Latin American contributions from the psychology of liberation. *Family Journal* 10, 334–343.

Hind B (2004) *CanSupport: Touching Lives*. New Delhi: CanSupport.

International Bank for Reconstruction and Development/The World Bank (2000). *World Development Report 2000/2001: attacking poverty*. New York: Oxford University Press.

Kimhi S, Shamai M (2004) Community resilience and the impact of stress: adult response to Israel's withdrawal from Lebanon. *Journal of Community Psychology* 32, 439–451.

Kumar S (2004) Learning from low income countries: what are the lessons? Palliative care can be delivered through neighbourhood networks. *British Journal of Medicine (Clinical Research edition)* 329, 1184.

Kumar S, Rajagopal MR (1996) Palliative care in Kerala. Problems at presentation in 440 patients with advanced cancer in a south Indian state. *Palliative Medicine* 10, 293–298.

Lee K, Zwi A (2003) A global political economy approach to AIDS: ideology, interests and implications. In: *Health Impacts of Globalization: towards global governance*, pp. 13–32 (ed. Lee K). Hampshire: Palgrave Macmillan.

Luthar SS, Cicchetti D, Becker B (2000) The construct of resilience: a critical evaluation and guidelines for future work. *Child Development* 71, 543–562.

Nakashima M, Canda ER (2005) Positive dying and resiliency in later life: a qualitative study. *Journal of Aging Studies* 19, 109–125.

NNPC (2005) *Neighbourhood Network in Palliative Care: what, how, why?* Calicut: Institute of Palliative Medicine, Medical College.

Rajagopal MR (2001) The challenges of palliative care in India. *The National Medical Journal of India* 14, 65–67.

Rajagopal MR, Palat G (2002) Kerala, India: status of cancer pain relief and palliative care. *Journal of Pain and Symptom Management* 24, 191–193.

Ramsey J, Blieszner R (1999) *Spiritual Resiliency in Older Women*. Thousand Oaks, CA: Sage.

Rutter M (1985) Resilience in the face of adversity. Protective factors and resilience to psychiatric disorder. *British Journal of Psychiatry* 147, 598–611.

Rutter M (1993) Resilience: some conceptual considerations. *Journal of Adolescent Health* 14, 626–631.

Sanders D, Chopra M (2003) Globalisation and the challenge of 'Health for All': a view from sub-Saharan Africa. In: *Health Impacts of Globalization: towards global governance*, pp. 105–119 (ed. Lee K). Hampshire: Palgrave Macmillan.

Seamark D, Ajithakumari K, Burn G, Saraswalthi DP, Koshy R, Seamark C (2000) Palliative care in India. *Journal of the Royal Society of Medicine* 93, 292–295.

Silbermann M (2001) Perspectives for cancer epidemiology research in the Middle East *Gastrointestinal Oncology* 4 (2–3), 181–181.

Sonn CS, Fisher AT (1998) Sense of community: community resilient responses to oppression and change. *Journal of Community Psychology* 26, 457–472.

Stjernswärd J, Clark D (2003) Palliative medicine—a global perspective. In: *Oxford Textbook of Palliative Medicine*, 3rd edn, pp. 1197–1224 (eds Doyle D, Hanks G, Cherny N, Calman K). Oxford: Oxford University Press.

Walter-Ginzburg A, Shmotkin D, Blumstein T, Shorek A (2005) A gender-based dynamic multidimensional longitudinal analysis of resilience and mortality in the old-old in Israel: the cross-sectional and longitudinal aging study (CALAS) *Social Science and Medicine* 60, 1705–1715.

Wisner B (2003) Disaster risk reduction in megacities: making the most of human and social capital. In: *Building Safer Cities. The future of disaster risk*, pp. 181–197 (eds Kreimar A, Arnold M, Carlin A). Disaster Risk Management Series No. 3. The World Bank.

WHO (2006a) *Country Cooperation Strategy for WHO and the occupied Palestinian Territory*. Regional Office for the Eastern Mediterranean, World Health Organization.

WHO (2006b) *Addressing the Health Situation in the Occupied Palestinian Territory*. World Health Organisation 'Health Action in Crisis'. http://www.who.int/hac/events/opt_2006/en/index.html.

Wright M, Clark D (2006) *Hospice and Palliative Care in Africa. A review of developments and challenges*. Oxford: Oxford University Press.

15

Resilience and creativity

Nigel Hartley

Introduction

> ... creativity is the doing that arises out of being ...
>
> *Winnicott (1971)*

It is common knowledge that many famous artists—painters, musicians, sculptors, poets—create in order to survive. Stories abound regarding a myriad of the great artworks relating their creation to the darkest of times for their creators. Serge Rachmaninov's famous second piano Concerto is the result of the composer working his way through the deepest of depressions (Rosen 1995), and reflections on the life of Vincent Van Gough (Meissner 1994) provide us with a paradoxical backdrop to his paintings, highlighting a struggle between beauty and angst, which introduce a man who lived a deeply complex inner emotional life. There are countless other examples.

These stories may seem far removed from our own lives and those around us, as anything more than observing great art and music from a distance will cause many to retreat in fear and panic. Creating art—hands in clay, paint on canvas, voice in song—is not an everyday occurrence for most people, so why in times of loss, trauma, and bereavement do the creative arts enable and inspire us simply to carry on?

Overarching problems with both examining and understanding creativity point us to a concept that is increasingly broad but sadly neglected by researchers and academics due to its intangible and complex nature. Every day most human beings will experience a number of what might be defined as 'creative moments'. Although these bear little relation to the creative arts as such, there are similarities in both their process and action. There is an increasing dialogue and debate related to the ways in which we think our way through everyday problems and act our way through everyday relationships that connect such things directly to the creative act and the creative process. Creative relationships, creative problem solving, creative management, and creative organisations all focus on the art of thinking 'outside of the box', of moving forward in a 'new way', of 'doing the next thing'. If something we do is truly creative, then every time we do it is a new event (May 1975) and we must therefore start afresh.

Motivation

Oliver Sacks, in his book 'A leg to stand on' (1994) tells us of a leg injury he sustained while on a walking holiday. During the recovery process he recounts how he used music by Mendelssohn in order to motivate himself to physically move one foot in front of the other and learn to walk again. If creativity is as Winnicott (1971) writes 'the doing that arises out of being', for many people in times of crisis and trauma, 'doing the next thing' will simply be forging the next step, taking the next breath, or speaking the next word. Life is diminished to its most basic level and the simplest of acts becomes both a struggle and a longing for survival. This concept of 'doing the next thing' puts the issue of motivation directly under the microscope. Simple acts are larger, louder, broader, and deeper than before and a more intense feeling of self-consciousness emerges. This forces the self into the open, exposed and witnessed as both raw and vulnerable.

There are few things in life that can enable us to embrace or move on from trauma. Psychological and psychotherapeutic theories and techniques provide frameworks for examination and change, but there are issues regarding both access to such interventions and the availability of such services in times of adversity. Questions may need to be asked about what we have readily available to us in these times of paralysis that is both accessible and easily available.

Hospices use the creative arts in a variety of ways. When attempts are made to articulate why the creative arts might be important as people approach death we hear talk of 'diversion', of 'taking one's mind off things' of 'having some time off one's illness'—the fact that being engaged with a simple artistic activity can give people some momentary relief or time-off from their dying. Such explanations, although true to a limited extent, sell the creative arts short of their true value and most central usefulness. Each of the major forms of art—painting, ceramics, poetry, music, dance, and drama—all contain in the fabric of their being unique motivational properties.

In painting, for example, one stroke of the brush leads to the next. Shapes and patterns are created and are governed by pre-existing systems and structures. We have little control over these systems and structures, as somehow we are controlled by them. A 40-year-old manual worker coming to St Christopher's Hospice for the first time presented as depressed and stuck. He told us of his serious financial problems that he was convinced would lead to him being homeless. He was adamant that he could not go to the bank to sort it all out. He felt paralysed. While at the hospice he found himself drawn into a painting session; picking up a brush he began and completed the most delicate of watercolours. Observing the creative process, one brush stroke led to another, colours merged, energy flowed. Once the painting was finished he told us of his surprise at what he had achieved and that he was now ready to face his bank. On the way home he stopped in at the bank to begin the job of sorting out his money problems.

In music, one beat of the drum follows another, one chord can do no less than move on to another pushing forward to its logical conclusion, '… and where music conveys this sense of rightness it helps us say 'yes' to life as we find it …' (Mayne 2002). An elderly woman on the hospice inpatient unit was deeply worried about leaving her husband alone with the burden of arranging her funeral when she died. A musician was visiting her and suggested that she might want to think about her funeral arrangements herself. Some days later when she died a nurse found in her locker instructions for her funeral and a list of the music she wanted as part of the service. There were also some words that she had written herself to be sung at her funeral to a well-known hymn tune. The words she had written expressed things that she had been unable to articulate to her husband during their life together.

The creative arts provide us with unique contexts within which we can 'do the next thing', but what do we need in order to take the first step?

Courage

Rollo May (1975) talks of the courage necessary to make *doing* possible. Artists working in healthcare have been reluctant to engage in research and evaluation processes focusing on their work. Healthcare institutions have been equally reluctant to fund such research initiatives and a search for proof of the efficacy of the creative arts used in healthcare provides us with a barren landscape. Yet we know of the power of the creative arts used with people in times of trauma and distress. Right through from the lives of the great artists to our experiences with those who are dying in hospices, we witness the motivational power of the creative arts when used in times of emotional paralysis. A major problem is that the creative arts are foreign to most people, and when times of crisis arrive there is a reluctance to engage with seemingly distant and meaningless concepts such as writing poetry, playing music or painting.

Doctors prescribe courses of medication in order that pain and symptoms can be managed. Sometimes people need to be guided and told what to do in order that problems might be solved. Do we need to move towards an environment in which people are prescribed a course of pottery, of painting, of music, because we *know* what is possible? Do we need to be more courageous in guiding people towards what we *know?* We have witnessed many experiences when peoples' lives and deaths have been changed through engaging in the creative arts. These go far beyond a diversion from the realities of trauma, ensuring that people make their way through, keep going and discover new ways of coping.

At St Christopher's Hospice we believe that offering a range of the creative arts to our users is important in providing them with a way through a potentially devastating time of life. Many are enabled to 'do the next thing' through the creative arts, to sing the next note, brush the next stroke, take the next step, and in doing so discover the resilience simply to live through it all.

By doing the next thing, and the next, one after the other in succession, process moves inevitably towards a product. The quality of the product is often surprising both to the creator and to those who observe. There are many examples of patients being surprised by their artistic efforts, giving them an unexpected feeling of self-worth as well as a new sense of meaning to both their living and dying. Family members, carers, and friends are surprised too. They see their loved ones in a new light, experiencing their relationship with them in a fresh and new way. At a 50-year-old woman's funeral, a tape recording of a piano duet improvised with a musician at the hospice where she was cared for was played during a time for reflection. The response from those present was overwhelming. A sense of awe, that at a time when her life was deteriorating due to a primary brain tumour, she was able to create something of such beauty and tenderness that it introduced her family and friends to a part of her they had never known.

When patients die, the art they create is given to their family members or friends or it hangs on the walls in the hospice reminding and motivating those of us who carry on living to do just that. The following stories bear testament to this.

Resilience

Music

Why do we sing?

In the late eighties, Estonia was one of a group of three Baltic States that rose up against the Soviet empire by whom they had been oppressed for centuries. In what has been called the 'Singing Revolution', hundreds of thousands of Estonians joined hands to form a human chain, and as they did so sang their national songs that had been banned for decades. As with the Negro Spirituals centuries before it was these folk songs that sustained such nations through years of oppression and in the end enabled them to claim back both their dignity and identity (Mayne 2002). Sabrina was 6 years old. Eight weeks previously her mother had died of an AIDS-related illness and Sabrina was now being cared for by a foster family. She was blind and HIV+ herself. During the weeks since her mother's death her teachers and foster parents noticed a withdrawal from life, a giving up. She spent most of the day curled up under the table, either in class or at home, and did not attempt to speak or engage in relationships in any noticeable way. A social worker referred her to a course of music sessions and her foster mother came with her to the first session. The musician took her by the hand and led her to sit with him at the piano, he lifted her right hand up and put it onto the keys explaining his actions to her. She played one note in the upper register of the piano and the musician began to accompany her. Her melody continued and developed weaving this way and that one note leading to the next as if it was meant to be and was well rehearsed. There were changes in dynamic and timing, an awareness of musical structure that was sophisticated and complete, and the quality of the sound she made demanded the attention of both the musician and her foster mother because it was mature and beyond the years of a 6 year old. When it came to an end there was silence, which was commanded by a tangible feeling of surprise. Eventually a voice emerged out of the silence—'Was that *really* me? …' There were three music sessions with Sabrina, culminating in a performance and recording of the song 'Over the rainbow'—her mother's favourite. During the weeks within which the sessions took place Sabrina became more communicative and her foster parents, teachers, and social worker were able to work with her towards a new future. The music gave her a possibility to 'do the next thing' and also to create a tangible product. '… **It is not us who play music, but we are played by it.**' (Pavlicevic 1999) She was able to embrace it, engage with it and rise above her traumatic circumstances. Ten years later Sabrina is alive, healthy, and confident. She has loving adoptive parents and is doing well at school. When she is at her most vulnerable and feeling low, she listens to the tape recordings of the music created in the music sessions from 10 years ago. She believes this inspires her to make it through these difficult times. Sabrina describes music as 'the best thing ever invented' and is determined to go to music college to study singing.

Poetry

Why do we write?

> … writing and reading decrease our sense of isolation…we are given a shot at clapping along with the absurdity of life, instead of being squashed by it over and over …
>
> Lamott (1995)

Simon lived in a care home in South East London. Bed-bound and blind he lived most of his days alone except for the healthcare professionals who nursed him. All his remaining family lived abroad and no friends came to call. After an initial visit by a Community Nurse Specialist, she was concerned about his mental state and his 'unbearable isolation'. Following discussion back at St Christopher's Hospice, a community artist visited him. During the first meeting Simon told her that he wanted to write something for his family to have after his death, but his increasing blindness made this impossible. He went on to ask her to place a video camera at the end of his bed so he could record himself speaking. He wanted to leave a recording behind for his family, indeed for the rest of the world to watch and pay attention to after he was gone. He was clear that although he wanted the artist to be present, he did not want her to speak, only to bear witness. The community artist visited a number of times during the last weeks of Simon's life; the following is the text of one of his recorded monologues:

> I've been that fat black kid in the corner all of my life and I'm gonna end it.
> Now I'm that fat black kid in the corner who can't see,
> Whose hands are always held out, always in need.
> When you're that fat black kid in the corner
> You learn not to need too much, you learn to get by.
> If a girl is willing to go with you, great guns!
> But if she suddenly changes her mind, no hardship!
> 'cos I've always been big, I've always been careful
> I'm no rapist, I'm no man who bullies his woman
> Although sometimes I wish I could,
> 'cos I see them leave me for other guys who hurt them.
> But I'm the fat black kid in the corner
> So I watch and philosophise, I stand on the side.
> Now I'm blind and I say 'How come I didn't grab one when I could see?
> Like all my friends told me to
> 'Grab her! She'll do all right, she really likes you, you're really in there son!
> Now I'm blind, where am I well in?
> I'm well out of everything.
> Lots of my friends, I've lost their telephone numbers
> 'cos I've lost my pieces of paper I used to write them down on
> And there's no-one to search out all these intimate little corners for me anymore.
> 'cos I was the fat black kid in the corner
> I did all of these things for myself
> I knew how to repair things
> I knew how to make things work
> Because that way I wouldn't have to beg anyone anything.
> I always stand in the corner and get by.
> Bye, Bye. Getting by
> Bye, Bye. Getting by
> The kid in the corner
> He'll get by.
> He's blind.
> He wants to cry.
> The end.

After Simon's death his family visited the hospice. The community artist met with them in order to show some of Simon's work. The content of the recordings work on many levels. One level appears to be how Simon was able to articulate his views on his own life, and in doing so lets us into his individual ways of coping. The structure of his monologues takes us into a world of language and poetry, but also into an inner emotional world that tells of Simon's struggles and the very human tools and resources he developed and used in order to get through and survive. Indeed we experience these tools and structures within the finished art form he has created.

Photography

Why do we capture images?

> Those people live again in print as intensely as when their images were captured … I am walking in their alleys, standing in their rooms and sheds and workshops, looking in and out of their windows. And they in turn seem to be aware of me.
>
> Adams (1947)

In terms of the creative arts we must be careful not to work to our own agenda. Just because a painting group or a certain type of craft work is available does not mean that it will always work or be something that each new patient will engage with. Flexibility has to be the key and artists who come with a range of skills and can be creative with their methods and usage are more likely to survive a landscape that can feel barren when we get stuck in a rut.

A group of elderly patients in the hospice wanted to learn how to use digital cameras in order to capture photographic portraits of themselves to give to their families. A community artist worked with them in order to teach them the possibilities when using such cameras, including how to choose an effective context when taking photographic portraits and the skills needed to download images on to a computer. The patients were motivated to learn quickly and efficiently and each patient took a photograph of another patient following a careful and meticulous selection of a backdrop. Within a short space of time, each photograph was downloaded and printed. While looking at the images following the photography shoot each patient made comments and captured some words in writing attempting to articulate what they saw. An elderly Jamaican gentleman looked out from his photograph, eyes shining and hands reaching forward. A fellow patient describes:

> Performing
> He expresses how happy happiness is
> He clasps his hands and sings
> And in an instant he is young again

Each patient gave their photograph to a relative, together with the words their fellow patients had created. Also copies of the photographs and words hang on one of the walls of the hospice corridors. As we stop to observe, in an instant we are with them in their world and they in turn seem to be aware of ours.

Community

Why is it important to create together?

> … for palliative care to be fully effective its practitioners must recognise that for its clients the meaning, experience and expression of their terminal illness is shaped and influenced by the communities within which they live …

Field (2000)

Hospices have a responsibility to work with their local communities in order to help them develop healthier attitudes towards death and dying. Sometimes, it is all too easy for hospices to remain isolated and in turn isolate those who are dying from the community they live in. A current major challenge for hospices is to engage with their local communities in new and creative ways in order to address the 'distant' nature and view of hospices. At St Christopher's we have developed a short programme with local primary schools in order to engage children, their parents and teachers, patients and families together in a creative way. The project lasts 4 weeks and includes four weekly meetings. To begin, the children are introduced to the hospice by a visit from hospice staff; this initial contact includes information regarding the history of St Christopher's as well as an opportunity for the children to raise and explore any questions. The children and their teachers then visit the hospice, which includes a meeting with a group of patients and tour of the building. Two more sessions follow where two of the hospice community artists work together with the children, their teachers and a group of patients to create some artwork. Normally a selection of big pieces are created developing themes chosen by the children as a response to having visited the hospice and having met the patients. One school developed a series of three large collages and mosaics focusing on the theme of trees. This work now adorns the reception area of their school. The project concludes with a celebration at the hospice where the artwork is displayed and the children, together with their parents and teachers, revisit the hospice. This might include a performance by the school choir or some readings from the children. Many of the patients will speak about the experience publicly and there will be visits from the local press. In this way the creative arts are useful in focusing a group of people—children and patients—in a positive and affirming way. Many of the parents are moved by the experience.

One parent, while visiting the hospice for the celebration told us that she had lived in the area all of her life, but had been always too afraid to enter the building. This project engages a component of our local community in a positive way and changes people's views of death and dying. The potential for such projects and the use of the creative arts as a central focus is enormous.

Primary schools and children are only a beginning.

Design

Why is it important to look and feel good?

Many hospices support their users through offering hairdressing and manicures. Most people would agree that looking good helps us to feel better during difficult times.

Some months ago a conversation was overheard between a group of young female patients each coming to the end of their lives. Their discussion was about body image and low self-esteem. Some had lost their hair due to treatment, others had undergone mastectomies, others had put weight on or lost weight due to medication. Generally they all felt bad about themselves and talked of the difficulties of looking and feeling good. They could not find clothes to fit them and if they visited shops on the high street they were too embarrassed to try clothes on, as they would have to undress and expose their vulnerability.

Overhearing their conversation, a community artist had the thought that someone should be able to do something about this. After some deliberation she decided to contact the London College of Fashion to tell them of the conversation she had overheard. She asked if they felt able to do something about it. What followed was something that had not been thought out or planned—a true, improvizational, creative process that unfolded over a period of weeks. A lecturer from the college and a group of students came to the hospice and met with the women. Following a discussion the women decided to design their own outfits. They were adamant that they did not want to design clothes that 'hid' their illness, rather they wanted to design clothes that 'expressed' it. Following the designing process, the women went along to the college with the students to create their outfits. The final piece of the jigsaw fell into place in the form of a celebration at the hospice. Each of the women invited friends and family to witness what they had achieved. A South American jazz band was hired and began playing in the centre of the building. Gradually, one by one, everyone in the building gravitated towards the music, some came to complain about the noise, others were intrigued by what they heard. Quickly the area where the band was playing became crowded, and at this moment the women appeared and walked down a catwalk. To conclude, they each spoke of their experiences. In the weeks that followed, the women worked with the artist to put together a slide show of photographs taken at the celebration. They chose the order of the photographs and the music which accompanied them, *Something Inside So Strong*, written and sung by Labi Siffre. Now over a year later each of the women has died. Each one of them was buried in the outfit they created.

The following poem was written and read out by one of the women at the end of the fashion show:

> I know I am beautiful
> Because my mum told me so
> I know I am beautiful
> Because he above said it was so.
> I was beautiful when my hair fell out
> His love for me helped it grow back
> A woman's vision from inside and out
> Knows what beauty is all about
> Our illness at times may make us low
> But we have been shown another way to go
> Our journey on this fashion show
> Has been a way to let us know
> That we are what our maker told us years ago
> Beautiful.

The impact of this experience was, and continues to be, widespread. Although it displayed the extraordinary capabilities for resilience of a specific group of women coming to the end of their lives, there were many other levels of impact. The students who were involved in this project were deeply affected by their experience and our connection with them remains. They also went on to win a major national award for their part in this work. Another important aspect was the way in which St Christopher's as an organization dealt with the experience of that final celebration. Such happenings can change the way in which communities of people think about themselves and act together for the future. Patients, carers, visitors, and staff joined together in such a public manner. In dealing with the experience and embracing it so creatively and intuitively, many people's lives were changed.

Conclusions

> The moving finger writes and having writ
> Moves on: nor all your Piety nor Wit
> Shall lure it back to cancel half a Line,
> Nor all your Tears wash out a Word of it

Omar Khayyam (1070)

A major challenge for the future development of the creative arts in hospices, indeed in healthcare generally, is to develop suitable research paradigms in order to examine the efficacy of the work. Engaging with local academic institutions and developing discourse with researchers will be vital if the true value of the arts in these kind of environments is to be secured. However, the examples of resilience we witness highlight the irrepressible nature of the human spirit and leave us with tangible proof of the extraordinary things achieved and the courage discovered during times of adversity. They also exhibit for us the motivational and inspirational properties of the creative arts that have the potential to inspire the individual to feel that life is worth living while impacting outwards into the family, the local community and the world at large. We also learn that the creative arts do not only provide a context for mere distraction.

There are two important points to be made with regard to the unique possibilities that the creative arts are able to offer those people facing the end-of-life.

First, the creative capacity of the arts offers a distinctive framework within which to 'do the next thing'. This is vital in that it gives a real possibility to move forward from the paralysis of shock, meaninglessness, fear, and loss. The creative arts *move* us, not only emotionally but also physiologically. Their unique properties and structures motivate both flesh and spirit into a future that not only seems possible but bearable. If we can do the next thing in music or poetry, then this can potentially inspire us to do the next thing in our every-day lives.

Secondly if the process of creating art is important then so too is the product that is created. Paintings, music, photographs, and poetry not only give the creator a sense of surprise and achievement on completion, but by the product existing long after the creator has gone they have an impact on those who remain. Patients who create the artwork are usually keen for it to be shared and witnessed, and with their permission, the work of art itself, the creation of which has given strength, inspiration, and courage to its creator, gives also strength, inspiration, and courage to those left behind.

The art created by these patients does not leave us with only a memory of something once experienced. These experiences are left in their actuality. These physical objects display a resilience that continues to inspire and impact far beyond their creation.

References

Adams A (1947) In: *Photographer and Citizen* (eds Alland A. Jacob A. Riis). New York: Aperture Foundation Inc. 1973.

Field D (2000) *What do we Mean by Psychosocial?* Briefing Paper No. 4. London: National Council for Palliative Care.

Khayyam O (1070) In: *The Nectar of Grace—Omar Khayyam's life and works* (ed. Tirtha SG). Allahbad, Kilabistan. 1941.

Lamott A (1995) *Bird by Bird*. London: Bantam.

May R (1975) *The Courage to Create*. New York: Norton.

Mayne M (2002) This intimate stranger. *Bulletin of the British Society for Music Therapy* **45**: 31–40.

Meissner WW (1994) Vincent Van Gogh as Artist—A psychoanalytic reflection. *Annual of Psychoanalysis* **22**: 111–141.

Pavlicevic M (1999) *Music Therapy—Intimate Notes*. London: Jessica Kingsley Publications.

Rosen C (1995) *The Romantic Generation*. M.A. U.S.A. Harvard University Press.

Sacks O (1994) *A Leg To Stand On*. New York: Perennial.

Winnicott DW (1971) *Playing and Reality*. London: Tavistock.

Afterword

The concept of resilience makes it clear that individual factors such as a sense of agency, seeing the world as understandable and having confidence in one's potential ability to manage situations, must be linked to positive family, community and cultural resources, values, and connections. Silverman, in her chapter in this book, quotes Borkman (1999), 'You alone can do it, but you cannot do it alone'. Both government and social commentators are expressing a growing unease about the limitations of a culture based on individual self-sufficiency and independence. Efforts to improve individual welfare cannot alone meet the aspirations of society in relation to high-quality, cost-effective and equitable care for all dying people. The growth of an individual sense of security and connectedness is inevitably mediated through relationships. Family, friendship and community networks and responses are profoundly important in the individual's experience of death and dying. The West has much to learn from the community-funded and volunteer-supported programmes of palliative care in resource-poor countries outlined by Bingley and McDermott in this book. Care cannot ultimately be defined as a commodity; a prescription created by professionals against assessed risks and predicted problems and anonymously paid for from a cash-strapped public purse. Care is centred in the relationships we make with one another and in the society we create together. We will all die, we will all be bereaved. At heart these are social experiences in which excellent physical care is profoundly important.

Research into resilience and working with resilience in practice is very much work in progress. There is much more to be understood about why some individuals have better than expected outcomes. We have to continue to find the balance between risk containment and risk taking. The potential research agenda is vast. Life experience tells us that two people with a very similar set of circumstances process the world in very different ways. Models of risk and resilience are inevitably complex and our understanding of what supports people needs to extend to viewing individuals as embedded in their social connections and to providing integrated interventions and models of service organization that operate across all levels. Resilience must not become a new orthodoxy. A simple view of resilience as ongoing coping and adaptation is not always desirable. We should focus not only on how people can thrive despite trauma, but also actively seek ways to reduce poverty, discrimination and depression (Boss 2002). Palliative care has been slow to respond to the challenges of meeting the needs of the excluded and disadvantaged: refugees, those with learning disabilities, prisoners, travellers, those with primary mental health problems and many others. Resilience must not become another set of tick boxes against which we measure potential. It would be possible, for example, to look at a child with learning disabilities against a general set of characteristics of resilient children and predict a negative outcome, yet much practice indicates that the opposite is often true. We should avoid categorizing particular 'populations' as resilient; each situation is unique and there are multiple paths to resilience. We must remain open to potential and the possibility of surprise. As St Exupéry reminds us in the *Little Prince* (Bluglass 2003) 'The meaning of things is not in things themselves, but in our attitude to them.'

Barbara Monroe and David Oliviere

Afterword references

Bluglass K (2003) *Hidden from the Holocaust: stories of resilient Hidden children who survived and thrived.* Westport, CT: Greenwood.

Borkman T (1999) *Understanding Self Help Mutual Aid: Experiential learning in the commons.* Camden, NJ: Rutgers University Press.

Boss P (2002). *Family Stress Management: A contextual approach*, 2nd edn. Thousand Oaks CA: Sage.

Index